Basic Concepts of Hemostasis and Thrombosis:

Clinical and Laboratory Evaluation of Thrombohemorrhagic Phenomena

Editors

Genesio Murano, Ph.D.
Physiologist
Bureau of Biologics
Food and Drug Administration
United States Department of Health, Education, and Welfare
Bethesda, Maryland

Rodger L. Bick, M.D.
Medical Director
San Joaquin Hematology and Oncology Medical Group
Bakersfield, California
Clinical Faculty
Division of Hematology-Oncology
School of Medicine
University of California
Los Angeles, California
Director of Hematology and Oncology
San Joaquin Community Hospital
Bakersfield, California

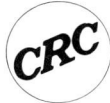

CRC Press, Inc.
Boca Raton, Florida

Library of Congress Cataloging in Publication Data

Main entry under title:

Basic concepts of hemostasis and thrombosis.

    Bibliography: p.
    Includes index.
    1. Hemorrhagic diseases. 2. Hemostasis.
3. Thrombosis. 4. Cancer—Complications and sequelae.
I. Murano, Genesio. II. Bick, Rodger L.
RC633.B37   616.1'5   79-19188
ISBN 0-8493-5393-9

This book represents information obtained from authentic and highly regarded sources. Reprinted material is quoted with permission, and sources are indicated. A wide variety of references are listed. Every reasonable effort has been made to give reliable data and information, but the author and the publisher cannot assume responsibility for the validity of all materials or for the consequences of their use.

All rights reserved. This book, or any part thereof, may not be reproduced in any form without written consent from the publisher.

Direct all inquiries to CRC Press, 2000 N.W. 24th Street, Boca Raton, Florida, 33431.

© 1980 by CRC Press, Inc.

International Standard Book Number 0-8493-5393-9

Library of Congress Card Number 79-19188
Printed in the United States

PREFACE

Since most physicians are frequently burdened with the awesome responsibility of diagnosing and treating thrombohemorrhagic syndromes, the consequences of such acute insults to normal body functions are all too well recognized. Not as well appreciated, however, are the delicately modulated interplays of various enzyme-inhibitor systems and the mechanism by which a variety of apparently unrelated disease processes precipitate sometimes catastrophic events: thrombosis / embolism or hemorrhage. Patients clot and/or bleed because of a variety of identifiable hemostatic abnormalities involving either the vasculature, the platelets, the plasma proteins, or any combination thereof. Logical and effective treatment depends upon the proper identification of the hemostatic compartment(s) involved and, when possible, the removal of the "triggering" process.

We have attempted a logical review of basic mechanisms of hemostasis and of diagnostic/therapeutic aspects of hemostatic dysfunction. The text is divided into three sections, the first of which briefly addresses the physiology and biochemistry of the vessel wall, the platelets, and pertinent plasma factors. The chapter on plasma proteins pays particular attention to biocybernetic principles (positive-negative feedback loops) and to the interrelationship of enzyme systems involved in coagulation, fibrino(geno)lysis, kinin generation, and complement activation.

The second section deals with the pathophysiology, clinical features, laboratory diagnosis and therapy of inherited and acquired disorders of hemostasis. Particular emphasis is placed on platelet disorders and syndromes of disseminated intravascular proteolysis.

In the third section, the subject of hypercoagulability and thrombosis is presented in terms of etiology, diagnosis, and therapy. The results obtained in some clinical trials are presented in support of the rationale (or lack thereof) for the use of oral anticoagulants, antiplatelet agents, and thrombolytic agents. The discussion on thrombolytic therapy with urokinase and streptokinase is limited to those indications in which safety and efficacy have been documented.

As frequently as possible, we have attempted to cross reference correlative information appearing throughout the text. However, each chapter or subsection thereof has addressed a respective topic, in most instances, as completely as possible. As a consequence, due to the similarity of the pathophysiology of some syndromes and the interrelationships of basic biochemical mechanisms, a certain element of repetition has been introduced. We are hopeful that this will benefit the reader who is primarily interested in a selected topic and not the entire text.

Progressive insights into the nature of biochemical mechanisms, the plethora of pathophysiologic interrelationships, clinical/laboratory diagnosis, and therapy in diseases of hemostasis have come about through the scholarly efforts and dedication of many investigators. In the text we have attempted to include as much as possible of the exemplary work performed in each discipline and to acknowledge it in the form of a reasonably extensive bibliography at the end of each chapter. In many instances, however, in the interest of brevity and clarity, the text presentation has been limited to most recent concepts and the reference material obligatorily selected and limited to recent (and review) articles. We apologize for omissions.

In summary, our book deals with the systematic and practical approach to the diagnosis and therapy of clotting and bleeding disorders. Although our remarks are aimed primarily at the clinical pathologist, the hematologist, and the medical technologist, those working in other disciplines (obstetrics, pediatrics, internal medicine), as well as medical and graduate students, should find the book interesting and, hopefully, instructive.

We thank our colleagues, Drs. Lowell E. McCoy, Raymond L. Henry, Douglas A. Triplett, and William L. Wilson, for their chapter contributions. We appreciate their promptness in furnishing their materials and we apologize for the delay in publication. We thank Dr. John Griffin of the Scripps Institute for reviewing the section on contact activation in Chapter 3. We thank our many A.S.C.P. workshop students for encouraging us to compile a text of this nature. We are grateful for the heroic efforts and tolerance of Julie Hainline and Sandra Fote-Philips in typing — and retyping ("... oh those references ...") — the manuscript. We are indebted to the publishers of *Seminars in Thrombosis and Hemostasis* and *Thrombosis and Hemostasis* for permission to use published figures. We are grateful to CRC Press for their assistance in completing this work and for their patience in dealing with our inability to meet certain deadlines.

Genesio Murano
and
Rodger L. Bick

THE EDITORS

Genesio Murano, Ph.D., is a physiologist at the Bureau of Biologics (FDA), Bethesda, Maryland and Associate Professor of Physiology, at the Uniformed Services University of Health Sciences, Bethesda, Maryland. He received his B.A. degree in zoology in 1964 from the University of Massachusetts, Amherst, Massachusetts, and his M.S. (1966) and Ph.D. (1968) degrees in physiology from Wayne State University, School of Medicine, Detroit, Michigan.

Dr. Murano is a member of the New York Academy of Sciences, the International Society of Thrombosis and Hemostasis, and the Federation for Advanced Education in the Sciences of the National Institutes of Health. His research interests have included the study of structural-functional characteristics of prothrombin and fibrinogen with much of the work performed at the Karolinska Institute, Stockholm, Sweden. Currently he is investigating the biochemical properties of fibrinolytic agents and of plasma protease inhibitors with potential therapeutic applications.

Rodger L. Bick, M.D., did his undergraduate work at University of California at Berkeley and obtained his M.D. degree from the University of California at Irvine in 1970. Following his medical internship and internal medicine residency, hematology/oncology as well as Hemostasis and Thrombosis Fellowships were obtained.

Dr. Bick is a National Hemostasis thrombosis Workshop/Seminar Director for the Council on Continuing Education of the American Society of Clinical Pathologists. He is a member of the American Society of Clinical Pathologists, American Society of Hematology, International Society on Thrombosis and Hemostasis, Thrombosis Council of the American Heart Association, and is a member of the Research Grant Peer Review Committee, California Heart Association.

Dr. Bick is the Director of Hematology and Oncology at San Joaquin Community Hospital, Medical Director of San Joaquin Hematology & Oncology Medical Group, and Director of San Joaquin Hematology & Oncology Laboratories. He is also a Clinical Faculty member of the Division of Hematology Oncology, UCLA Center for the Health Sciences, Los Angeles, California, Associate Professor of Allied Health Professions, California State College at Bakersfield, and Adjunct Associate Professor of Physiology, Wayne State University School of Medicine, Detroit, Michigan. His current research interests include clinical disorders of hemostasis and thrombosis, especially alterations of hemostasis associated with cardiopulmonary bypass, alterations of hemostasis associated with malignancy, and the role of hemostasis and thrombosis in atherogenesis; additional special interests are in the nature of antithrombin III and its alterations in various disease states.

CONTRIBUTORS

Raymond L. Henry, Ph.D.
Professor of Physiology
Wayne State University
  School of Medicine
Detroit, Michigan

Lowell E. McCoy, Ph.D.
Professor of Physiology
Wayne State University
  School of Medicine
Detroit, Michigan

Douglas Triplett, M.D.
Director
Hematology Department
Ball Memorial Hospital
Director
Muncie Center for Medical Education
Associate Professor of Pathology
Indiana University School of Medicine
Muncie, Indiana

William L. Wilson, M.D.
Bay Area Hematology Oncology
Santa Monica, California

DEDICATION

To my mother Michelina and my father Gerardo

                                            Genesio Murano

To my daughter Michelle and my mother Pauline

                                            Rodger L. Bick

TABLE OF CONTENTS

PHYSIOLOGY AND BIOCHEMISTRY OF HEMOSTASIS

Introduction
The Three Hemostatic Compartments 3
Genesio Murano

Chapter 1
Vascular Function in Hemostasis. 5
Lowell E. McCoy

Chapter 2
Platelet Function in Hemostasis 17
Raymond L. Henry

Chapter 3
Plasma Protein Function in Hemostasis 43
Genesio Murano

CLINICAL DISORDERS OF HEMOSTASIS

Chapter 4
A Systematic Approach to the Diagnosis of Bleeding Disorders. 81
Rodger L. Bick

Chapter 5
Vascular Disorders 89
Rodger L. Bick

Chapter 6
Platelet Disorders 95
Douglas Triplett

Chapter 7
Hereditary Plasma Protein Disorders 149
Rodger L. Bick

Chapter 8
Disseminated Intravascular Coagulation (DIC) and Related Syndromes 163
Rodger L. Bick

Chapter 9
Primary Hyperfibrino(geno)lytic Syndromes 181
Rodger L. Bick and Genesio Murano

Chapter 10
Acquired Circulating Anticoagulants and Defective Hemostasis in Malignant Paraprotein Disorders 205
Rodger L. Bick

Chapter 11
Alterations of Hemostasis Associated with Malignancy 213
Rodger L. Bick

Chapter 12
Malignancy and Anticoagulation 227
William L. Wilson

HYPERCOAGULABILITY, THROMBOSIS, AND THERAPY

Chapter 13
Hypercoagulability and Thrombosis 237
Rodger L. Bick

Chapter 14
Anticoagulant and Antiplatelet Therapy 245
Rodger L. Bick

Chapter 15
Thrombolytic Therapy 259
Genesio Murano and Rodger L. Bick

Glossary 269

Index 271

Physiology and Biochemistry of Hemostasis

INTRODUCTION

THE THREE HEMOSTATIC COMPARTMENTS

Genesio Murano

The property of the circulation whereby the blood is maintained fluid within the vessels and the ability of the system to prevent excessive blood loss upon injury is referred to as *hemostasis*. To accomplish this function, the body depends on a delicate interplay of three anatomic compartments, namely: *tissues, blood cells* and *plasma*. The relative importance of each hemostatic component varies in different species and, in man, depends upon the size of the blood vessel involved.

Upon injury, the vascular wall has the ability to constrict and to contribute a variety of platelet and plasma protein activators. The platelets, by the process of adhesion and cohesion, provide another physical means of arresting blood loss. With their disruption (viscous metamorphosis), a variety of compounds are released that further promote platelet aggregation, vascular constriction, and "activation" of coagulation components. The plasma proteins, once activated, serve to impart solidity to the "platelet plug" at the site of injury and contribute to the ensuing tissue repair processes. A variety of chemical signals, designed to initiate and terminate various events, serve as a system of checks and balances to modulate the responses leading to the maintenance of blood fluidity and the prevention of blood loss. Any disturbance in the balance of this highly integrated system leads to inappropriate responses and, depending on the nature of the abnormality, predisposes either to thrombosis or hemorrhage.

In order to appreciate the plethora of details regarding the inter- and intracompartmental interactions, the normal hemostatic aspects of the vessel wall, the platelets, and the plasma proteins are discussed separately in the ensuing three chapters of this section. The reader is instructed, however, to maintain a perspective of integrated function, since this constitutes the basis for a proper and efficient diagnosis of hemostatic dysfunction and for the institution of appropriate forms of therapy.

Chapter 1

VASCULAR FUNCTION IN HEMOSTASIS

Lowell E. McCoy

TABLE OF CONTENTS

I.	Introduction	6
II.	Vascular Structure	6
	A. Vascular Tree	6
	B. Vascular Wall	6
III.	Vascular Function in Hemostasis	7
	A. Endothelium in Hemostasis	7
	B. Subendothelium in Hemostasis	9
IV.	Vascular-Platelet Interaction	9
	A. Endothelial Support	9
	B. Subendothelium-Platelet Interaction	10
	C. Vascular Prostaglandin-Platelet Interaction	11
V.	Summary	11
References		13

I. INTRODUCTION

All components of the hemostatic system are confined within a closed network of vessels in the body, that is, the vascular tree. This system of arteries, capillaries, and veins was originally thought to function simply as conduits for the transport of blood,[1] and vasoconstriction,[2] a means of maintaining the blood within the system. This response to trauma was attributed to the inherent irritability[3] of living tissues and/or their response to "vasoactive" substances.[4] Current reports indicate that vascular contribution to the hemostatic process is more complex than simple vasoconstriction in response to trauma. The endothelial lining of the system acts as an inert shield between the potentially thrombotic blood proteins and platelets and the procoagulant-acting subendothelial layers. Traumatic disruption of this barrier permits contact between blood and the subendothelium, which, in addition to vasoconstriction, stimulates the processes of platelet aggregation and coagulation. This chapter briefly details current knowledge of vascular function as it relates to hemostasis.

II. VASCULAR STRUCTURE

A. Vascular Tree

The vertebrate circulatory system is composed of three interconnecting types of vessels: arteries, veins, and capillaries. The arterial, high-pressure side of the system, is composed of conical, thick-walled, multilamellar, smooth muscle-containing vessels that have progressively smaller diameters as they near the peripheral tissues. Veins originate at the tissue level and become progressively larger and fewer in number as they near the heart. Physiologically, veins are known as the compliance vessels of the cardiovascular system[5] because of their elasticity and the capacity to contain large volumes of blood. Blood pressure in the venous side of the system is less than one tenth of that observed in the arteries.[6] The histologic structure of veins and arteries are similar in that both are multilayered, each having a smooth muscle layer. However, the venous walls are thinner, less rigid, and contain a smaller *muscularis* layer than arteries.

Interconnecting these vessels is a network of unilamellar capillaries, through which blood flows intermittently in close proximity to the tissues. The pressures in this system are lower than those observed in either arteries or veins.[6] Capillaries are lined with a single layer of endothelial cells.

Blood flow in the system is greatest in the arteries (30 to 230 cm/sec), slower in veins (8 to 50 cm/sec), and slowest in capillaries (0.5 cm/sec).[6] Resistance to flow is inversely proportional to vessel diameter. The capillary bed, having the greatest resistance to flow, has the lowest flow velocity in the system.[6] Stasis and low flow conditions within capillaries and veins may result in endothelial trauma induced by oxygen deprivation, which can cause cellular sloughing and exposure of the underlying subendothelium. This can result in thrombosis.[7]

B. Vascular Wall

Vascular wall substructure is divided into (1) endothelial and (2) subendothelial areas,[8] with the endothelium being the innermost layer of cells. It forms a contiguous lining for the arteries, capillaries, and veins. This layer is normally inert with respect to the platelets and coagulation proteins in blood.[9] The subendothelium includes all tissue layers external to the endothelium. Capillary endothelium is bounded externally by a discrete basement membrane (BM), the outermost layer of which contains collagen fibers.[10] In arteries and veins this membrane is less distinct, or absent. In the larger vessels it is replaced by an internal elastic lamina (IEL). The IEL also contains collagen and elastin. External to the IEL is a tissue layer containing elastin fibers intermingled with circumferential and longitudinally arrayed smooth muscle cells. This layer composes most of the arterial wall, is less pronounced in veins, and absent in capillaries. In both arteries and veins this layer is innervated by the autonomic nervous system (ANS). Vasoconstriction in response to the ANS and to mechanical or chemical stimulation has been observed.[11] Capillaries, which lack smooth muscle cells and innervation, will nevertheless constrict in response to mechanical and chemical stimuli.[12] In large arteries the muscle layer is surrounded by a layer of longitudinal elastic fibers, the external elastic lamina (EEL). External to this, and surrounding the entire vessel, is a layer of densely packed collagen fibers (Figure 1).[8]

III. VASCULAR FUNCTION IN HEMOSTASIS

As pointed out in the introduction, vascular function in hemostasis was initially thought to involve only the constrictive capabilities of arteries and veins. This characteristic of the muscular arteries and veins is required for normal hemostasis.[13] However, results of current vascular function studies indicate that each vessel layer has a specific function or contains materials that are vital to normal hemostasis.[9]

A. Endothelium in Hemostasis

Microscopic examination of longitudinal endothelial preparations that have been stained with silver salts[14] reveals a continuous sheet of cells having distinct, darkly stained boundaries, with bridge-like interconnections between adjacent cells.[15] Individual cells appear spindle shaped, with their long axes parallel to the direction of flow (Figure 2).[16] Cellular dimension varies with the state of vascular contraction.[17] In the unconstricted state, the cells approximate 50×10 μ and extend into the lumen 2 to 5 μ.[18] In areas of trauma and exposure of the subendothelium, a layer of platelets can be seen adhering to the site of injury (Figure 3).[16] In cross section, the luminal surface of the endothelial cell appears to be covered with a 500 to 1000 Å coat of ruthenium red staining (possibly mucopolysaccharide) material.[19] This coat appears to penetrate the space between adjacent endothelial cells[20] and may represent the inert boundary between blood and the vessel wall cells.

Functionally, endothelial cells throughout the vascular system appear to be capable of contraction when stimulated by histamine, serotonin, and bradykinin.[21] Cellular turnover rates appear to be extremely slow[17] except at arterial bifurcations,[22] in growing animals,[23] at points of injury,[24] and in malignancy.[25] The enhanced turnover at bifurcation sites may be a response to sheer stress erosion caused by the hydrodynamics of the system. This turbulence continually denudes areas at bifurcations, exposing the subendothelium, resulting in thrombosis; thus the predilection toward arteriosclerosis observed at these points.[9]

In addition to the above considerations, endothelial cells are the site of Factor VIII antigen synthesis and release.[26] Capillary, venous, and pulmonary endothelial cells, excluding arterial endothelium, are capable of releasing a plasminogen activator.[27-30] In addition to retention of ABO blood group antigenicity and the immunologic presence of thrombosthenin,[9] tissue cultures of endothelial cells[31] also have demonstrated the capability of synthesis and release of Factor VIII antigen,[26] the presence of which is required for normal intrinsic blood coagulation.[32] Of further significance is the observation[33] and subsequent confirmation[34,35] that tissue factor is a lipoprotein. The protein moiety has been isolated[37,38] and found to be located on the surface of endothelial cells.[39] The endothelium also appears to share antigenicity with platelets[9] and with smooth muscle cells.[40] The presence of common antigens implies a direct relationship between these cells and the other components of hemostasis.

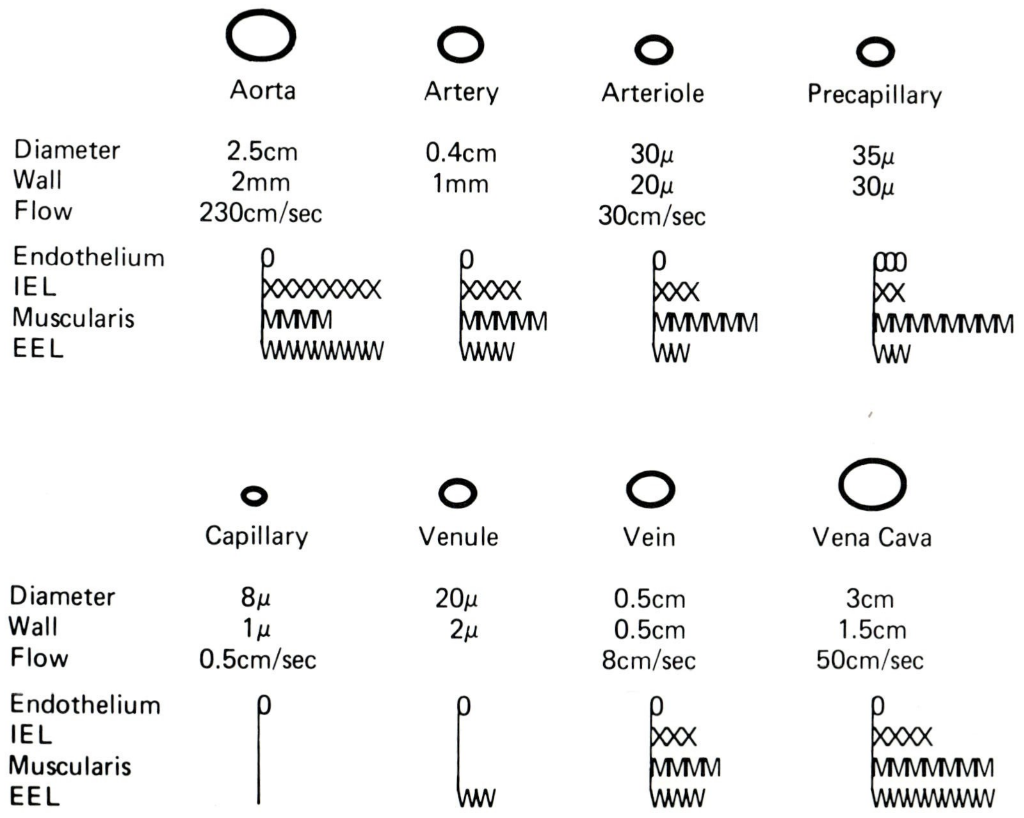

FIGURE 1. Comparative schematic depicting vascular diameter, blood flow, and wall lamellar relationships for arteries, capillaries, and veins. IEL = internal elastic lamina. Muscularis = smooth muscle lamina. EEL = external elastic lamina.

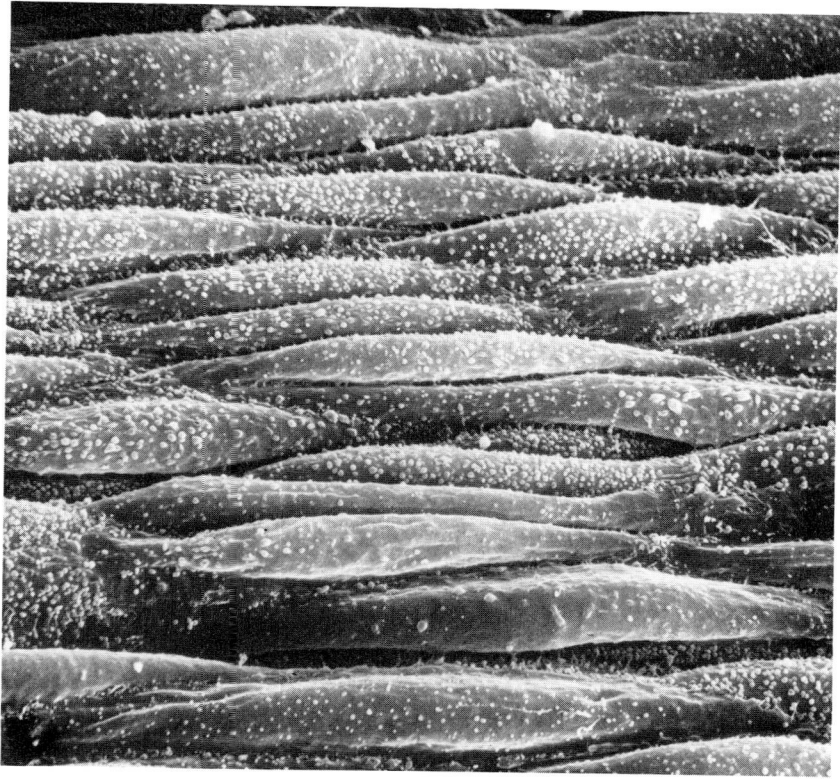

FIGURE 2. Endothelium of normal umbilical vein perfused with heparinized Dulbecco's phosphate buffered saline at pH 7.3 for 30 min at 37°C. Note tightness of endothelial cell junctions and abundant microvilli typical of this full-term vessel. (Magnification × 3340.) (Courtesy of Dr. M. I. Barnhart, Wayne State University, Detroit, Mich. With permission.)

B. Subendothelium in Hemostasis

Minor trauma is known to damage the endothelium, causing cellular destruction and/or contraction, leaving gaps between the cells.[41] This exposes the basement membrane[42] to which the platelets are preferentially attracted[43] (Figure 3). Severe trauma results in platelet adhesion to the damaged endothelial cells,[44] without the usual membrane responses characteristic of platelet adhesion.[45] If trauma is sufficiently severe to cause endothelial detachment, the initial processes of platelet adhesion[46] occur virtually simultaneously with those of vasoconstriction.[42] Platelets appear to enter sites of damage even at the capillary level.[47] The material within the basement membrane to which platelets adhere was initially thought to be collagen.[48] Subsequent electron microscopic examination failed to confirm the presence of characteristic collagen fibers.[49] It may be that platelet adhesion to subendothelial lamina involves not only the presence of distinct fibrous collagen[50] with microscopic periodicity of 640 Å, but also a soluble monomeric form or a completely different structural protein. In addition to serving as a stimulus for aggregation, collagen also activates Factor XII.[51]

IV. VASCULAR-PLATELET INTERACTION

A. Endothelial Support

The involvement of platelets in the maintenance of vascular integrity was initially

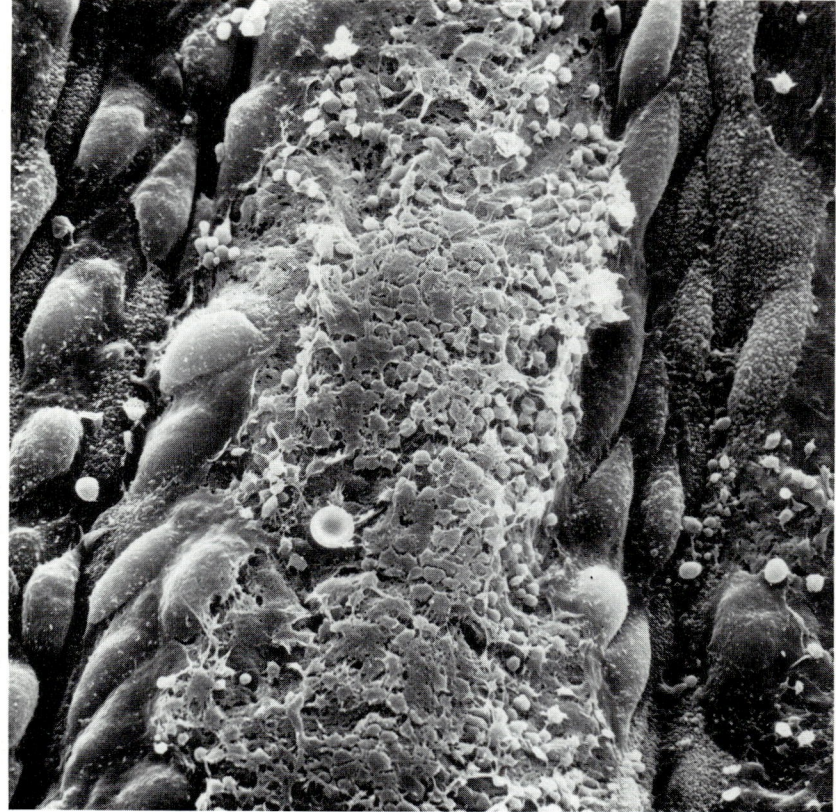

FIGURE 3. Pavement of platelets adherent to umbilical vein subendothelium exposed during enzyme induced injury, prior to perfusion with platelet-rich plasma. Platelets are in various stages of activation, illustrating their attempt to seal the injured vessel wall. Note erythrocyte (discocyte) for size reference. (Magnification × 1040.) (Courtesy of Dr. M. I. Barnhart, Wayne State University, Detroit, Mich. With permission.)

observed in edematous and hemorrhagic states in thrombocytopenic animals.[52] The direct inclusion of platelets into endothelial cell layers has been observed.[52] Electron microscopic examination has revealed platelet adhesion to collagen fibers of the exposed basement membrane.[53] The stickiness of platelets to foreign surfaces has been attributed, in part, to a mosaic of clumped positive and negative charges on the platelet surface, complementary to those on the surface of the foreign material.[54] This phenomenon may explain the interaction of platelets with other blood or vessel wall cells[55] and with basement membrane collagen.[56] The latter reaction is preferential for platelets[54] and is independent of calcium ions.[56] The mosaic of surface charge may also explain the apparent repulsion between normal platelets and between platelets and normal endothelium.[54]

B. Subendothelium-Platelet Interaction

As indicated above, exposure of the subendothelium results in exposure of collagen to which platelets adhere with particular affinity.[43] Although species differences in platelet-collagen interaction have been related to platelet responsiveness[57] or to collagen structure differences,[58] there is general agreement that collagen induces the adhesion/aggregation reaction in platelets.[59]

Several theories have been advanced with regard to the mechanism of this induction.

To date, no single theory completely explains the process. The physical configuration of collagen (fibrous, microcrystalline,[60] or vitreous[61]) may reflect unique induction properties. Biochemically, an enzyme-acceptor complex[62] has been proposed in which certain platelet membrane glycosyl transferases may attach to incomplete galactosyl-hydroxylysine groups of collagen. This observation has resulted in extensive research on the role of carbohydrate in platelet aggregation,[63] although some forms of collagen[64] induce aggregation after carbohydrate modification. Free sulfhydryl groups also appear to be required for aggregation.[65] Collagen has also been implicated in the direct activation of platelet-bound Factor XI in the absence of Factor XII.[66]

C. Vascular-Prostaglandin-Platelet Interaction

Recent studies of arterial wall prostaglandins has led to the discovery of prostacyclin (PGI_2),[67] which relaxes arterial strips and inhibits platelet aggregation.[68] PGI_2 is synthesized by arterial microsomes from prostaglandin endoperoxides PGG_2 and PGH_2.[67] These endoperoxides are synthesized from arachidonic acid by the arterial microsomes or provided by adjacent circulating platelets.[68] PGI_2 is an extremely potent inhibitor of platelet aggregation. This may account for the nonthrombogenicity (neutrality, inertness) of certain arterial beds, but does not account for the thrombogenic potential of the capillary and venous systems, unless these latter vessels lack the capability of PGI_2 synthesis.

In contrast to arterial PGI_2 synthesis, platelets have been found to utilize PGG_2 and PGH_2 as precursors for thromboxane (TXA_2) synthesis,[69] which is a potent platelet aggregator. The compounds PGI_2 and TXA_2, although having opposing actions, have parallel synthesis pathways, resulting in the production of two compounds that regulate hemostasis in arteries (Figure 4). Arterial wall injury results in decreased PGI_2 synthesis, with consequent platelet thrombosis. Aspirin has been found to inhibit TXA_2 synthesis at a step prior to formation of the endoperoxide intermediates and thus decreases or abolishes platelet aggregation.[70] Certain lipoperoxides of arachidonic acid have been found to inhibit PGI_2 synthesis.[71] This may be predisposing to thrombosis and atherogenesis.

V. SUMMARY

Vascular involvement in hemostasis has proven to be more complex than vasoconstriction alone. Although vasoconstriction is required for normal hemostasis, interaction of endothelial and subendothelial tissue components with plasma proteins and platelets is also required if normal platelet aggregation and coagulation are to occur. The presence of Factor VIII antigen in endothelial cells and collagen activation of platelet-borne Factor XI, coupled with the delicate balance between platelet TXA_2 and arterial PGI_2 serve to highlight the fact that normal hemostasis is dependent upon the complementary interaction of the vasculature, the platelets, and the appropriate plasma proteins.[72-74]

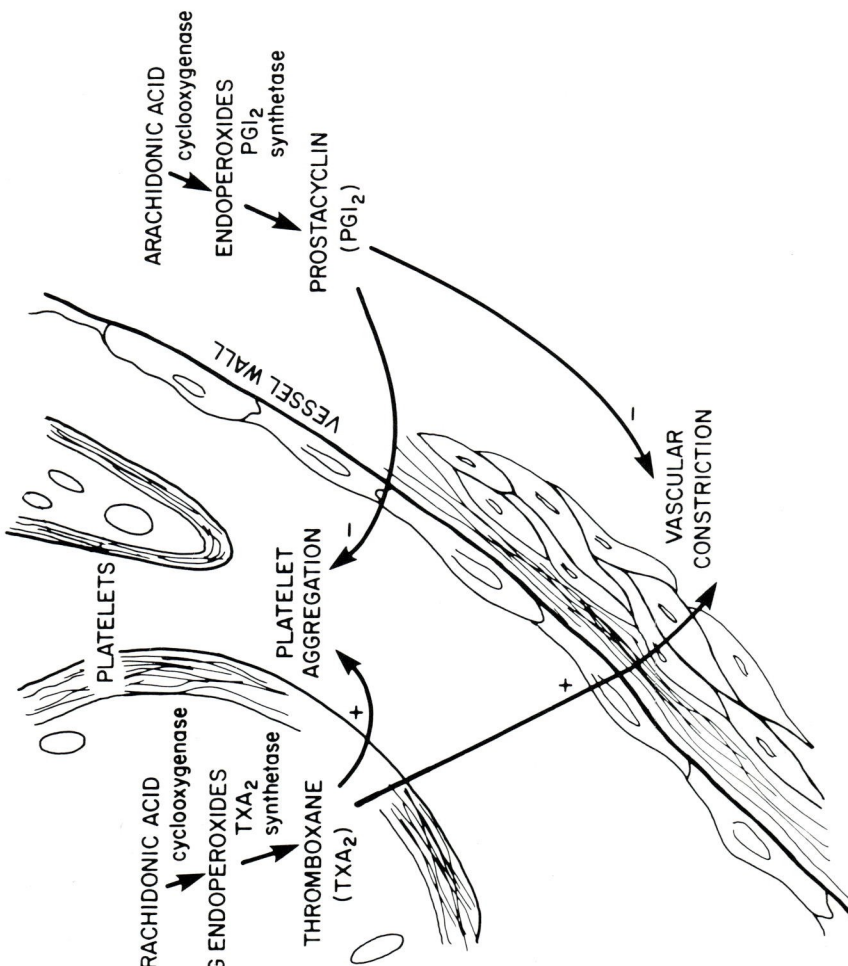

FIGURE 4. Schematic of arterial and platelet prostaglandin synthesis pathways. Thromboxane and prostacyclin are synthesized from prostaglandin endoperoxides by specific platelet and vascular wall synthetases, respectively. Thromboxane stimulates (+) platelet aggregation and vasoconstriction, while prostacyclin inhibits (−) these responses. Based on the work of Moncada et al.[71]

REFERENCES

1. **Harvey, W.**, *Exercitatio Anatomica de Motu Cordis et Sanguinis in Animalibus*, Frankfurt, 1628.
2. **Zucker, M. B.**, Platelet agglutination and vasoconstriction as factors in spontaneous hemostasis in normal, thrombocytopenic, heparinized and hypothrombinemic rats, *Am. J. Physiol.*, 148, 245, 1947.
3. **Harris, A. K.**, Cell surface movements related to cell locomotion, *Ciba Found. Symp.*, 14, 3, 1973.
4. **Roskam, J.**, Du role de la paroi vasculaire dans l'Hemostase spontanee et la pathogenie des etats hemorrhagiques, *Thromb. Diath. Haemorrh.*, 12, 338, 1964.
5. **Guyton, A. C.**, The venous system and its role in the circulation, *Mod. Concepts Cardiovasc. Dis.*, 27, 483, 1958.
6. **Alexander, R. S.**, The systemic circulation, *Ann. Rev. Physiol.*, 25, 213, 1963.
7. **Stehbins, W. E.**, Reaction of venous endothelium in injury, *Lab. Invest.*, 14, 449, 1965.
8. **Kitchin, A. H. and Julian, D. G.**, The cardiovascular system, in *A Companion to Medical Studies*, Vol. 1, Passmore, R. and Robson, J. S., Eds., F. A. Davis, Philadelphia, 1968, chap. 28.
9. **Stemerman, M. B.**, Vascular intimal components: precursors of thrombosis, in *Progress in Hemostasis and Thrombosis*, Vol. 2, Spaet, T. H., Ed., Grune & Stratton, New York, 1974, chap. 1.
10. **Majno, G.**, Ultrastructure of the vascular membrane, in *Handbook of Physiology*, Vol. 3, Hamilton, W. F. and Dow, H., Eds., American Physiological Society, Washington, D.C., 1965, 2293.
11. **Ganong, W. F.**, *Review of Medical Physiology*, 3rd ed., Lange, Los Altos, Calif., 1967, 472.
12. **Majno, G., Shea, S. M., and Leventhal, M.**, Endothelial contraction induced by histamine-type mediators. An electron microscopic study, *J. Cell. Biol.*, 42, 647, 1969.
13. **Henry, R. L. and Steiman, R. H.**, Mechanisms of hemostasis, *Microvasc. Res.*, 1, 68, 1968.
14. **Lautsch, E. V., McMillian, G. C., and Duff, G. L.**, Techniques for the study of the normal and atherosclerotic arterial intima from its endothelial surface, *Lab. Invest.*, 2, 397, 1953.
15. **Shimamoto, T. and Sunaga, T.**, Contraction of endothelial cells as a key mechanism in atherogenesis, *Proc. Jpn. Acad.*, 48, 633, 1972.
16. **Chen, S. and Barnhart, M. I.**, Platelet-vessel wall interaction after glycohydrolase treatment, *Scanning Electron Micros.*, 2, 485, 1977.
17. **Altschul, R.**, *Endothelium: Its Development, Morphology, Function and Pathology*, Macmillan, New York, 1954.
18. **Smith, U., Ryan, J. W., Mickie, D. D., and Smith, D. S.**, Endothelial projections as revealed by scanning electron microscopy, *Science*, 173, 925, 1971.
19. **Luft, J. H.**, Fine structure of capillary and endothelial layer as revealed by ruthenium red, *Fed. Proc.*, 25, 1773, 1966.
20. **Copley, A.L. and Scheinthal, B. M.**, Nature of the endothelial layer as demonstrated by ruthenium red, *Exp. Cell. Res.*, 59, 491, 1970.
21. **Becker, C. G. and Murphy, G. E.**, Demonstration of contractile protein in endothelium and cells of the heart valves, endocardium, intima, arteriosclerotic plaques and Aschoff bodies of rheumatic heart disease, *Am. J. Pathol.*, 55, 1, 1969.
22. **Payling-Wright, H.**, Endothelial mitosis around aortic branches in normal guinea pigs, *Nature (London)*, 220, 78, 1968.
23. **Payling-Wright, H.**, Endothelial turnover, *Thromb. Diath. Haemorrh.*, 40, 79, 1970.
24. **Spaet, T. H. and Lejnieks, L.**, Mitotic activity of rabbit blood vessels, *Proc. Soc. Exp. Biol. Med.*, 125, 1197, 1967.
25. **Algire, G. H. and Chalkney, H. W.**, Vascular reactions of normal and malignant tissues in vivo. I. Vascular reactions of mice to wounds and to normal and neoplastic transplants, *J. Natl. Cancer Inst.*, 6, 73, 1945.
26. **de los Santos, R. P. and Hoyer, L. W.**, Antihemophiliac factor in tissue: localization by immunofluorescence, *Fed. Proc.*, 31, 279, 1972.
27. **Todd, A. S.**, Histological localization of fibrinolysis activator, *J. Pathol. Bacteriol.*, 78, 281, 1959.
28. **Astrup, T.**, Tissue activators of plasminogen, *Fed. Proc.*, 25, 42, 1966.
29. **Pecket, L.**, Fibrinolysis, *N. Engl. J. Med.*, 273, 966, 1965.
30. **Kwaan, H. C. and Astrup, T.**, Fibrinolytic activity in thrombosed veins, *Circ. Res.*, 17, 477, 1965.
31. **Jaffe, E. A., Nachman, R. L., and Gecker, C. G.**, Culture of human endothelial cells derived from umbilical cord veins, *Abstr. 3rd Congr. Int. Soc. Thromb. Haemostasis*, 1972, 366.
32. **Patek, A. J., Jr. and Taylor, F. H. L.**, Hemophilia. II. Some properties of a substance obtained from normal human plasma effective in accelerating the coagulation of hemophilic blood, *J. Clin. Invest.*, 16, 113, 1937.
33. **Cohen, S. S. and Chargaff, E.**, Studies on the chemistry of blood coagulation. IX. The thromboplastic protein from lung, *J. Biol. Chem.*, 136, 243, 1940.

34. Deutsch, E., Irsigler, K., and Lomoschitz, H., Studien uber gewebethromboplastin, *Thromb. Diath. Haemorrh.*, 12, 12, 1964.
35. Irsigler, K., Human brain tissue thromboplastin, *Thromb. Diath. Haemorrh. Suppl.*, 13, 433, 1964.
36. Hvatum, M. and Prydz, H., Studies on tissue thromboplastin. 1. Solubilization with sodium deoxycholate, *Biochim. Biophys. Acta*, 130, 92, 1966.
37. Nemerson, Y. and Pitlick, F. A., Purification and characterization of the protein component of tissue factor, *Biochemistry*, 9, 5100, 1970.
38. Bjorklid, E. and Storm, E., Purification and some properties of the protein component of tissue thromboplastin from human brain, *Biochem. J.*, 165, 89, 1977.
39. Zeldes, S. M., Nemerson, Y., Pitlick, F., and Lentz, T., Tissue factor (thromboplastin). Localization to plasma membrane by peroxidase-conjugated antibodies, *Science*, 175, 766, 1972.
40. Becker, C. G. and Nachman, R. L., Contractile proteins of endothelial cells, platelets and smooth muscle cells, *Am. J. Pathol.*, 71, 1, 1973.
41. Wessler, S. and Yin, E. T., On the mechanism of thrombosis, in *Progress in Hematology*, Vol. 4, Brown, E. B. and Moore, C. V., Eds., Grune & Stratton, New York, 1969, 201.
42. Majno, G. and Palade, G. E., Studies on inflammation. 1. The effect of histamine and serotonin on vascular permeability. An electron microscopic study, *J. Biophys. Biochem. Cytol.*, 11, 571, 1961.
43. Sheppard, B. L. and French, J. E., Platelet adhesion in the rabbit abdominal aorta following the removal of the endothelium: a scanning and transmission electron microscopical study, *Proc. R. Soc. London, Ser. B.*, 176, 427, 1971.
44. O'Brien, J. R., The adhesiveness of native platelets and its prevention, *J. Clin. Pathol.*, 14, 140, 1961.
45. Baumgartner, H. R., Platelet interaction with vascular structures, *Thromb. Diath. Haemorrh. Suppl.*, 43, 161, 1971.
46. French, J. E., McFarlane, R. G., and Sanders, A. G., The structure of haemostatic plugs and experimental thrombi in small arteries, *Br. J. Exp. Pathol.*, 45, 467, 1964.
47. Tranzer, J. P. and Baumgartner, H. R., Filling gaps in the vascular endothelium with blood platelets, *Nature (London)*, 216, 1126, 1967.
48. Kjaerheim, A. and Hovig, T., The ultrastructure of haemostatic blood platelet plugs in rabbit mesenterium, *Thromb. Diath. Haemorrh.*, 7, 1, 1962.
49. Baumgartner, H. R., Stemerman, M. B., and Spaet, T. H., Adhesion of blood platelets to subendothelial surface: distinct from adhesion to collagen, *Experientia*, 27, 283, 1971.
50. Hodge, A. J., Structure at the electron microscopic level, in *Treatise on Collagen*, Gould, B. S., Ed., Academic Press, New York, 1967, 185.
51. Wilner, G. D., Nossel, H. L., and LeRoy, E. C., Activation of Hageman factor by collagen, *J. Clin. Invest.*, 47, 2608, 1968.
52. Wojcik, J. D., Van Horn, D. L., Webber, A. J., and Johnson, S. A., Mechanism whereby platelets support the endothelium, *Transfusion (Philadelphia)*, 9, 324, 1969.
53. Weiss, H. J., Platelets and their role in hemostasis, *Ann. N. Y. Acad. Sci.*, 201, 3, 1972.
54. Holmsen, H., The platelet: its membrane, physiology and biochemistry, *Clin. in Haematol.*, 1, 325, 1972.
55. Seaman, G. V. F., Surface potential and platelet aggregation, *Thromb. Diath. Haemorrh. Suppl.*, 26, 53, 1967.
56. Wilner, G. D., Nossel, H. L., and Procupec, T. C., Aggregation of platelets by collagen: polar active sites of insoluble human collagen, *Am. J. Physiol.*, 220, 1074, 1971.
57. Mason, R. G. and Read, M. S., Platelet response to six agglutinating agents: species similarities and differences, *Exp. Mol. Pathol.*, 6, 370, 1967.
58. Jaffe, R. and Deykin, D., Evidence for a structural requirement for the aggregation of platelets by collagen, *J. Clin. Invest.*, 53, 875, 1974.
59. Cooper, H. A., Mason, R. G., and Brinkhous, K. M., The platelet: membrane and surface reactions, *Annu. Rev. Physiol.*, 38, 501, 1976.
60. Mason, R. G. and Read, M. S., Some effects of a microcrystalline collagen preparation on blood, *Haemostasis*, 3, 31, 1974.
61. Swann, D. H., The role of vitreous collagen in platelet aggregation in vitro and in vivo, *J. Lab. Clin. Med.*, 84, 264, 1974.
62. Barber, A. J. and Jamison, G. A., Platelet collagen adhesion: characterization of collagen glycosyltransferase of plasma membranes of human blood platelets, *Biochim. Biophys. Acta*, 253, 533, 1971.
63. Chesney, C. M., Harper, E., and Coleman, R. W., Critical role of the carbohydrate side chains of collagen in platelet aggregation, *J. Clin. Invest.*, 51, 2693, 1972.
64. Pruett, D., Wasserman, B. K., Ford, J. D., and Cunningham, L. W., Collagen-mediated platelet aggregation. Effects of collagen modification involving the platelet and carbohydrate moieties, *J. Clin. Invest.*, 52, 2495, 1973.

65. **Robinson, C. W., Mason, R. G., and Wagner, R. H.**, Effect of sulfhydryl inhibitors on platelet agglutinability, *Proc. Soc. Exp. Biol. Med.*, 113, 857, 1963.
66. **Walsh, P.**, The effect of collagen and kaolin on the intrinsic coagulant activity of platelets. Evidence for an alternative pathway in intrinsic coagulation not requiring Factor XII, *Br. J. Haematol.*, 22, 393, 1972.
67. **Gryglewski, R. J., Bunting, S., Moncada, S., Flower, R. J., and Vane, J. R.**, Arterial walls are protected against deposition of platelet thrombi by a substance (Prostaglandin X) which they make from prostaglandin endoperoxides, *Prostaglandins*, 12, 685, 1976.
68. **Bunting, S., Gryglewski, R., Moncada, S., and Vane, J. R.**, Arterial walls generate from prostaglandin endoperoxides a substance (Prostaglandin X) which relaxes strips of mesenteric and coeliac arteries and inhibits platelet aggregation, *Prostaglandins*, 12, 897, 1976.
69. **Hamberg, M., Svensson, J., and Samuelsson, B.**, Thromboxanes: a new group of biologically active components derived from prostaglandin endoperoxides, *Proc. Natl. Acad. Sci. U.S.A.*, 72, 2994, 1975.
70. **Day, C. E.**, On the newly discovered role of prostaglandins in arteries and its implications for the control of atherosclerosis, platelets, and thrombosis, *Artery*, 2, 480, 1976.
71. **Moncada, S., Gryglewski, R., Bunting, S., and Vane, J. R.**, A lipid peroxide inhibits the enzyme in blood vessel microsomes that generate from prostaglandin endoperoxides the substance (Prostaglandin X) which prevents platelet aggregation, *Prostaglandins*, 12, 715, 1976.
72. **Barnhart, M. I. and Baechler, C. A.**, Endothelial cell physiology, perturbations and responses, *Semin. Thromb. and Hemos.*, 5, 50, 1979.
73. **Nalbandian, R. M. and Henry, R. L.**, Platelet-endothelial cell interactions: metabolic maps of structures and actions of prostaglandins, prostacycline, thromboxane, and cyclic-AMP, *Semin. Thromb. and Hemos.*, 5, 87, 1979.
74. **Barnhart, M. I. and Chen, S. T.**, Vessel wall models for studying interaction capabilities with blood platelets, *Semin. Thromb. and Hemos.*, 5, 112, 1979.

Chapter 2

PLATELET FUNCTION IN HEMOSTASIS

Raymond L. Henry

TABLE OF CONTENTS

I. Introduction 18

II. Platelet Morphology 18
    A. Peripheral Zone 18
        1. Glycocalyx 18
            a. Coagulation Proteins and Platelet Factors 19
            b. Molecules Related to the Complement System 20
        2. Plasma Membrane 21
            a. Morphology 21
            b. Biochemical Properties 21
            c. Surface Charge 23
            d. Platelet Receptors 23
                1. ADP Receptors 23
                2. Thrombin Receptors 24
                3. Epinephrine Receptors 24
                4. Serotonin Receptors 25
        3. Open Canalicular System 25
    B. Sol-Gel Zone 25
        1. Microtubules and Microfilaments 25
        2. Dense Tubular System 25
        3. Thrombosthenin 25
    C. Organelle Zone 27
        1. Dense Bodies 27
        2. Mitochondria 28
        3. α-Granules 28

III. Platelet Adhesion and Cohesion 28
    A. Collagen 29
    B. Shape Change 29
    C. ADP 29

IV. Platelet Production, Storage, and Destruction 30
    A. Megakaryocytopoiesis 30
    B. Platelet Age and Size 32

V. Summary 32

References 33

I. INTRODUCTION

Platelets are structural complex elements of the blood, which circulate in disc form averaging 3 μ in diameter and 1 μ in thickness (Figure 1). Their volume is approximately 6 μm^3. Platelets contain dense bodies, alpha granules, mitochondria, vacuoles, microtubules, vesicles, microfilaments, lysosomes, glycogen granules, a dense tubular system, Golgi apparatus, cytosol, plasma membrane, and a glycocalyx. The Golgi complex and endoplasmic reticulum (dense tubular system) are rarely seen. Platelets are anucleate since their origin is by pinching off of megakaryocyte cytoplasm. The purpose of this discussion is to examine the relationship of these structures and their contents to platelet function. Interrelationships with the blood vessel wall and blood plasma compartment will not be discussed in detail in this section, except where necessary to describe specific platelet functions, such as platelet factor 3 (PF-3) and its location, release, and interaction with blood coagulation. Platelet constituents, such as coagulation proteins and molecules of the complement system, will be discussed in relation to platelet morphology. Their generation, activation, and interrelated function are dealt with in Chapter 3. Abnormalities of platelet function, hereditary and acquired, are presented in Chapter 6.

II. PLATELET MORPHOLOGY

Platelet structure can arbitrarily be viewed in terms of a peripheral zone, a sol-gel zone, and an organelle zone. There are obvious morphologic and functional interrelations of these three zones. However, this compartmentalization has been helpful in the examination of location and specific functional characteristics of constituents of the various platelet structures (Figure 1).

A. Peripheral Zone

The peripheral zone contains an exterior coat (glycocalyx), the plasma membrane with its submembrane area, and an open canalicular system. The glycocalyx (fluffy coat) is peculiar to the platelet among the cellular elements of the blood. The plasma membrane, like other cell membranes, is a triple-layered structure of 70 Å to 90 Å in thickness. The open canalicular system traverses the plasma membrane and glycocalyx and represents a channel for platelet pickup and release of various materials.

The peripheral zone represents that aspect of platelets first to respond to external stimuli. Since it serves as a physical barrier between the intracellular constituents and extracellular environment, the peripheral zone must undergo change for the platelet functions of adhesion, cohesion, and the release reaction. The glycocalyx undoubtedly accounts for the unusual stickiness of the platelet surface, but it must be enhanced by external stimulation. The membrane must change its shape, likely by movement of glycoproteins and lipoproteins in the membrane lipid matrix, to reassemble and magnify receptor areas that are intimately linked to membrane and submembrane biochemical processes that evoke the typical platelet response of contraction with centralization of vacuoles, pseudopod formation, and the release mechanisms. The open canalicular system fuses with granular membranes, in response to the triggering of intracellular biochemical events, and allows for extrusion of granular contents to the exterior. When the platelet response is severe, lysosomal enzymes are released, and the morphological integrity of the peripheral zone is lost.

1. Glycocalyx

The glycocalyx contains plasma proteins, carbohydrates, and a number of molecules

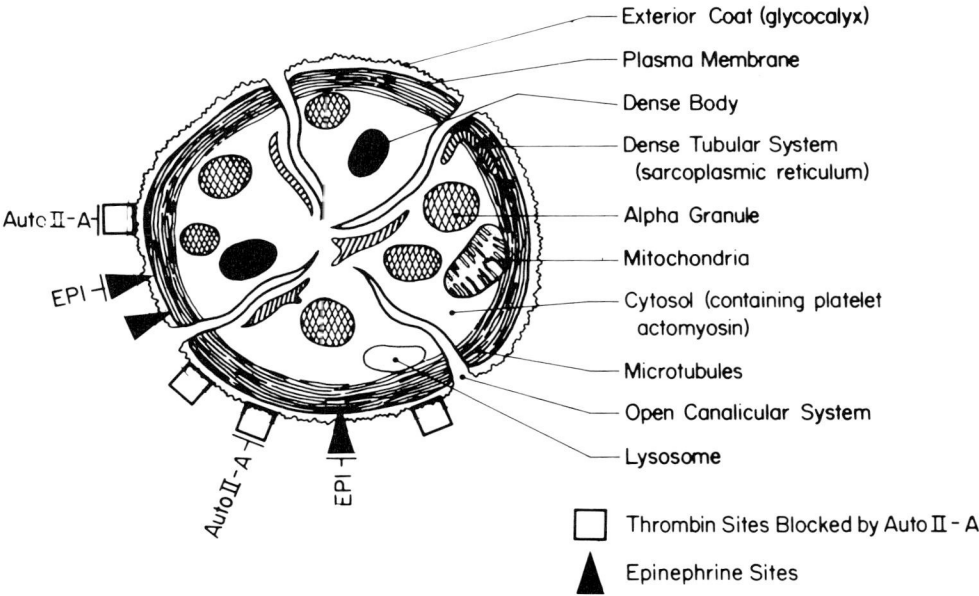

FIGURE 1. Composite diagramatic representation of platelet structural constituents taken from electron micrographs. Presumed receptor sites for thrombin and epinephrine, for examples, are shown. Other vitamin K-dependent proteins are known to function at thrombin receptor sites. Here, autoprothrombin II-A is shown at the thrombin receptor sites.

related to the complement, coagulation, and fibrinolytic systems. This "plasmatic atmosphere" was early described by Roskam.[1] Although the presence of a plasmatic atmosphere has been confirmed, only some of the constituents adsorbed to the surface can be removed by gel filtration or simple washing.[2,3] Others, although present as adsorbed constituents, are also bound in some manner to internal membranes. There are notable examples. Factor V (PF-1)* is firmly bound to platelet particles.[4] Freeze-thawing with homogenization and extraction procedures does not remove PF-1 activity from the platelet particles. No acceleration of thrombin activity is found with the supernatants. PF-3 is found associated with platelet membrane fractions.[5,6] However, some PF-3 activity can be found in solution following platelet aggregation.[7-11] PF-4 is located in platelet-dense bodies, but is readily released during platelet activation.[12-14] Fibrinogen, although adsorbed onto the platelet surface, is also found in the platelet interior.

a. Coagulation Proteins and Platelet Factors

Vitamin K-dependent Factors II, VII, IX, and X, as well as Factor VIII, are closely associated with platelet membranes.[15,16] The platelet aggregating component of the Factor VIII complex is responsible for ristocetin-induced platelet aggregation.[17,18] Presence of these procoagulant factors undoubtedly accounts for much of the local platelet function, both in normal hemostasis and abnormal thrombosis. Four of the seven platelet factors are intimately involved with platelet function.[19] Although they are found principally in the platelet interior, release allows for interaction with the glycocalyx and plasma components (Table 1).

PF-2 (fibrinoplastic substance) accelerates thrombin's ability to clot fibrinogen.[20] PF-4 enhances fibrin monomer polymerization[21] and inhibits heparin. PF-3 (lipopro-

---

* PF = Platelet factor.

TABLE 1

Platelet Factors and Their Function

	Factors	Function
PF-1:	Platelet accelerator globulin (Factor V)	Accelerates conversion of prothrombin to thrombin
PF-2:	Fibrinoplastic substance	Enhances thrombin clotting of fibrinogen
PF-3:	Lipoprotein thromboplastin (phospholipoprotein)	Accelerates intrinsic pathway and common pathway of thrombin formation
PF-4:	Antiheparin factor	Neutralizes heparin activity
PF-5:	Fibrinogen, clotting factor	May function in platelet adhesiveness
PF-6:	Antifibrinolytic principle	Inhibits plasmin—noncompetitively
PF-7:	Platelet cothromboplastin	Assists thromboplastin in complete conversion of prothrombin to thrombin

tein platelet thromboplastin) is required in the intrinsic (platelet-plasma) coagulation system. It is the phospholipid that complexes with F-XII* and F-XI to yield active products; with F-IXa + F-VIII + F-X + Ca^{++} to yield F-Xa; and with F-Xa + F-V + F-II + Ca^{++} to yield thrombin. The resultant enzyme, thrombin, forms fibrin to firm up the platelet aggregate and, in addition, induces further release of adenine nucleotides, platelet factors, lysosomal enzymes, and intraplatelet procoagulants such as F-XIII, the fibrin-stabilizing factor.[22] Among the platelet factors released is PF-6, an antiplasmin (antifibrinolysin) that further prevents dissolution of the fibrin-firmed plug.[19,23]

Thus the glycocalyx is intimately involved in the interdependent functions of platelets with the coagulation system. Platelets are necessary for the intrinsic coagulation systems that ultimately produce thrombin. Thrombin firms up the platelet mass with fibrin, degrades the platelet with secondary complete release of platelet constituents, including fibrin-stabilizing substances, antifibrinolytic agents, and vasoactive material.

b. Molecules Related to the Complement System

Naturally occurring macromolecules that are involved in platelet aggregation include fibrinogen, von Willebrand factor, and aggregated immunoglobulin G (IgG). Others are also known, such as polylysine[24] and platelet-aggregating factor (PAF).[25]

The aggregated subclasses of IgG (IgG1, IgG2, IgG3, and IgG4) induce the platelet release reaction and aggregate platelets.[26] Other immunoglobulins in the aggregated form (IgA, IgA2, IgD, IgE, and IgM) do not mediate platelet aggregation.[27] Heterologous antibodies, in the absence of complement, will induce release of serotonin without cytolysis. In the presence of complement, complete release occurs. Complement-fixing platelet isoantibodies will bring about platelet release and aggregation, but non-complement-fixing isoantibodies cause some release without platelet aggregation.[28]

Since F (ab) 2 fragments do not participate in IgG-induced platelet aggregation, while Fc fragments do, there is likely an Fc receptor on the platelet membrane or within the glycocalyx to directly accept the Fc portion of IgG.[29] The Fc binding site is likely exposed by the formation of immune complexes by aggregated IgG, since native 7s

---

* F = Plasma factor.

antibody does not bind to the receptor.[30]

Another mechanism to account for IgG platelet-aggregating function could be the presence of the Cl component on the platelet membrane or absorbed in the platelet plasmatic atmosphere. Since serum and Clq inhibit the release reaction by IgG,[26,27] and since the Fc fragment contains the binding site for Cl, the Fc receptor could actually be the Cl component of complement.

Calcium ions are essential for activity of the Cl complex. Chelating agents prevent platelet aggregation, but aggregated IgG can still elicit the release reaction. Furthermore, periodate oxidation of the carbohydrate portion of IgG abolishes its platelet-aggregating capability.[30] In addition, IgG4 does not bind complement, but it does induce platelet aggregation. Peculiarities of this type make it difficult to sort out the role of complement in platelet aggregation.

2. Plasma Membrane
a. Morphology

Platelet plasma membranes are 70 Å to 90 Å and, like other cell membranes, have a triple layer. Although lipids, lipoproteins, and glycoproteins are present, they are not arranged in a strict tri-layered form. Some of the proteinaceous molecules likely are free to migrate within the lipid matrix.[31] Others, the membrane structural proteins primarily, are fixed in position.

b. Biochemical Properties

Numerous enzymes are associated with platelet membranes. Methods to separate enzymes belonging to the plasma membrane from those belonging to intraplatelet membranes are not discriminatory. However, platelet plasma membranes appear to be rich in glycosyl transferases.[32] One such transferase, an ectoenzyme, transfers amino-sugar residues to collagen or glycoprotein and may be involved in platelet adhesion to collagen.[33,34]

Another ectoenzyme of special interest is "ecto-ATPase". Since it is inhibited by ADP, it may participate in platelet aggregation induced by ADP.[35] The ecto-ATPase may be necessary to maintain the platelet in a nonadhesive state. In addition, ecto-ATPase has antithrombosthenin properties and may function in preventing surface responses of this contractile protein.[36] However, antibodies to thrombosthenin do not prevent platelet aggregation by various inducers.[37]

Other molecules of platelet membranes include phosphodiesterases (likely an intraplatelet membrane enzyme), acid and alkaline phosphatases, nucleotidases besides ATPase, hexokinases, and adenylate cyclase.[38]

Activation of the membrane enzyme adenylate cyclase converts ATP to cyclic AMP (cAMP) (Figure 2). Evidence exists to implicate cAMP as a central figure in platelet responsiveness.[39-43] Increased intraplatelet levels of cAMP are associated with inhibition of platelet aggregation, while decreased levels are related to activation of platelets.[40,41,44] These observations are not conclusive since they are not consistent in all instances of either activation or inhibition.

Phosphodiesterase (PDE), an intraplatelet enzyme, degrades cAMP to the inert form, 5'AMP (Figure 2). Inhibitors of PDE, such as the methylxanthines, affect mechanisms directed at inhibition of platelet aggregation with an increase in cAMP by-product inhibition.[45,46,47]

Various platelet functions are directed by the phosphorylated protein enzymes induced by cAMP (Figure 2). An example of one such function is related to the calcium chelator properties of the phosphorylated protein kinase.[48] Calcium ions are required for most forms of platelet aggregation. Calcium chelators (sodium citrate, EDTA, etc.) inhibit platelet aggregation. An excess of chelator, such as in blood collection sampling

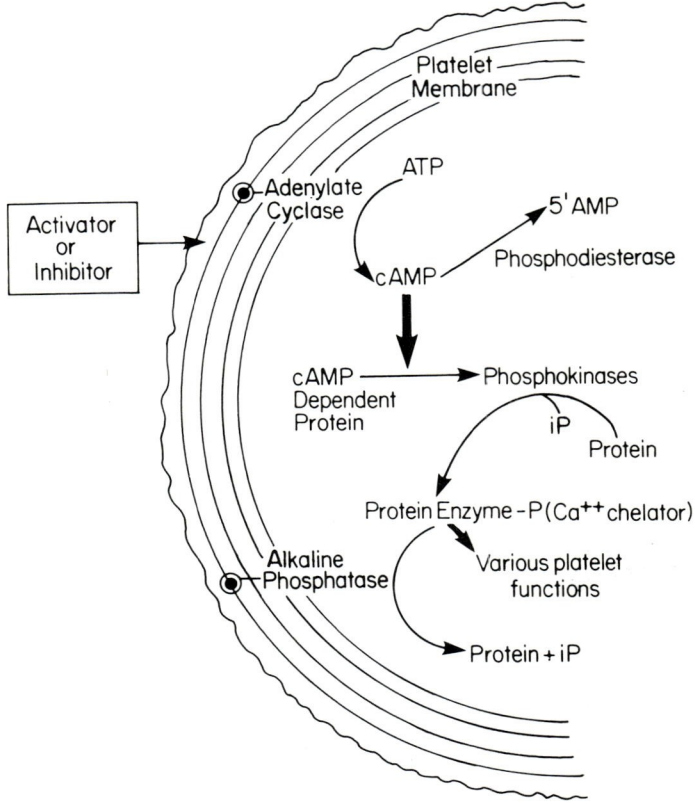

FIGURE 2. Representation of the biochemical reactions involving cyclic-AMP that can be activated or inhibited. Activation of adenylate cyclase or inhibition of phosphodiesterase increases cAMP levels, which is consistent with inhibited platelet aggregation. Activation of the membrane-bound alkaline phosphatase reduces the phosphorylated protein enzyme, and Ca^{++} are free to enhance platelet aggregation.

errors, profoundly affect platelet aggregometry studies for assessment of platelet responsiveness. Heparin, only a mild chelator of Ca^{++}, can be used as the anticoagulant when such sampling errors are suspected. Increased uptake of Ca^{++} occurs by the sarcoplasmic reticulum of skeletal and cardiac muscle in the presence of cAMP.[49,50] The dense tubular system of platelets functions as a sarcoplasmic reticulum, and it is believed that cAMP functions in platelets by directing uptake of Ca^{++}.[51] Therefore, an increase in cAMP would inhibit platelet responsiveness.

Since the phosphorylated protein enzyme is a divalent cation chelator, phosphate acceptor molecules should enhance platelet function by competing for phosphate, so that the chelator complex cannot be formed, allowing more Ca^{++} to remain free. Thrombin platelet aggregation may be accounted for by this mechanism.[48] However, thrombin may also inhibit adenylate cyclase.[52,53]

Alkaline phosphatase, an enzyme probably attached to the inner aspect of the plasma membrane, dephosphorylates the protein Ca^{++} chelator and thereby releases Ca^{++} (Figure 2). Some aggregating agents could function by activation of the phosphatase, while some inhibitors of platelet aggregation could function by inhibition of the enzyme.

c. Surface Charge

Platelets are negatively charged in plasma. Platelet electrophoretic mobility is decreased after exposure to most aggregating agents. This normal net charge becomes more negative when platelets are exposed to ADP.[54-59] ADP may uncover phospholipids of the platelet plasma membrane and allow formation of Ca^{++} bridges between platelets. This may be one means to account for increased stickiness of stimulated platelets. However, there are many other molecules in the membrane and within the plasmatic atmosphere that could also account for increased stickiness upon activation.

Sialic acid residues on the platelet surface appear to account for about one half of the surface charge because treatment of platelets with neuraminidase decreases both charge and electrophoretic ability by at least 45%.[60] It has been calculated, by content of N-acetyl neuraminic acid released, that platelets have about 11 times more sialic acid residues per square micrometer than red blood cells.[61] Perhaps this could account for the great difference between the two cell types in ability to form a sticky surface.

Other molecules or side groups of molecules that could take part in the development of a sticky membrane, or at least the surface charge, include phosphate, sulfate, carboxyl groups, and various receptor binding sites. Whether these charges are simply uncovered or bound by a platelet activator or whether the membrane and fluffy coat receive signals from the platelet interior is not known. Both negative and positive charges are scattered over the entire surface. The net charge is negative and so is that of vascular endothelium. Platelets become more negative upon stimulation and endothelium becomes more positive (yet still net negative) upon damage. It is likely that the relative difference allows for attraction and adhesion. Cohesion, however, probably depends upon released materials, such as ADP.

d. Platelet Receptors

There are many types of receptors on the platelet membrane or within the plasmatic atmosphere (Figure 1). Complement receptors have already been discussed (see above, Section II.A.1.b). Others to be discussed here include receptors for ADP, thrombin, epinephrine, and serotonin.

1. ADP Receptors

Platelet aggregation is inhibited by nucleotides other than ADP.[62] However, ATP and AMP likely must be degraded to adenosine for this inhibitory effect.[63] Papaverine blocks adenosine uptake by platelets, but enhances inhibition of aggregation. In addition, aggregation inhibition remains after adenosine deamination. Adenosine likely acts as an intraplatelet inhibitor, rather than binding to an ADP site on the membrane.

Adenine nucleotides with unequal charges (ADP, adenosine tetraphosphate) are the nucleotides that induce platelet activation.[64] ADP may function by forming bridges with Ca^{++} or by product inhibition of an ATPase on the membrane. The ATPase may be necessary to maintain the platelet in a nonadhesive state.[35,36]

Repeated or prolonged exposure of platelets to ADP renders them insensitive to further additions of ADP.[65-67] However, these desensitized platelets will still aggregate with epinephrine and collagen.[67,68] It is likely that ADP does not deplete all endogenous stores of release materials.

Platelet aggregation by ADP requires Ca^{++}, fibrinogen, and intraplatelet metabolic ATP. Magnesium ions will not substitute for Ca^{++} and, in fact, inhibit platelet aggregation by ADP.[69,70] If glycolysis and oxidative phosphorylation are blocked with reduction or depletion of metabolic ATP, or if platelets are suspended in a glucose-free medium for several hours, ADP will not induce aggregation.[71,72]

Fibrinogen has been suggested as a requirement for ADP platelet aggregation.[70,73-77] Washed or gel-filtered platelets will not respond to ADP unless fibrinogen is added back.[75] These platelets, however, will respond with collagen or thrombin.[77] Since the intracellular fibrinogen is not removed by washing, release by the potent activators collagen and thrombin may account for these observations.[78-80]

2. Thrombin Receptors

Thrombin activation of platelets is complete and irreversible. ADP is likely required at some step because adenosine block of the release reaction or apyrase removal of ADP both inhibit thrombin-induced platelet aggregation.[74,81,82] That thrombin produces fibrin on the platelet surface to account for platelet aggregation is doubtful in view of these observations.[83,84] In addition, snake venoms and staphylococcal coagulase will clot fibrinogen without platelet aggregation.[85,86] These clots will not retract, indicating lack of platelet function at that physiologic level.

Thrombin aggregates platelets made refractory to ADP, so release of materials other than ADP may be involved in the thrombin response. Thrombin's phosphate receptor activity and resultant competition for phosphate with intraplatelet proteins that act as Ca^{++} chelators may represent primary mechanisms for the platelet response to thrombin (Figure 2).[87]

Molecules similar to thrombin compete for the thrombin sites on the platelet membrane. Autoprothrombin II-A* and Factor X_a depress thrombin platelet aggregation and yet are mild aggregators themselves.[88-90] When autoprothrombin II-A reacts with the thrombin sites, epinephrine-induced platelet aggregation is potentiated. Dog platelets, for example, respond to an intermediate optimal concentration of epinephrine. They do not aggregate with higher or lower concentrations unless a molecule like thrombin, autoprothrombin II-A, or Factor X_a interact with thrombin receptor sites.[88] With excess epinephrine, addition of autoprothrombin II-A enables it to occupy the thrombin sites and, in addition, develop complexes (epinephrine with some released constituent) that have a predilection for epinephrine receptors previously distorted by overload. With epinephrine saturation and excess epinephrine molecules, autoprothrombin II-A can be added before or after epinephrine, since complexes can form in either case with free epinephrine molecules. In the case of low quantities of epinephrine, complexes can only form when autoprothrombin II-A is added first, because platelet release must take place before or when free epinephrine molecules are within the platelet atmosphere.

3. Epinephrine Receptors

Epinephrine functions primarily through an alpha receptor on the platelet membrane. It ordinarily induces a biphasic platelet aggregation pattern.[91] The second phase can be blocked with aspirin and, therefore, likely depends on activation of the platelet release reaction.[92] The second wave may develop because of the potentiating effect of epinephrine on ADP, serotonin, or thrombin-induced platelet aggregation.[93,94] The release, however, is not related to constituents of the alpha granules, so that epinephrine's potentiation of the thrombin effect is less likely than potentiation of materials released from other nonmetabolic sites. PF-4 is released with high levels of epinephrine,[95] and up to 55% of platelet ADP and 30% of platelet ATP are released.[96] This equals the entire nonmetabolic storage levels of the adenine nucleotides. That ADP is involved in epinephrine platelet aggregation is supported by the observation that ADPase inhibits both aggregation waves.[82]

Epinephrine likely binds to its alpha site and then functions through inhibition of cAMP.[97] Some epinephrine diffuses into the platelet, and this uptake is related to beta receptor activity, since propranolol, a beta blocker, inhibits epinephrine uptake. This

---

* Active Protein-C (see Chapter 3).

inhibition is additive to that obtained with the alpha blocker, phentolamine.[53,94] Phentolamine does not allow the decrease in cAMP induced by epinephrine. The epinephrine effect on cAMP likely accounts for its ability to potentiate collagen- and thrombin-mediated platelet aggregation.[98,99]

4. Serotonin Receptors

About 90% of the body stores of serotonin are carried by platelets in the dense bodies. Uptake is by way of a facilitated diffusion transport mechanism, the serotonin receptor. Uptake can be inhibited by imipramine and reserpine[60] and destroyed by neuraminidase. Transport of serotonin in or out of the platelet by its receptor mechanism is not related to the much faster mechanism of serotonin release through the open canalicular system. However, uptake may be related to some ADP release, since a weak aggregation occurs if platelets are stirred during serotonin uptake. Serotonin potentiates ADP aggregation, but the second phase level of platelet aggregation and release is never achieved.[60]

3. Open Canalicular System

Platelets have two tubular systems.[101] One system contains dense material and, hence, is called the dense tubular system (Figure 1). These tubular structures are thought to function as a sarcoplasmic reticulum for Ca^{++} sequestration (see below). The open canalicular system is believed to be the channel for transport of released intraplatelet constituents to the platelet exterior.[102] Storage granules have been seen intact within the open canalicular system when platelets were allowed to take up polylysine and then activated.[103,104] When the open canalicular system is treated with thrombin following platelet release, electron-dense material similar to fibrin appears, supporting the idea that fibrinogen is released through this tubular system.[105]

B. Sol-Gel Zone

The sol-gel zone is that area of the platelet containing molecules and structures involved in the formation of the contractile protein, thrombosthenin, and its interaction with microtubules. The dense tubular system, or sarcoplasmic reticulum, is important for the source of Ca^{++} necessary for the contractile mechanism to function.

1. Microtubules and Microfilaments

Microtubules seem to form a skeleton framework on which thrombosthenin can function.[106] Microtubules are preserved by cytochalasin B stabilization, and the platelet discoid shape is preserved upon chilling.[107] Pseudopod formation occurs upon chilling if the microtubules are not stabilized. In this case, the microtubules dissolve, releasing subcomponents that retain Ca^{++}-chelating properties.

2. Dense Tubular System

The dense tubular system functions like the sarcoplasmic reticulum of muscle tissue and sequesters Ca^{++}.[102] Dense granules also contain Ca^{++}, which is released when platelets are activated.[108] These calcium ions are likely extruded to the platelet exterior through the open canalicular system. Ionophores, such as A23187 and X537A, will free Ca^{++} from the dense tubular system.[49,109,110] These calcium ions are thought to be the trigger for contraction of thrombosthenin.[111]

3. Thrombosthenin

Thrombosthenin, a contractile protein like actomyosin of muscle, is related to microtubules of the sol-gel zone of platelets. The microtubular skeleton ring is retracted toward the platelet center, trapping components of the organelle zone (Figure 3). In

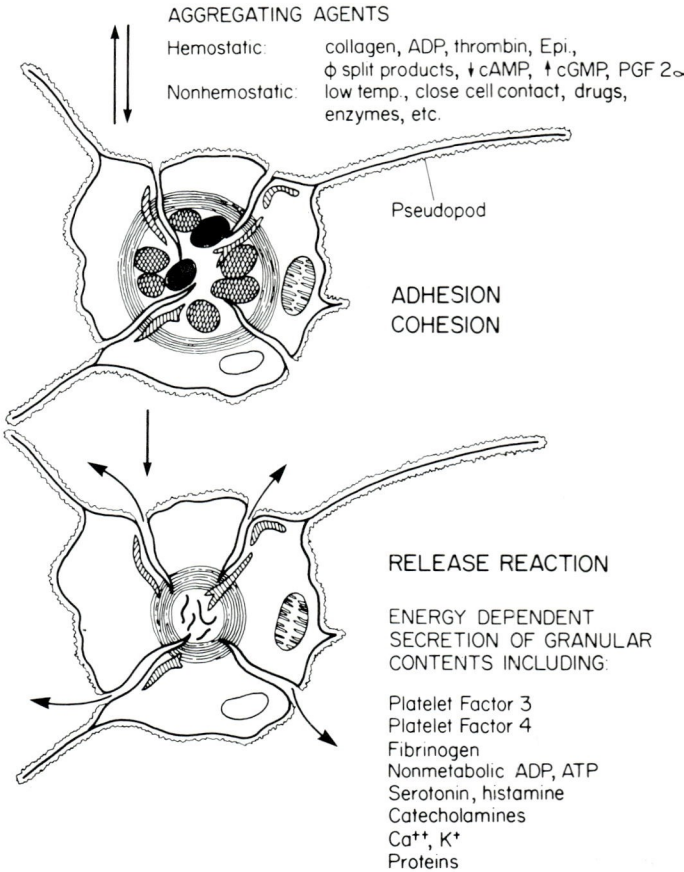

FIGURE 3. Diagramatic representation of platelet structural changes during organelle retraction and the release reaction. These are reversible events until α-granules are released leading to complete platelet destruction.

addition, microfilaments of thrombosthenin appear to project outward and assist in the formation of pseudopods similar to that observed in other cells (Figure 4).[31] Microfilaments within the pseudopod and at nodal points of the plasma membrane may also be involved in surface receptor modification by directing movements of proteinaceous molecules through the lipid matrix of the platelet plasma membrane.[30,31]

Thrombosthenin accounts for nearly 15% of the total platelet protein.[112,113] It requires Ca^{++} for contractile activity and development of ATPase function.[114-116] Within the platelet, contractile activity is related to retraction of the microtubular system and release of stored granular constituents.[112] When released from platelets by thrombin, thrombosthenin functions to retract the clot consisting of fibrin, platelets, and other trapped cellular elements, with expression of serum.[119,120] Clot retraction is ordinarily abnormal in thrombasthenia.[121-124] However, thrombosthenin contraction within platelets is often found to be normal in thrombasthenic states.[125,126] Dysfunction of some other platelet component with subsequent faulty release of thrombosthenin must be involved.[122,125,127] In thrombasthenia, storage and release of nucleotides are abnormal, but platelet aggregation by ADP, serotonin, collagen, or thrombin is normal.[122,123,126] PF-4 release by collagen and PF-3 generation of thromboplastic activity are also nor-

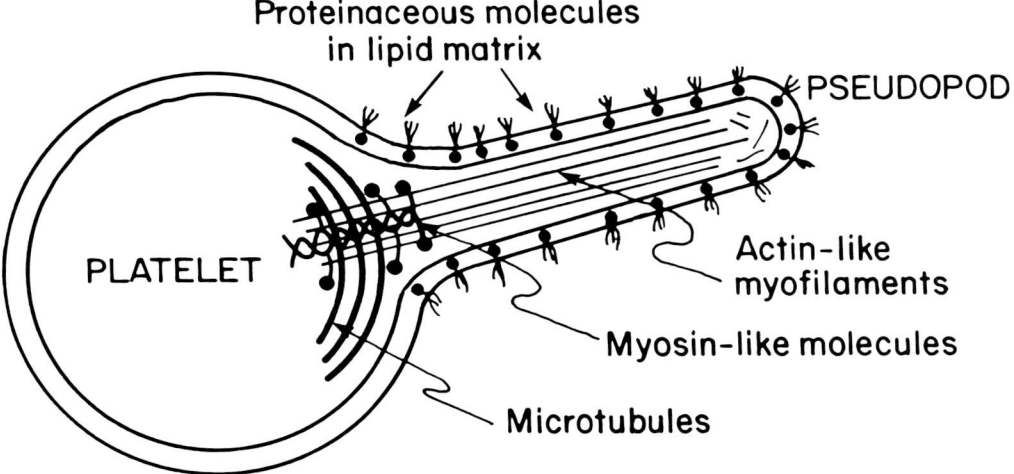

FIGURE 4. Contractile platelet protein (thrombosthenin) function in the formation of pseudopods. In the presence of Ca^{++}, the actin-myosin-like molecules, attached to microtubules, deform the platelet membrane in addition to retracting microtubules to entrap organelles in the platelet interior.

mal.[122,128] Apparently, release of thrombosthenin is independent of other platelet release mechanisms.

C. Organelle Zone

Platelet release reactions ordinarily take place following retraction of the micotubular structure by the contractile mechanism (Figure 3). There occurs a relation and fusion of granule membranes with the open canalicular system to release granule contents to the platelet exterior. Platelet release then requires induction, intracellular transmission, and extrusion from the platelet.[60,111] Substances capable of platelet aggregation also induce release of some constituents from normal platelets. ADP, epinephrine, norepinephrine serotonin, and other lowmolecular weight substances induce release by activation of specific membrane receptors (see above). Thrombin, trypsin, snake venom, papain, and other proteolytic enzymes could induce release by proteolysis of membrane proteins, although other mechanisms have also been proposed (see above).[129,132] Endotoxins, viruses, latex, fatty acids, collagen, and other particulate materials probably induce release of platelet constituents by platelet phagocytosis and membrane surface distortion.[60] Ristocetin, a small peptide antibiotic derived from actinomycetes,[133] likely mediates platelet aggregation by interaction with a component of the Factor VIII complex, since antisera to Factor VIII eliminates ristocetin platelet aggregation.[134-136] Platelets prepared by formaldehyde fixation retain ability to aggregate by ristocetin, but not with usual platelet aggregating agents that also induce the release reaction.[137]

1. Dense Bodies

Each platelet contains two to ten dense bodies surrounded by a membrane and variably filled with grains of osmiophilic electron-dense material.[138,139] These organelles are quite labile and may disappear during preparation for electron microscopic observation. Substances contained in dense bodies that are released through the open canalicular system when platelets are activated include nonmetabolic ATP and ADP, calcium, serotonin, catecholamines, and PF-4.[101,102,140-142]

Release of dense body constituents requires energy through an ATP-dependent reaction. Much attention has been given to the cAMP-dependent protein kinase system to direct the release reaction (see above). ATP energy source is generated from the platelet glycolytic pathway, as well as the tricarboxylic acid cycle, in approximately equal amounts in nonstimulated platelets.[143-145]

2. Mitochondria

Mitochondria of platelets have double membranes, but are smaller and have fewer cristae than mitochondria of other cells.[60] There are 10 to 60 mitochondria per normal platelet. They are located in the organelle zone and are the principal site for platelet metabolism. Glucose is the prime substrate for platelet metabolism, although anaerobic metabolism can occur in absence of fatty acids.[141] Glucose, stored as glycogen in granules of the organelle zone, becomes readily available for platelet metabolism.[60]

Although ATP is produced in about equal amounts from glycolysis and oxidative phosphorylation in normal nonstimulated platelets, the process of glycolysis accounts for about 80% of ATP production during platelet activation.[143-145]

The adenine nucleotides, ATP and ADP, exist in two different compartments or pools within the platelet.[146-148] About two thirds of the total platelet ADP appears in a nonmetabolic pool, but ATP is divided in about equal amounts between the metabolic and nonmetabolic pool.[141] About 2% of metabolic ATP is utilized during the primary phase of platelet aggregation, and probably no more than 10% to 50% is degraded during activation of the release reaction and secondary aggregation. However, nearly 100% of nonmetabolic ADP and ATP are extruded during full release reactions. These differences in nucleotide depletion have been used to measure the degree of storage pool contents, as well as the efficiency of the release reaction.[149] Some metabolic ATP is bound to thrombosthenin and may account for the increased utilization during microtubule retraction and activation of the release reaction.[150] Other metabolic ATP molecules are located in the platelet cytoplasm and are under a constant state of turnover in viable platelets.[148] Nonmetabolic nucleotides are complexed with serotonin in platelet-dense body granules.[151,152]

3. α-Granules

Platelet α-granules are round, triple-layered membrane organelles located in the cytoplasm. There are 20 to 200 α-granules per platelet, containing electron-dense grains often eccentrically positioned within the granules.

Release of material from α-granules occurs during release phase II by strong platelet aggregation inducers such as thrombin, collagen, or latex particles. Fibrinogen and lysosomal enzymes are the primary constituents released. The concentration of fibrinogen released is considerably lower than that of plasma, but may be magnified in importance when released locally within interstices of the platelet mass, especially since PF-4 (antiheparin),[20,21] PF-2 (fibrinoplastic substance), PF-3 (platelet thromboplastin),[153-155] PF-6 (antiplasmin),[19,23] and a substance to activate Factor XIII for fibrin stabilization[22] are also released.

Lysosomal enzymes released from α-granules are acid hydrolases that include β-N-acetylglucosaminidase, β-glucuronidase, β-galactosidase, arylsulphatase, cathepsins, and pro-elastinase.[60] These enzymes probably induce further complete destruction of platelet morphology with release of PF-3 and potassium and may be involved in clot lysis.[142]

III. PLATELET ADHESION AND COHESION

Adhesion of platelets refers to their ability to react and stick to any surface other than another platelet. In vivo, during hemostasis, platelets adhere to exposed subendothelial collagen and possibly also components of the ground substance.[156-158] Adhesion to collagen does not require calcium or other divalent cations.[69]

A. Collagen

Collagen suspensions used in vitro for aggregometry testing of platelet adhesive capability lose effectiveness if aged. It has also been noted that collagen from older human or animal sources is less active in mediating platelet aggregation and release.[159,160] Collagen also loses effectiveness if heated[161] or treated with collagenase enzymes.[161,162] Studies on structural aspects of collagen reveal that epsilon amino acid groups of lysine are important for platelet adhesion to the collagen surface, while carboxyl-exposed groups are not.[161] Platelets will adhere to the primary structure of collagen monomers, but molecules consisting of the polymer collagen form are necessary for induction of platelet aggregation.[163-165] These observations infer that simple adhesion is a surface phenomenon that does not induce even phase I release from platelet-dense bodies. However, when adhesion to collagen polymers occurs, there is sufficient stimulation for release.

Aspirin diminishes collagen-induced platelet aggregation, suggesting that the release reaction is essential for a full collagen response.[166-168] However, ADP, although contributory, is not the essential component released to account for collagen-induced platelet aggregation. Platelets made refractory to ADP, by repeated exposure to small quantities of ADP, still respond to collagen.[169] In addition, receptor-blocking agents that interfere with ADP aggregation do not alter the collagen-induced reaction.[170] There is some evidence that collagen can activate Factor XI on the platelet surface and assist in activation of the intrinsic coagulation mechanism at the site of platelet adherence.[171]

B. Shape Change

Cohesion, or platelet to platelet sticking, follows the adhesion reaction (Figure 3). A shape change from the resting disc form of platelets to a spiny sphere form is mediated by almost all inducers of platelet aggregation, with the notable exception of epinephrine.[60] It is interesting to note that epinephrine will aggregate platelets made insensitive to ADP.[67,68] Inhibitors of the platelet release reaction usually also inhibit the shape change. However, shape change on aggregometry tracings is made manifest by complete chelation of calcium ions in the presence of platelet activators because, without aggregation, the decreased light transmission (resulting from formation of spherical platelets) is not masked.

C. ADP

Nearly all inducers of platelet aggregation also bring about the release of ADP. Platelet aggregation by ristocetin,[17,18] epinephrine,[67,68] and collagen[169,170] may not require ADP. However, epinephrine is known to potentiate low levels of ADP.[233,234] Platelets exposed to ADP, exogenously or released from endogenous platelet stores, undergo a shape change.[65,112,119,172-177] This ADP-induced shape change is not dependent on calcium ions[175,178,179] or stirring of the platelet suspension.[180] ADP induces the shape change without subsequent platelet aggregation in the cold, at low pH, or with high chelator concentration.[172,181]

Platelet aggregation by ADP may be reversible or irreversible, depending on the concentration of inducer used.[182] Intermediate levels of the ADP inducer will result in a biphasic pattern of platelet aggregation similar to that obtained with epinephrine.[183] The second wave, or late irreversible phase, is due to activation of the release reaction with release of intraplatelet constituents, such as ATP, serotonin, PF-4, and PF-

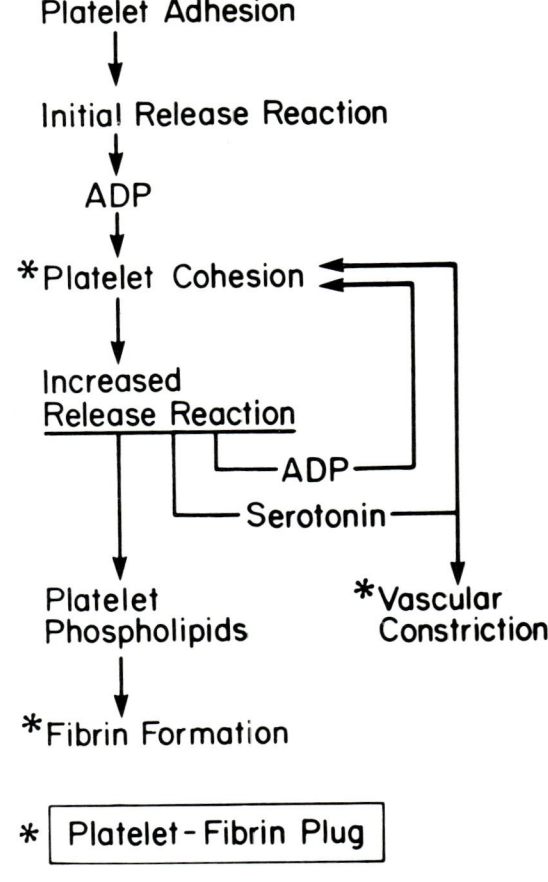

FIGURE 5. Summary of platelet function in hemostasis.

3.[12,13,183-188] Figure 5 summarizes and Figure 6 illustrates platelet function in hemostasis.

IV. PLATELET PRODUCTION, STORAGE, AND DESTRUCTION

Platelets split off from cytoplasm of megakaryocytes found principally in bone marrow.[189-191] These large platelet producing cells develop by nuclear division and cytoplasmic maturation from precursor cells. Diffuse granulation delineated by demarcation zones mark the final stages of megakaryocyte maturation. The demarcation zones represent formation of platelet plasma membranes. The number of platelets split off from a megakaryocyte is directly related to the quantity of the mother cell cytoplasm.

A. Megakaryocytopoiesis

Megakaryocytopoiesis appears to be controlled by thrombopoietin.[192,193] The source of this plasma humoral factor, or whether only one factor exists, is not known. Evidence for the existence of such a humoral factor was suggested from early studies of thrombocytopenia and thrombocytosis.[194,195] Changes in megakaryocyte numbers was used as the measure of effect. Other methods utilized measurement of radioactivity in platelets following incorporation of radioactive labels in megakaryocytes.[196,197] Measurement of changes in DNA synthesis were also followed.[198,199] Precursor megakary-

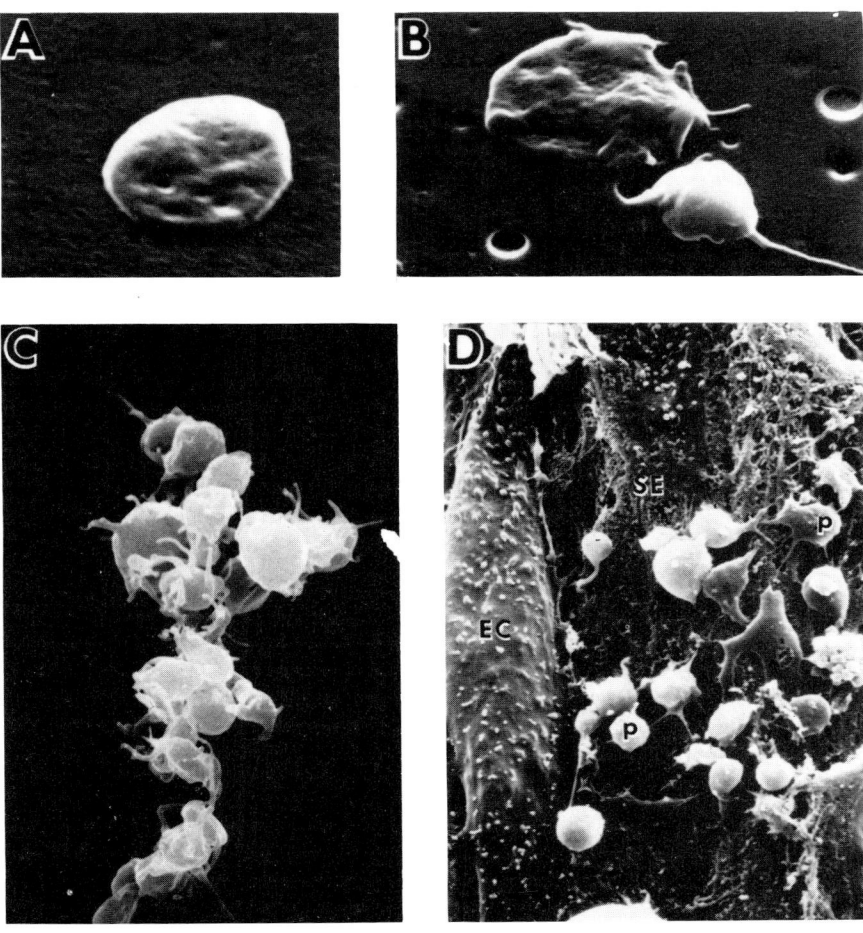

FIGURE 6. Composite illustration of platelet responsiveness. (A) Unactivated platelet simulates the circulating blood platelet, which exists normally in the thin disc form. (Magnification × 10000.), (B) platelets activated by surface contact (adhesion). Note large spread form and another less activated platelet that is swollen and has long pseudopods. (Magnification × 10000.), (C) platelet aggregate illustrating platelet cohesion. (Magnification × 5000.), (D) platelet interaction with injured vessel wall. Endothelial cell (EC) detachment exposes fibrillar and collagenous subendothelium (SE). Circulating platelets (p) adhere to and activate on the exposed subendothelium in an attempt to seal vessel wall. (Magnification × 5000.) (Courtesy of Dr. Marion I. Barnhart, Wayne State University School of Medicine, Detroit. With permission.)

ocyte cells reduplicate and undergo cytoplasm mass increase following accelerated peripheral platelet destruction.[44] These new megakaryocytes proceed to cytoplasmic maturation and platelet release. Thrombocytosis was found to have opposite effects.[198-202]

Survival of platelets in plasma in man is 9 to 12 days, as measured by labeling studies.[198,200,203,204] Non-viable or aged platelets are removed primarily by the spleen and liver.[205] Their removal and destruction appears to be by both senescence and by random selection. Naturally, platelets are utilized in hemostatic and thrombotic processes. In these physiologic and pathologic situations, increased random destruction appears to predominate.[206-209] Thrombocytopenias with intrinsic platelet abnormalities are marked by shortened platelet survival.[210,211]

B. Platelet Age and Size

Platelets from circulating blood can be separated by oil or sucrose gradients. Although a number of populations can be obtained, it is generally agreed that at least large and small platelets exist. Most studies of platelet function concerning size density, and age have dealt with the largest and smallest populations.

Large platelets are approximately 2.5 times larger than small platelets. The large platelet population composes about 18% of the total number, while the small platelets account for about 17%.[212] The large platelets, per unit size, contain more nucleotides, protein, phospholipid, and glycogen.[213,214] Their glycolytic rate is greater, and both protein and glycogen synthesis is greater.[213,215] In addition, the large platelets have greater resistance to osmotic shock.[216]

Platelets decrease in size as they age in the circulation.[217,218] Platelets become less dense as they age and decrease in size.[219] Aggregation of larger, more dense platelets is better with epinephrine, serotonin, collagen, and thrombin, but show no selective adhesion to glass beads.[220] Labeling studies have indicated that the younger large platelets prefer to adhere to collagen both in vivo and in vitro, but show no preferential aggregation by ADP.[221] Adhesiveness to glass, however, is unaffected by age.[222] Measurements of ATP content, O_2 consumption, and size are not altered after passing through a glass bead column, so there is no preferential selection by the column.[223] However, washed platelets resuspended in EDTA show preferential adhesion of the younger population to glass, collagen, or Dacron.®[224] These large platelets must have the ability to release the necessary constituents needed for adhesion that have been washed away from the surface. It is known that the release of PF-4, ADP, and ATP (mediated by thrombin, ADP, or epinephrine) is greater for large young platelets.[225] These materials are all dense-body constituents. Curiously, serotonin uptake is greater for older, smaller, less dense platelets.[226] Serotonin is believed to be taken up by an active energy-dependent mechanism against a concentration gradient, and this mechanism can be blocked by metabolic inhibitors.[226] The decrease in metabolic activity of older platelets must preferentially be related to other mechanisms.

V. SUMMARY

Much evidence points to cAMP as a key chemical in platelet responsiveness. Increased intraplatelet levels appear to be related to inhibition of platelet aggregation, while decreased levels are related to activation of platelets. These events can be generated by activation or inhibition of adenylate cyclase, which induces production of cAMP from ATP or by an effect on phosphodiesterase, which normally degrades cAMP. Cyclic AMP directs the activity of dependent kinases for specific cellular functions. One such kinase mediates the complexing of inorganic phosphate with a protein to form a chelator of calcium ions. Alkaline phosphatase in the platelet membrane dephosphorylates the complex; calcium is then released, and platelet aggregation is enhanced.

Platelet aggregating agents could activate alkaline phosphatase, thereby releasing calcium ions and reducing cAMP levels by mass action. Aggregating agents could also compete with the cAMP-dependent protein system for phosphate and thereby allow free calcium to trigger platelet aggregation.

Inhibitors of platelet aggregation can stimulate adenylate cyclase, inhibit phosphodiesterase, inhibit alkaline phosphatase, or function at some other point within this system, resulting in increased levels of cAMP, increased levels of the phosphorylated protein-calcium complex, and decreased availability of calcium ions. In addition, inhibiting agents may also interfere with the prostaglandin pathway, leading to reduced capability of thromboxane production (Chapter 1).

Other kinases are likely activated to induce the release reaction. Many substances are released from granules following thrombosthenin function to concentrate these granules. Among the agents released, ADP from nonmetabolic stores is important. This further promotes cohesive platelet aggregation by forming ADP-Ca^{++} bridges between platelets. Pseudopod formation, blebs, and thin filaments appear to be important for increased platelet "stickiness". Another important substance released is platelet factor 3. Along with the plasma cofactors, Factor VIII, and Factor V, blood clotting can be initiated to form fibrin in the interstices of the platelet aggregate, resulting in irreversible aggregation and total platelet destruction (viscous metamorphosis). Anticoagulants can function at this point, but do not affect initial reversible platelet aggregation. Serotonin is also released. Its vasoconstrictive properties may have significant relevance to hemostasis.

Platelet surface charges, plasma cofactors, platelet membrane changes, antigen-antibody reactions, nucleotide storage functions, thrombosthenin function, and other parameters must be considered when contemplating quantitative or qualitative platelet dysfunction. Evaluation of platelet dysfunction by analysis of platelet aggregometry curves is difficult and should be used only in conjunction with other tests, since only platelet cohesion is involved in a limited sample of platelets ex vivo. Determination of platelet adherence to foreign surfaces, such as glass beads, can be helpful. Measurement of substances released is still a modality limited to the research laboratory; however, simple procedures, such as PF-4 determination by radioimmunoassays, are becoming available and can give a good picture of the "intactness" of the platelet release reaction. When platelet function at the molecular level is more clearly defined, assays for diagnosing each disease state can be developed. Most likely, a battery of platelet function tests will be necessary to assess the "healthiness" of platelets or the effectiveness of drugs in thromboembolic and other abnormal conditions.

REFERENCES

1. **Roskam, J.**, Contribution of l'étude de la physiologie normale et pathologique du globulin (plaquettes de Bizzozero), *Arch. Int. Physiol.*, 20, 241, 1923.
2. **Kinlough-Rathbone, R. L., Chahil, A., Packham, M. A., Reimers, H. J., and Mustard, J. F.**, Effect of ionophore A 23 187 on thrombin-degranulated washed rabbit platelets, *Thromb. Res.*, 7, 435, 1975.
3. **Tangen, O. and Bygdeman, S.**, Study of the clotting, esterase and platelet aggregating activities of thrombin, acetylated thrombin, and reptilase, *Scand. J. Haematol.*, 9, 333, 1972.
4. **Fell, C. and Seegers, W. H.**, Platelet factor 1 related to prothrombin activation, *Can. J. Biochem. Physiol.*, 36, 645, 1958.
5. **Marcus, A. J., Zucker-Franklin, D., Safier, L. B., and Ullman, H. L.**, Studies on human platelet granules and membranes, *J. Clin. Invest.*, 45, 14, 1966.
6. **Penner, J. A. and Seegers, W. H.**, Activation of prothrombin, *Am. J. Physiol.*, 186, 343, 1956.
7. **Hardisty, R. M. and Hutton, R. A.**, Platelet aggregation and the availability of platelet factor 3, *Br. J. Haematol.*, 12, 764, 1966.
8. **Horowitz, H. I. and Papayoanou, M. F.**, Release of nonsedimentable platelet factor 3 during coagulation *J. Lab. Clin. Med.*, 69, 1003, 1967.
9. **O'Brien, J. R.**, The platelet like activity of serum, *Br. J. Haematol.*, 1, 223, 1955.
10. **White, J. G. and Krivit, W.**, The ultrastructural localization of platelet lipids, *Blood*, 27, 167, 1966.
11. **Wolf, P.**, The nature and significance of platelet products in human plasma, *Br. J. Haematol.*, 13, 269, 1967.
12. **O'Sullivan, E. F., Hirsh, J., McCarthy, R. A., and de Gruchy, G. C.**, Heparin in the treatment of venous thrombo-embolic disease. Administration, control, and results, *Med. J. Aust.*, 2, 153, 1968.

13. **Thomas, D. P., Niewiarowski, S., and Ream, V. J.**, Release of adenosine nucleotides and platelet factor 4 from platelets of man and four other species, *J. Lab. Clin. Med.*, 75, 607, 1970.
14. **Day, H. J., Stormorken, H., and Holmsen, H.**, Subcellular Localization of Platelet Factor 3 and Platelet Factor 4, 12th Congr. Int. Soc. Hematol., New York, 1968, 172.
15. **Seegers, W. H.**, *Prothrombin*, Harvard University Press, Cambridge, Mass., 1962, 267.
16. **Nachman, R. L.**, Platelet proteins, *Semin. Hematol.*, 5, 18, 1968.
17. **Gangarosa, E. J., Johnson, T. R., and Ramos, H. S.**, Ristocetin-induced thrombocytopenia: site and mechanism of action, *Arch. Intern. Med.*, 105, 83, 1960.
18. **Howard, M. A. and Firkin, B. G.**, Ristocetin—a new tool in the investigation of platelet aggregation, *Thromb. Diath. Haemorrh.*, 26, 362, 1971.
19. **Ardlie, N. G. and Han, P.**, Enzymatic basis for platelet aggregation and release: the significance of the "platelet atmosphere" and the relationship between platelet function and blood coagulation, *Br. J. Haematol.*, 26, 331, 1974.
20. **Ware, A. G., Fahey, J. L., and Seegers, W. H.**, Platelet extracts, fibrin formation and interaction of purified prothrombin and thromboplastin, *Am. J. Physiol.*, 154, 140, 1948.
21. **Niewiarowski, S., Poplawski, A., Lipinski, B., and Farbiszewski, R.**, The release of platelet factor 4 and ADP during platelet aggregation, *Nature (London)*, 222, 1269, 1969.
22. **Karpatkin, M. H. and Karpatkin, S.**, In vivo and in vitro binding of factor VIII to human platelets, *Thromb. Diath. Haemorrh.*, 21, 129, 1969.
23. **Joist, J. H., Niewiarowski, S., and Mustard, J. F.**, Release of antiplasmin during thrombin or collagen induced platelet aggregation, in *Thrombolytic Therapy*, Mammen, E. F., Anderson, G. F., and Barnhart, M. I., Eds., Schattauer, Stuttgart, 1971, 113.
24. **Jenkins, C. S. P., Packham, M. A., Kinlough-Rathbone, R. L., and Mustard, J. F.**, Interactions of polylysine with platelets, *Blood*, 37, 395, 1971.
25. **Griggs, T. R., Cooper, H. A., Webster, W. P., Wagner, R. H., and Brinkhous, K. M.**, Plasma aggregating factor (bovine) for human platelets: a marker for study of antihemophilic and von Willebrand factors, *Proc. Natl. Acad. Sci. U.S.A.*, 70, 2814, 1973.
26. **Henson, P. M. and Spiegelberg, H. L.**, Release of serotonin from human platelets induced by aggregated immunoglobulins of different classes and subclasses, *J. Clin. Invest.*, 52, 1282, 1973.
27. **Pfueller, S. L. and Luscher, E. F.**, The effects of aggregated immunoglobulins on human blood platelets in relation to their complement-fixing abilities. I. Studies of immunoglobulins of different types, *J. Immunol.*, 109, 517, 1972.
28. **Shulman, N. R., Lange, R. F., Tomasulo, P. A., and Coleman, C. N.**, Antibodies and platelet membranes, *Thromb. Diath. Haemorrh. Suppl*, 54, 261, 1973.
29. **Israels, E. D., Nisli, G., Paraskevas, F., and Israels, L. G.**, Platelet Fc receptor as a mechanism for Ag-Ab complex-induced platelet injury, *Thromb. Diath. Haemorrh.*, 29, 434, 1973.
30. **Cooper, H. A., Mason, R. G., and Brinkhous, K. M.**, The platelet: membrane and surface reactions, *Am. Rev. Physiol.*, 38, 501, 1976.
31. **Nicolson, G. L. and Poste, G.**, The cancer cell: dynamic aspects and modifications in cell-surface organization, *N. Engl. J. Med.*, 295, 197, 1976.
32. **Jamieson, G. A., Urban, C., and Barber, A. J.**, An enzymatic basis for platelet:collagen adhesion, Int. Soc. Thrombosis Haemostasis, 2nd Congr., Oslo, (Abstr.,) 1971, 220.
33. **Barber, A. J. and Jamieson, G. A.**, Isolation and characterisation of plasma membranes from human blood platelets, *J. Biol. Chem.*, 245, 6357, 1970.
34. **Bosmann, B. B.**, Platelet adhesiveness and aggregation: the collagen: glycosyl, polypeptide: N-acetylgalactosaminyl and glycoprotein: galactosyl transferases of human platelets, *Biochem. Biophys. Res. Commun.*, 43, 1118, 1971.
35. **Salzman, E. W., Chambers, D. A., and Neri, L. L.**, Possible mechanism of aggregation of blood platelets by adenosine diphosphate, *Nature (London)*, 210, 167, 1966.
36. **Chambers, D. A., Salzman, E. W., and Neri, L. L.**, Characterization of "ecto-ATPase" of human blood platelets, *Arch. Biochem. Biophys.*, 119, 173, 1967.
37. **Nachman, R. L. and Marcus, A. J.**, Immunological studies on protein associated with the subcellular fractions of thrombosthenic and afibrinogenaemic platelets, *Br. J. Haematol.*, 15, 181, 1968.
38. **Holmsen, H., Day, H. J., and Pimentel, M. A.**, Adenine nucleotide metabolism of blood platelets. V. Subcellular localization and kinetics of some related enzymes, *Biochim. Biophys. Acta*, 186, 244, 1969a.
39. **Haslam, R. J. and Taylor, A.**, Role of cyclic 3', 5'-adenosine monophosphate in platelet aggregation, in *Platelet Aggregation*, Caen, J., Ed., Masson et Cie, Paris, 1971, 85.
40. **Brodie, G. N., Bienziger, N. L., and Chase, L. R.**, The effects of thrombin on adenyl cyclase activity and a membrane protein from human platelets, *J. Clin. Invest.*, 51, 81, 1972.
41. **Salzman, E. W.**, Cyclic AMP and platelet function, *N. Engl. J. Med.*, 286, 358, 1972.

42. Droller, M. J. and Wolfe, S. M., Thrombin-induced increase in intracellular cyclic 3', 5'-adenosine monophosphate in human platelets, *J. Clin. Invest.*, 51, 3094, 1972.
43. Haslam, R. J., Interactions of the pharmacological receptors of blood platelets with adenylate cyclase, *Ser. Haematol.*, 6, 333, 1973.
44. Hirsh, J. and Doery, J. C. G., Platelet function in health and disease, *Prog. Haematol.*, 7, 185, 1971.
45. Horlington, M. and Watson, P. A., Inhibition of 3' 5'-cyclic-AMP phosphodiesterase by some platelet aggregation inhibitors, *Biochem. Pharmacol.*, 19, 955, 1970.
46. Cole, B., Robison, G. A., and Hartman, R. C., Effects of prostaglandin E_1 and theophylline on aggregation and cyclic AMP levels of human blood platelets, *Fed. Proc.*, 29, 316, 1970.
47. Mills, D. C. B. and Smith, J. B., The influence on platelet aggregation of drugs that affect the accumulation of adenosine 3' 5'-cyclic monophosphate in platelets, *Biochem. J.*, 121, 185, 1971.
48. Booyse, F. M., Hoveke, T. P., Kisieleski, D., and Rafelson, M. E., Mechanism and control of platelet-platelet interaction. I. Effects of inducers and inhibitors of aggregation, *Microvasc. Res.*, 4, 179, 1972.
49. White, J. G., Rao, G. H. R., and Gerrard, J. M., Effects of the ionophore A 23187 on blood platelets. I. Influence on aggregation and secretion, *Am. J. Pathol.*, 77, 135, 1974.
50. Morkin, E. and la Raia, P. J., Biochemical studies on the regulation of myocardial contractility, *N. Engl. J. Med.*, 290, 445, 1974.
51. Weise, H. J., Platelet physiology and abnormalities of platelet function, *N. Engl. J. Med.*, 293, 531, 1975.
52. Salzman, E. W., Inhibition of platelet aggregation by cyclic AMP and dibutryl cyclic AMP, *Fed. Proc.*, 29, 316, 1970.
53. Marquis, N. R., Becker, J. A., and Vigdahl, R. L., Platelet aggregation. III. An epinephrine induced decrease in cyclic AMP synthesis, *Biochem. Biophys. Res. Commun.*, 39, 783, 1970.
54. Abramson, H. A., The elecrophoresis of the blood platelets of the horse with reference to their origin and to thrombus formation, *J. Exp. Med.*, 47, 677, 1928.
55. Hampton, J. R. and Mitchell, J. R. A., Effect of aggregating agents on the electrophoretic mobility of human platelets, *Br. Med. J.*, 1, 1074, 1966.
56. Seaman, G. V. F., Surface potential and platelet aggregation, *Thromb. Diath. Haemorrh. Suppl.*, 26, 53, 1967.
57. Betts, J. J., Betts, J. P., and Nicholson, J. T., Significance of ADP, plasma and platelet concentration in platelet electrophoretic studies, *Nature (London)*, 219, 1280, 1968.
58. Grottum, K. A., Influence of aggregating agents on electrophoretic mobility of blood platelets from healthy individuals and from patients with cardiovascular disease, *Lancet*, 1, 1406, 1968.
59. Rutty, D. and Vine, T. L., Electrokinetic mobility of blood platelets, *Lancet*, 1, 206, 1969.
60. Holmsen, H., The platelet: its membrane, physiology and biochemistry, *Clin. Haematol.*, 1, 235, 1972.
61. Grottum, K. A., Electrophoretic investigations of blood platelets, in *Platelet Aggregation*, Caen, J., Ed., Masson et Cie, Paris, 1971, 199.
62. Born, G. V. R., The platelet membrane and its function, in, *Plenary Session Papers*, 12th Congr. Int. Soc. Hematology, New York, 1968, 95.
63. Rozenberg, M. C. and Holmsen, H., Adenine nucleotide metabolism of blood platelets. II. Uptake of adenosine and inhibition of ADP-induced platelet aggregation, *Biochim. Biophys. Acta*, 155, 342, 1968a.
64. Gaarder, A. and Laland, S., Hypothesis for the aggregation of platelets by nucleotides, *Nature (London)*, 202, 909, 1964.
65. O'Brien, J. R., Effects of adenosine diphosphate and adrenalin on mean platelet shape, *Nature (London)*, 207, 306, 1965.
66. Packham, M. A., Ardlie, N. G., and Mustard, J. F., Effect of adenine compounds on platelet aggregation, *Am. J. Physiol.*, 217, 1009, 1969.
67. Scarborough, D. E., Mason, R. G., Dalldorf, F. G., and Brinkhous, K. M., Morphologic manifestations of blood-solid interface reactions. A scanning and transmission electron microscopic study, *Lab. Invest.*, 20, 164, 1969.
68. Doery, J. C. G. and Hirsh, J., Aspirin and salicylate: divergent effects on platelet glucose metabolism and function, *Experientia*, 27, 533, 1971.
69. Hovig, T., The effect of calcium and magnesium on rabbit blood platelet aggregation in vitro, *Thromb. Diath. Haemorrh.*, 12, 179, 1964.
70. Mustard, J. F. and Packham, M. A., Factors influencing platelet function—adhesion, release and aggregation, *Pharmacol. Rev.*, 22, 97, 1970.
71. Muёr, E. H., Hellem, A. J., and Rozenberg, M. C., Energy metabolism and platelet function, *Scand. J. Clin. Lab. Invest.*, 19, 280, 1967.

72. Kinlough-Rathbone, R. L., Packham, M. A., and Mustard, J. F., The effect of glucose on adenosine diphosphate induced platelet aggregation, *J. Lab. Clin. Med.*, 75, 780, 1970.
73. Hellem, A. J., Platelet adhesiveness, *Ser. Haematol.*, 1, 99, 1968.
74. Haslam, R. J., Role of adenosine diphosphate in the aggregation of human platelets by thrombin and by fatty acids, *Nature (London)*, 202, 765, 1964.
75. McLean, J. R., Maxwell, R. E., and Herther, D., Fibrinogen and adenosine diphosphate induced aggregation of platelets, *Nature (London)*, 202, 605, 1964.
76. Cross, M. J., Effect of fibrinogen on the aggregation of platelets by adenosine diphosphate, *Thromb. Diath. Haemorrh.*, 12, 524, 1964.
77. Solum, N. O. and Stormorken, H., Influence of fibrinogen on the aggregation of washed human blood platelets induced by adenosine diphosphate, thrombin, collagen and adrenalin, *Scan. J. Clin. Lab. Invest.*, 17 (Suppl. 84), 170, 1965.
78. Grette, R., Studies on the mechanism of thrombin-catalysed hemostatic reactions in blood platelets, *Acta Physiol. Scand.*, 56, (Suppl. 15), 5, 1962.
79. Castaldi, P. A. and Caen, J., Platelet fibrinogen, *J. Clin. Pathol.*, 18, 579, 1965.
80. Nachman, R. L., Marcus, A. J., and Zucker-Franklin, D., Immunologic studies of proteins associated with subcellular fractions of normal human platelets, *J. Lab. Clin. Med.*, 69, 651, 1967.
81. Ireland, D. M., Effect of thrombin on radioactive nucleotides of human washed platelets, *Biochem. J.*, 105, 857, 1967.
82. Haslam, R. J., Mechanisms of blood platelet aggregation, in *Physiology of Hemostasis and Thrombosis*, Johnson, S. A. and Seegers, W. H., Eds., Charles C Thomas, Springfield, Ill., 1967, 88.
83. Schmid, J. H., Jackson, D. P., and Conley, C. L., Mechanism of action of thrombin on platelets, *J. Clin. Invest.*, 41, 543, 1962.
84. Morse, E. E., Jackson, D. P., and Conley, C. L., Role of platelet fibrinogen in the reactions of platelets to thrombin, *J. Clin. Invest.*, 44, 809, 1965.
85. Davey, M. G. and Lüscher, E. F., Action of some coagulant snake venoms upon blood platelets, *Nature (London)*, 207, 730, 1965.
86. Soulier, J. P., Prou-Wartelle, O., and Halle, L., Study of thrombin coagulase, *Thromb. Diath. Haemorrh.*, 17, 321, 1967.
87. Seegers, W. H., Hassouna, H. I., Hewett-Emmett, D., Walz, D. A., and Andary, T. J., Prothrombin and thrombin: selected aspects of thrombin formation, properties, inhibition, and immunology, *Sem. Thromb. Hemostas.*, 1, 211, 1975.
88. Herman, G. E., Seegers, W. H., and Henry, R. L., Effects of autoprothrombin II-A on epinephrine induced platelet aggregation of normal and coumadin treated dogs, *Thromb. Haemostas.*, 40, 61, 1978.
89. Seegers, W. H., McCoy, L. E., Groben, H. D., Sakuragawa, N., and Agrawal, B. B. L., Purification and some properties of autoprothrombin II-A: an anticoagulant perhaps also related to fibrinolysis, *Thromb. Res.*, 1, 443, 1972.
90. Seegers, W. H., Novoa, E., Henry, R. L., and Hassouna, H. I., Relationship of "new" vitamin K-dependent protein C and "old" autoprothrombin II-A, *Thromb. Res.*, 8, 543, 1976.
91. O'Brien, J. R., Some effects of adrenaline and anti-adrenaline on platelets in vitro and in vivo, *Nature (London)*, 200, 763, 1963.
92. Smith, J. B., Ingerman, C., and Kocsis, J. J., Formation of an intermediate in prostaglandin biosynthesis and its association with the platelet release reaction, *J. Clin. Invest.*, 53, 1468, 1974.
93. Ardlie, N. G., Glew, G., and Schwartz, C. J., Influence of catecholamines on nucleotide-induced platelet aggregation, *Nature (London)*, 212, 415, 1966.
94. Mills, D. C. B. and Roberts, G. C. K., Effects of adrenalne on human blood platelets, *J. Physiol.*, 193, 443, 1967.
95. Niewiarowski, S., Poplawski, A., Lipinski, B., and Farbiszewski, R., The release of platelet clotting factors during aggregation and viscous metamorphosis, *Exp. Biol. Med.*, 3, 121, 1968.
96. Youssef, A. and Barkham, P., Release of platelet factor 4 by adenosine diphosphate and other platelet aggregating agents, *Br. Med. J.*, 1, 746, 1968.
97. Salzman, E. W. and Neri, L. L., Profiles of activity in rodents of some narcotic and narcotic antagonist drugs, *Nature (London)*, 224, 610, 1969.
98. Thomas, D. P., The role of platelet catecholamines in the aggregation of platelets by collagen and thrombin, *Exp. Biol. Med.*, 3, 129, 1968.
99. Thomas, D. P., Effect of catecholamines on platelet aggregation by thrombin, *Nature (London)*, 215, 298, 1967.
100. Wooley, D. W. and Goumi, B. W., Serotonin receptors. V. Selective destruction by neuraminidase plus EDTA and reactivation with tissue lipids, *Nature (London)*, 202, 1074, 1964.
101. White, J. G., Identification of platelet secretion in the electron microscope, *Ser. Haematol.*, 6, 429, 1973.

102. **White, J. G.**, Interaction of membrane systems in blood platelets, *Am. J. Pathol.*, 66, 295, 1972.
103. **White, J. G.**, Effects of cationic polypeptides on thrombasthenic and afibrinogenemic blood platelets, *Am. J. Pathol.*, 68, 447, 1972.
104. **White, J. G.**, Exocytosis of secretory organelles from blood platelets incubated with cationic polypeptides, *Am. J. Pathol.*, 69, 41, 1972.
105. **Droller, M. J.**, Ultrastructure of the platelet release reaction in response to various aggregating agents and their inhibitors, *Lab. Invest.*, 29, 595, 1973.
106. **White, J. G.**, Shape change, *Thromb. Diath. Haemorrh.*, 60, 159, 1974.
107. **White, J. G. and Krumwiede, M.**, Influence of cytochalasin B on the shape change induced in platelets by cold, *Blood*, 41, 823, 1973.
108. **Martin, J. H., Carson, F. L., and Race, G. J.**, Calcium-containing platelet granules, *J. Cell Biol.*, 60, 775, 1974.
109. **Feinman, R. D. and Detwiler, T. C.**, Platelet secretion induced by divalent cation ionophores, *Nature (London)*, 249, 172, 1974.
110. **Gerrard, J. M., White, J. G., and Rao, G. H. R.**, Effects of the ionophore A 23187 on blood platelets. II. Influence on ultrastructure, *Am. J. Pathol.*, 77, 151, 1974.
111. **Day, J. H. and Holmsen, H.**, Concepts of the blood platelet release reaction, *Semin. Hematol.*, 4, 3, 1971.
112. **White, J. G.**, Fine structural alterations induced in platelets by adenosine diphosphate, *Blood*, 31, 604, 1968.
113. **Zucker-Franklin, D. and Bloomberg, N.**, Microfibrils of blood platelets: their relationship to microtubules and the contractile protein, *J. Clin. Invest.*, 48, 167, 1969.
114. **Bettex-Galland, M. and Lüscher, E. F.**, Thrombosthenin—a contractile protein from thrombocytes. Extraction from human blood platelets and some of its properties, *Biochim. Biophys. Acta*, 49, 536, 1961.
115. **Davey, M. G. and Lüscher, E. F.**, Release reactions of human platelets induced by thrombin and other agents, *Biochim. Biophys. Acta*, 165, 490, 1968.
116. **Nachman, R. L., Marcus, A. J., and Safier, L. B.**, Platelet thrombosthenin: subcellular localization and function, *J. Clin. Invest.*, 46, 1380, 1967.
117. **Booyse, F. M. and Rafelson, M. E.**, Cell-free synthesis of contractile protein of human platelets: its location and role in cellular adhesiveness, *Blood*, 30, 553, 1967.
118. **Booyse, F. M. and Rafelson, M. E.**, Studies on human platelets. I. Synthesis of platelet protein in a cell-free system, *Biochim. Biophys. Acta*, 166, 689, 1968.
119. **Hovig, T.**, The ultrastructure of blood platelets in normal and abnormal states, *Ser. Haematol.*, 2(1), 3, 1968.
120. **Booyse, F. M. and Rafelson, M. E.**, Studies on human platelets. III. A contractile protein model for platelet aggregation, *Blood*, 33, 100, 1969.
121. **Alkjaersig, N., Abe, T., and Seegers, W. H.**, Purification and quantitative determination of platelet factor 3, *Am. J. Physiol.*, 181, 304, 1955.
122. **Caen, J., Castaldi, J., Ledere, S., Inceman, S., Larrieu, M., Probst, M., and Bernard, J.**, Congenital bleeding disorders with long bleeding time and normal platelet count. I. Glanzmann's thrombasthenia (report of 15 patients), *Am. J. Med.*, 41, 4, 1966.
123. **Zucker, M. B., Pert, J., and Hillgartner, M.**, Platelet function in a patient with thrombasthenia, *Blood*, 28, 524, 1966.
124. **Hardisty, R. M., Dormandy, K. M., and Hutton, R. A.**, Thrombasthenia: studies on three cases, *Br. J. Haematol.*, 10, 371, 1964.
125. **Mason, R. G., Read, M. S., and Brinkhous, K. M.**, Effect of fibrinogen concentration on platelet adhesion to glass, *Proc. Soc. Exp. Biol. Med.*, 137, 680, 1971.
126. **Weiss, H. J. and Kochwa, S.**, Studies of platelet function and proteins in three patients with Glanzmann's thrombasthenia, *J. Lab. Clin. Med.*, 71, 153, 1968.
127. **Löhr, G. W., Waller, H. O., and Gross, R.**, Beziehugen zwischen Plattchenstoffwechsel und Retraktion des Blutgerinnsels unter besonderer Berucksichtigung der thrombopathic Glanzmann-Naegeli, *Dtsch. Med. Wochenschr.*, 86, 897, 1961.
128. **Kubisz, P., Sultan, Y., Delobel, J., and Caen, J.**, Mesure de la liberation du factor plaquettaire 4 (FP_4) dans des thrombopathies constitutionelles et acquises, *Eur. J. Clin. Biol. Res.*, 15, 698, 1970.
129. **Phillips, D. R.**, Effect of trypsin on the exposed polypeptides and glycoproteins in the human platelet membrane, *Biochemistry*, 11, 4582, 1972.
130. **Barber, A. J. and Jamieson, G. A.**, Isolation of glycopeptides from high and low density platelet plasma membranes, *Biochemistry*, 10, 4711, 1971.
131. **Jamieson, G. A., Fuller, N. A., Barber, A. J., and Lombart, C.**, Membrane glycoproteins of human platelets, *Ser. Haematol.*, 4(1), 125, 1971.

132. **Phillips, D. R. and Agin, P. P.,** Thrombin substrates and proteolytic site of thrombin action on human-platelet plasma membranes, *Biochim. Biophys. Acta,* 352, 218, 1974.
133. **Romansky, M. J., Limson, B. M., and Hawkins, J. E.,** Ristocetin: a new antibiotic-laboratory and clinical studies, *Antibiot. Annu.,* p. 706, 1956.
134. **Olson, J. D., Fass, D. N., Bowie, E. J. W., and Mann, K. G.,** Ristocetin-induced aggregation of gel filtered platelets. A study of von Willebrand's disease and the effect of aspirin, *Thromb. Res.,* 3, 501, 1973.
135. **Weiss, H. J., Rogers, J., and Brand, H.,** Defective ristocetin-induced platelet aggregation in von Willebrand's disease and its correction by factor VIII, *J. Clin. Invest.,* 52, 2697, 1973.
136. **Meyer, D., Dreyfus, M. D., and Larrieu, M. J.,** Willebrand factor: immunological and biological study, *Pathol. Biol.,* 21, 66, 1973.
137. **Brinkhous, K. M., Graham, J. E., Cooper, H. A., Allain, J. P., and Wagner, R. H.,** Assay of von Willebrand factor in von Willebrand's disease and hemophilia: use of a macroscopic platelet aggregation test, *Thromb. Res.,* 6, 267, 1975.
138. **Schulz, H.,** *Thrombozyten und Thrombose in elektromikroskopischen Bild.,* Springer-Verlag, Stuttgart, 1968.
139. **White, J. G.,** *The Circulating Platelet,* Johnson, S. A., Ed., Academic Press, New York, 1971, 46.
140. **Droller, M. J.,** Ultrastructure of the platelet release reaction in response to various aggregating agents and their inhibitors, *Lab. Invest.,* 29, 595, 1973.
141. **Stuart, M. J.,** Inherited defects of platelet function, *Semin. Hematol.,* 12, 233, 1975.
142. **Schneider, M. D.,** Preparative technique for platelet preservation for SEM, *Scanning Electron Microsc.,* 2, 343, 1972.
143. **Karpatkin, S.,** Studies on human platelet glycolysis. Effect of glucose, cyanide, insulin, citrate, and agglutination and contraction on platelet glycolysis, *J. Clin. Invest.,* 46, 409, 1967.
144. **Doery, J. C. G., Hirsh, J., and Cooper, I.,** Energy metabolism in human blood platelets. Interrelationship between glycolysis and oxidative metabolism, *Blood,* 36, 159, 1970.
145. **Detwiler, T. C. and Zivkovic, R. V.,** Control of energy metabolism in platelets. A comparison of aerobic and anaerobic metabolism in washed rat platelets, *Biochim. Biophys. Acta,* 197, 117, 1970.
146. **Holmsen, H.,** Platelet adenine nucleotide metabolism and platelet malfunction, in *Platelet Aggregation,* Caen, J., Ed., Masson et Cie, Paris, 1971, 109.
147. **Holmsen, H.,** Adenine nucleotide metabolism in platelets and plasma, in *Biochemistry of Blood Platelets,* Kowalski, E. and Niewiarowski, S., Eds., Academic Press, New York, 1967, 81.
148. **Holmsen, H., Day, H. J., and Storm, E.,** Adenine nucleotide metabolism of blood platelets. VI. Subcellular localization of nucleotide pools with different functions in the platelet release reaction, *Biochim. Biophys. Acta,* 186, 254, 1969.
149. **White, J. G. and Witkop, C. J.,** Effects of normal and aspirin platelets on defective secondary aggregation in the Hermansky-Pudlak syndrome. A test for storage pool deficient platelets, *Am. J. Pathol.,* 68, 57, 1972.
150. **Holmsen, H., Storm, E., and Day, H. J.,** Protein bound ADP in platelets: a possible function in the release reaction, *Fed. Proc.,* 29, 316, 1970.
151. **Da Prada, M. and Pletscher, A.,** Isolated 5-hydroxytryptamine organelles of rabbit blood platelets: physiological properties and drug induced changes, *Br. J. Pharmacol.,* 34, 591, 1968.
152. **Weber, E., Towliati, H., and Schmidt, B.,** Untersuchungen an frahtionierten Plattchen-homogenaten. IV. Quantitative Bezichungen bei der Freisetzung von strukturgebundenen ATP und serotonin, *Biochem. Pharmacol.,* 19, 1943, 1970.
153. **Seegers, W. H.,** *Prothrombin,* Harvard University Press, Cambridge, Mass., 1962, 268.
154. **Mammen, E. F.,** Physiology and biochemistry of blood coagulation, in *Thrombosis and Bleeding Disorders,* Bang, N. U., Beller, F. K., Deutsch, E., and Mammen, E. F., Eds., Georg Thieme Verlag, Stuttgart, 1971, 1.
155. **Packham, M. A. and Mustard, J. F.,** Platelet reactions, *Semin. Hematol.,* 8, 30, 1971.
156. **Bounameaux, Y.,** L'accolement des plaquettes aux fibres sous endotheliales, *C. R. Soc. Biol.,* 153, 865, 1959.
157. **Hughes, J.,** Accolement des plaquettes aux structures conjonctives perivasculaires, *Thromb. Diath. Haemorrh.,* 8, 241, 1962.
158. **Baumgartner, H. R. and Haudenschild, C.,** Adhesion of platelets to subendothelium, *Ann. N.Y. Acad. Sci.,* 201, 22, 1972.
159. **Bankowski, E., Niewiarowski, S., and Galasinski, W.,** Platelet aggregation by human collagen in relation to its age, *Gerontologia,* 13, 319, 1967.
160. **Legrand, Y., Caen, J., and Robert, L.,** Effect of glucosamine on platelet collagen reaction, *Proc. Soc. Exp. Biol. Med.,* 127, 941, 1968.
161. **Wilner, G. D., Nossel, H. L., and LeRoy, E. C.,** Aggregation of platelets by collagen, *J. Clin. Invest.,* 47, 2616, 1968.

162. **Zucker, M. B. and Borelli, J.**, Platelet clumping produced by connective tissue suspensions and by collagen, *Proc. Soc. Exp. Biol. Med.*, 109, 779, 1962.
163. **Puett, D., Wasserman, B. K., Ford, J. D., and Cunningham, L. W.**, Collagen-mediated platelet aggregation. Effects of collagen modification involving the platelet and carbohydrate moieties, *J. Clin. Invest.*, 52, 2495, 1973.
164. **Jaffe, R. and Deykin, D.**, Evidence for a structural requirement for the aggregation of platelets by collagen, *J. Clin. Invest.*, 53, 875, 1974.
165. **Brass, L. and Bensusan, H.**, The platelet: collagen interaction, *Fed. Proc.*, 34, 241, 1975.
166. **Hirsh, J., Street, D., Cade, J. F., and Amy, H.**, Relation between bleeding time and platelet connective tissue reaction after aspirin, *Blood*, 41, 369, 1973.
167. **Green, D., Dunne, B., Schmid, F. R., Rossi, E. C., and Louis, G.**, A study of the variable response of human platelets to collagen: relation to aspirin-induced inhibition of aggregation, *Am. J. Clin. Pathol.*, 60, 920, 1973.
168. **MacKenzie, R. D., Thompson, R. J., and Gleason, E. M.**, Evaluation of a quantitative platelet-collagen adhesiveness test, *Thromb. Res.*, 5, 99, 1974.
169. **Nunn, B.**, The role of adenosine diphosphate (ADP) in collagen-induced platelet aggregation, *Br. J. Pharmacol.*, 46, 579P, 1972.
170. **Kubisz, P. and Suranova, J.**, The effect of alpha- and beta-receptor blocking agents on collagen-induced platelet release reaction (a comparison with ADP-induced release), *Thromb. Diath. Haemorrh.*, 27, 278, 1972.
171. **Walsh, P. N.**, The effect of collagen and kaolin on the intrinsic coagulant activity of platelets. Evidence for an alternative pathway in intrinsic coagulation not requiring factor XII, *Br. J. Haematol.*, 22, 293, 1972.
172. **Bull, B. S., and Zucker, M. B.**, Changes in platelet volume produced by temperature, metabolic inhibitors and aggregating agents, *Proc. Soc. Exp. Biol. Med.*, 120, 296, 1965.
173. **Hovig, T.**, The ultrastructure of rabbit blood platelet aggregation, *Thromb. Diath. Haemorrh.*, 8, 455, 1962.
174. **Karpatkin, S. and Siskind, G. W.**, Effect of antibody binding and agglutination on human platelet glycolysis: comparison with thrombin and epinephrine, *Blood*, 30, 617, 1967.
175. **O'Brien, J. R. and Heywood, J. B.**, Effect of aggregating agents and their inhibitors on the mean platelet shape, *J. Clin. Pathol.*, 19, 148, 1966.
176. **Zucker, M. B. and Zaccardi, J. B.**, Platelet shape change by adenosine diphosphate and prevented by adenosine monophosphate, *Fed. Proc.*, 23, 299, 1964.
177. **Reddick, R. L. and Mason, R. G.**, Freeze-etch observations on the plasma membrane and other structures of normal and abnormal platelets, *Am. J. Pathol.*, 70, 473, 1973.
178. **Skoza, L., Zucker, M. B., Jerushalmy, Z., and Grant, R.**, Kinetic studies of platelet aggregation induced by adenosine diphosphate and its inhibition by chelating agents, guanidino compounds and adenosine, *Thromb. Diath. Haemorrh.*, 18, 713, 1967.
179. **Zucker, M. B. and Jerushalmy, Z.**, Studies on platelet shape and aggregation: effect of inhibitors on these and other platelet characteristics, in *Physiology of Haemostasis and Thrombosis*, Johnson, S. A. and Seegers, W. H., Eds., Charles C Thomas, Springfield, Ill., 1967, 249.
180. **Skjørten, F.**, Studies on the ultrastructure of pseudopod formation in human blood platelets. I. Effect of temperature, period of incubation, anticoagulants and mechanical forces, *Scand. J. Haematol.*, 5, 401, 1968.
181. **McLean, J. R. and Veloso, H.**, Change of shape without aggregation caused by ADP in rabbit platelets at low pH, *Life Sci.*, 6, 1983, 1967.
182. **Born, G. V. R. and Cross, M. J.**, The aggregation of blood platelets, *J. Physiol.*, 168, 178, 1963.
183. **MacMillan, D. C.**, Secondary clumping effect in human citrated platelet-rich plasma produced by adenosine diphosphate and adrenoline, *Nature (London)*, 211, 140, 1966.
184. **Zucker, M. B. and Peterson, J.**, Serotonin, platelet factor 3 activity and platelet aggregating agent released by adenosine diphosphate, *Blood*, 30, 556, 1967.
185. **Zucker, M. B. and Peterson, J.**, Inhibition of adenosine diphosphate-induced secondary aggregation and other platelet functions by acetysalicylic acid ingestion, *Proc. Soc. Exp. Biol. Med.*, 127, 547, 1968.
186. **Mills, D. C. B., Robb, I. A. and Roberts, G. C. K.**, The release of nucleotides 5-hydroxytryptamine and enzymes from human blood platelets during aggregation, *J. Physiol.*, 195, 715, 1968.
187. **Horowitz, H. I. and Papayoanou, M. F.**, Activation of platelet factor 3 by adenosine 5'diphosphate, *Thromb. Diath. Haemorrh.*, 19, 18, 1968.
188. **Bygdeman, S. and Johnson, O.**, Studies on the effect of adrenergic blocking drugs on catecholamine-induced platelet aggregation and uptake of noradrenaline and 5-hydroxytryptamine, *Acta Physiol. Scand.*, 75, 129, 1969.

189. Wright, J. H., The origin and nature of the blood platelets, *Boston Med. Surg. J.*, 154, 643, 1906.
190. Odell, T. T., Jackson, C. W., and Gosslee, D. G., Maturation of rat megakaryocytes studied by spectrophotometric measurement of DNA, *Proc. Soc. Exp. Biol. Med.*, 119, 1194, 1965.
191. Pennington, D. G. and Olsen, T. E., Megakaryocytes in states of altered platelet production, *Br. J. Haematol.*, 18, 447, 1970.
192. Cooper, G. W., The regulation of thrombopoiesis, in *Regulation of Hematopoiesis*, Gordon, A. S., Ed., Appleton-Century-Crofts, New York, 1970, 1611.
193. Keleman, E., Cserhati, I., and Tanos, B., Demonstration of some properties of human thrombopoietin in thrombocythemic sera, *Acta Hematol.*, 20, 350, 1958.
194. Corn, M., Effects of thrombin, adenosine diphosphate, connective tissue and endotoxin on platelet glycolysis, *Nature (London)*, 212, 508, 1966.
195. de Gabriele, G. and Pennington, D. G., Physiology of the regulation of platelet production, *Br. J. Haematol.*, 13, 202, 1967.
196. Pennington, D. G., Assessment of platelet production with ^{75}Se selenomethionine, *Br. Med. J.*, 4, 782, 1969.
197. Evatt, B. L. and Levin, J., Measurement of thrombopoiesis in rabbits using ^{75}selenomethionine, *J. Clin. Invest.*, 48, 1615, 1969.
198. Odell, T. T., Jackson, C. W., Friday, T. J., and Charsha, D. E., Effect of thrombocytopenia on megakaryocytopoiesis, *Br. J. Haematol.*, 17, 91, 1969.
199. Rolovic, Z., Baldini, M., and Dameshek, W., Megakaryocytopoiesis in experimentally induced immune thrombocytopenia, *Blood*, 35, 173, 1970.
200. Harker, L. A., Megakaryocyte quantitation, *J. Clin. Invest.*, 47, 452, 1968.
201. Harker, L. A., Regulation of thrombopoiesis, *Am. J. Physiol.*, 218, 1376, 1970.
202. Cronkite, E P., Bond, V. P., Fliedner, T. M., Paglia, D. A., and Adamik, E. R., Studies on the origin, production and destruction of platelets, in *Blood Platelets*, Johnson, S. A., Monto, R. W., Rebuck, J. W., and Horn, R. C., Eds., Little, Brown, Boston, 1961, 595.
203. Odell, T. T., McDonald, T. P., and Asano, M., Response of rat megakaryocytes and platelets to bleeding, *Acta Haematol.*, 27, 171, 1962.
204. Ebbe, S., Stohlman, F., Overcash, J., Donovan, J., and Howard, D., Megakaryocyte size in thrombocytopenic and normal rats, *Blood*, 32, 383, 1968.
205. Aster, R. H., Studies of the fate of platelets in rats and men, *Blood*, 34, 117, 1969.
206. Harker, L. A. and Finch, C. A., Thrombokinetics in man, *J. Clin. Invest.*, 48, 963, 1969.
207. Adelson, E., Rheingold, J. J., Parker, O., Buenaventura, A., and Crosby, W. H., Platelet and fibrinogen survival in normal and abnormal states of coagulation, *Blood*, 17, 267, 1961.
208. Baldini, M., Idiopathic thrombocytopenic purpura, *N. Engl. J. Med.*, 274, 1245, 1966.
209. O'Neill, B. and Firkin, B., Platelet survival studies in coagulation disorders, thrombocythemia, and conditions associated with atherosclerosis, *J. Lab. Clin. Med.*, 64, 188, 1964.
210. Gröttum, K. A., Hovig, T., Holmsen, H., Abrahamsen, A. F., Jeremic, M., and Seip, M., Wiskott-Aldrich syndrome: qualitative platelet defects and short platelet survival, *Br. J. Haematol.*, 17, 373, 1969.
211. Baldini, M., Kim, B., and Steiner, M., Metabolic platelet defect in Wiskott-Aldrich syndrome, *Pediatr. Res.*, 3, 377, 1969.
212. Karpatkin, S. and Charmatz, A., Heterogeneity of human platelets. III. Glycogen metabolism in platelets of different sizes, *Br. J. Haematol.*, 19, 135, 1970.
213. Karpatkin, S. and Strick, N., Heterogeneity of carbohydrate enzymes in platelets, *Clin. Res.*, 18, 407, 1970.
214. Ginsburg, A. D. and Aster, R. H., Changes associated with platelet aging, *Clin. Res.*, 17, 325, 1969.
215. Steiner, M. and Baldini, M., Protein synthesis in aging blood platelets, *Blood*, 33, 628, 1969.
216. Weber, E., Towliati, H., and Schmidt, B., Untersuchungen an fraktionierten Plattchenhomogenaten. IV. Quantitative Beziehungen bei der Freisetzung von strukturgebundenen ATP und serotonin, *Biochem. Pharmacol.*, 19, 1943, 1970.
217. Detwiler, T. C., Odell, T. T., and McDonald, T. P., Platelet age, ATP content and clot retraction in relation to platelet size, *Am. J. Physiol.*, 203, 107, 1962.
218. McDonald, T. P. Odell, T. T., and Gosslee, D. G., Platelet size in relation to platelet age, *Proc. Soc. Exp. Biol. Med.*, 115, 684, 1964.
219. Minter, N. and Ingram. M., Density distribution of platelets, *Blood*, 30, 551, 1967.
220. Mannucci, P. M. and Sharp, A. A., Platelet volume and shape in relation to aggregation and adhesion, *Br. J. Haematol.*, 13, 604, 1967.
221. Hirsh, J., Glynn, M. F., and Mustard, J. F., The effect of platelet age on platelet adherence to collagen, *J. Clin. Invest.*, 47, 466, 1968.
222. Rolovic, Z. and Baldini, M., Studies of platelet adhesiveness with references to platelet age, *Scand. J. Haematol.*, 6, 25, 1969.

223. **Melchinger, D. and Nemerson, Y.**, Randomness of platelet adhesiveness with respect to their ATP, O_2 consumption and size, *J. Appl. Physiol.*, 22, 197, 1967.
224. **Evans, G. and Mustard, J. F.**, Platelet surface reactions and thrombosis, *Surgery*, 64, 274, 1968.
225. **Karpatkin, S.**, Heterogeneity of human platelets. II. Functional evidence suggestive of young and old platelets, *J. Clin. Invest.*, 48, 1083, 1969.
226. **Kamoun, P., Lafourcade, G., and Jerome, H.**, Serotonin uptake by various human blood platelets, *Scand. J. Haematol.*, 16, 266, 1976.
227. **Hardisty, R. M. and Stacey, R. S.**, 5-hydroxytryptamine in normal human platelets, *J. Physiol.*, 130, 711, 1955.

Chapter 3

PLASMA PROTEIN FUNCTION IN HEMOSTASIS

Genesio Murano

TABLE OF CONTENTS

I. Introduction 44

II. Coagulation..44
    A. Fibrin Formation 46
        1. Proteolytic Phase 46
        2. Polymerization Phase 47
        3. Stabilization Phase..48
    B. Thrombin Formation 49
    C. Factor X_a Formation 52
        1. Extrinsic Pathway — Rapid Formation of Factor X_a..........54
        2. Intrinsic Pathway — Slow Formation of Factor X_a...........55
    D. Factor IX_a Formation 56
    E. The Early Steps in Coagulation..56
    F. Inhibitory Mechanisms 59
        1. Nonproteolytic Activation of Factors XII and VII............59
        2. Factor X_a as an Inhibitor 60
        3. Thrombin as an Inhibitor 60
        4. Generation of Activated Protein-C 60
        5. Stoichiometric Requirements 60
        6. Antithrombin III 61
        7. Fibrin(ogen) as an Inhibitor 61
        8. Fibrin(ogen) Degradation Products 61

III. Fibrino(geno)lysis..61
    A. Plasmin Formation..63
    B. Mechanism of Fibrin Dissolution 65
    C. Chemistry and Function of Fibrin(ogen) Degradation
       Products (FDP)..65

IV. Kinin Generation 66

V. Complement Activation..67
    A. Classic Mechanisms..67
    B. The Hageman (Factor XII) Connection............................68

VI. Concluding Remarks 71

References...71

I. INTRODUCTION

In the preceding two chapters, we have observed that, upon injury, the vessel wall and the platelets play a major role in the maintenance of hemostasis. However, vasoconstriction and the formation of the "platelet plug" are not adequate in achieving permanent hemostasis. For this, a series of coagulation (plasma) proteins must be activated, finally resulting in the formation of a fibrin network. It is at this point that, technically, permanent hemostasis is achieved. However, this does not represent the termination of the sequence of events. In the process of activating the coagulation system, other systems involved in (1) the destruction of the fibrin clot (lysis), (2) the generation of kinins, and (3) immunologic defense, although to a variable extent, are simultaneously activated. Based on experimental data obtained in the laboratory and various clinical observations, these four apparently separate systems have been demonstrated to be interrelated. Each system will be discussed separately. Their interrelationships will become evident as the discussion proceeds.

II. COAGULATION

Basically, clot formation consists of the conversion of fibrinogen to fibrin by the enzyme thrombin (Figure 1). The latter exists in plasma as a zymogen (prothrombin). The potential resources for thrombin formation reside in (1) the plasma, (2) the platelets, and (3) the tissue cells. This distribution guarantees ready availability of "activators" providing a perpetual sentinel service always ready to prevent hemorrhage from the site of injury.

The exact sequence of chemical events preceding fibrin formation has been a subject of dispute since the description of the first coagulation theory of Morawitz[1] in 1904. He stated that prothrombin was converted to thrombin by tissue thrombokinase (thromboplastin) and calcium ions. Thrombin, in turn, converted fibrinogen to fibrin.

The work of Brinkhous[2] provided the evidence for a pathway in coagulation not involving tissue thromboplastin. Investigating the delayed thrombin production in hemophilic plasma, Brinkhous observed that tissue thromboplastin would normalize thrombin formation. This observation established the presence of a hitherto unrecognized clotting factor, subsequently called antihemophilic factor (AHF, Factor VIII, platelet cofactor). These developments were basic to the understanding of prothrombin activation via the "extrinsic pathway" involving tissue thromboplastin and the "intrinsic pathway" involving plasma constituents and platelets.

In the following years, additional coagulation factors were recognized mainly through clinical observation of various bleeding disorders. When the defect was characterized by substantial differences from previously recognized disorders, it was presumed that the patient's plasma was lacking a hitherto unrecognized factor. Based on this logic, several deficiencies* were characterized: Factor V,[3] Factor VII,[4] Factor IX,[5] Factor X,[6] Factor XI,[7] Factor XII,[8] and Factor XIII.[9] Table 1 correlates the various Roman numerals assigned to clotting factors (by the International Nomenclature Committee) with the most common synonyms.

A number of schemes have been proposed to explain the interactions of the various clotting factors in fibrin formation. The "cascade"[10] or "waterfall"[11] hypothesis of fibrin formation states that clotting factors (Factors I to XII) are distinct entities in

---

* Presently, the term "deficiency" is under scrutiny. It has been demonstrated in several cases that a bleeding problem need not be characterized by the absence of a clotting factor. Rather, the presence of the same component as a structural variant—consequently, biologically partially or totally inactive—or the presence of a specific inhibitor may result in the same pathology.

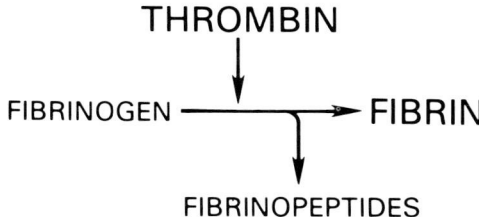

FIGURE 1. The conversion of fibrinogen to fibrin by the enzyme thrombin, releasing fibrinopeptides.

TABLE 1

Coagulation Factors and Synonyms

Factor	Synonyms
Factor I	Fibrinogen
Factor II	Prothrombin
Factor III	Tissue thromboplastin
Factor VI	Calcium ions
Factor V	Accelerator globulin, Ac-globulin, proaccelerin, labile factor
Factor VI	—[a]
Factor VII	Serum prothrombin, conversion accelerator (SPCA), proconvertin, autoprothrombin I
Factor VIII	Antihemophilic factor (AHF), antihemophilic globulin (AHG), platelet cofactor
Factor IX	Christmas factor, plasma thromboplastin component (PTC), autoprothrombin II
Factor X	Stuart-Prower factor, thrombokinase, autoprothrombin III
Factor XI	Plasma thromboplastin antecedent (PTA)
Factor XII	Contact factor, Hageman factor
Factor XIII	Fibrin stabilizing factor, protransglutaminase, fibrinase, fibrinoligase (active form)

[a] Probably responsible for all "false positive" results in the clinical laboratory.

plasma, synthesized independently, and present in the circulation as inactive precursors (zymogens). Generally, each factor is converted to its enzymatic form by the preceding one in a sequence of events best described as a chain reaction, ultimately resulting in the formation of fibrin. Hageman factor (Factor XII), a surface-sensitive protein, becomes activated—initiating the intrinsic sequence—upon contact with foreign surfaces. Tissue thromboplastin, released from injured tissue, together with Factor VII, initiates the extrinsic activation pathway by directly activating Factor X, bypassing the "contact phase", which involves Factors XII_a, XI_a, IX_a, and VIII.*

Other studies have established that all of the clotting factors do indeed participate in the generation of the enzyme thrombin, but not in the mode outlined by the "cascade" hypothesis. In both the intrinsic and extrinsic system, a series of complexes are formed involving zymogens, cofactors, calcium ions, and phospholipids prior to the formation of thrombin. A series of reviews have been written on this topic.[12-20]

* The subscript letter "a" following the Roman numeral is used to designate the active form of the respective factor.

In order to facilitate our understanding of the complex sequence of reactions, the outline is developed around five basic reactions that are best viewed from the end result (fibrin formation) and proceeds backwards to the initiating events. The reactions are

1. The formation of fibrin
2. The formation of thrombin (Factor II_a)
3. The formation of Factor X_a
4. The formation of Factor IX_a
5. The early steps in coagulation

The enzymes—thrombin, Factor X_a, Factor IX_a (as well as Factor VII and a newly recognized factor, "Protein-C")[21,22]—are synthesized in the liver parenchymal cells in precursor forms by a vitamin K-dependent process.[21,23] The function of vitamin K is to attach calcium-binding prosthetic groups, postribosomally, on the amino terminal regions of these factors. The process involves the introduction of an extra COOH group on the side chain of several glutamic acid residues. The modified amino acid is called γ-carboxyglutamic acid (Figure 2).[24]

In the absence of vitamin K or, in the case of anticoagulant therapy with vitamin K antagonists, Factors II, VII, IX, and X are synthesized but are incomplete, lacking the special calcium-binding γ-carboxyglutamic acids, and appear in the plasma as abnormal nonfunctional factors, unable to adequately bind calcium ions.;[24,44] These factors are known as PIVKA (protein induced by vitamin K absence/antagonism).

A. Fibrin Formation

The sequence of events in fibrin formation may be subdivided in three phases: (1) proteolysis, (2) polymerization and (3) stabilization (Figure 3). The fibrinogen (Factor I) molecule, a protein synthesized in the liver parenchymal cells[25] is soluble in plasma. Its concentration is about 300 mg/dl, and its biologic half-life is about 3 days. The molecule is composed of three (most likely, independently synthesized)[26] pairs of polypeptide chains: $[A\alpha, B\beta, \gamma]_2$.[27,28] The molecular size of the dimeric structure is about 340,000. Disulfide bridges link the three chains together, as well as the dimer (Figure 4).[28]

1. Proteolytic Phase

In the proteolytic phase, the enzyme thrombin[29] attacks the amino terminal region of Aα and Bβ chains, splitting specific arginyl-glycine peptide bonds, releasing a pair of peptides, A and B.[27] The γ chain is not involved in this process. The resulting molecule, i.e., fibrinogen minus peptides A and B, is called fibrin monomer.* Peptide A is removed most rapidly. Peptide B is removed more slowly, and this latter reaction is likely dependent upon a specific steric rearrangement of the molecule prior to the removal of the B peptide.

Studies on the structure of fibrinopeptides A and B from various species have shown that their carboxy terminal amino acid residue is always arginine.[27] Furthermore, the area immediately adjacent and to the left of the arginyl-glycine bond cleaved by thrombin has been strongly selected for during evolution, and a portion of this area, in all species studied, is hydrophobic in nature and is an ordered structure.[30] Positions 6 to 8 to the right of the arginyl-glycine bond also has a restricted amino acid sequence.[13,31] This may reflect, in part, the restricted specificity of the enzyme thrombin on fibrinogen (see Section II.B).

---

* Fibrin monomer refers to the fibrinogen molecule (which in its native form is a dimer) minus fibrinopeptides A and B. This is in distinction from fibrin, and fibrin, that are polymers of the basic fibrin monomer subunit.

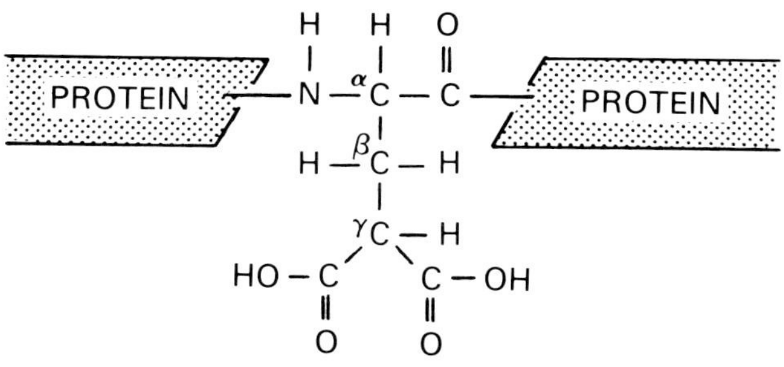

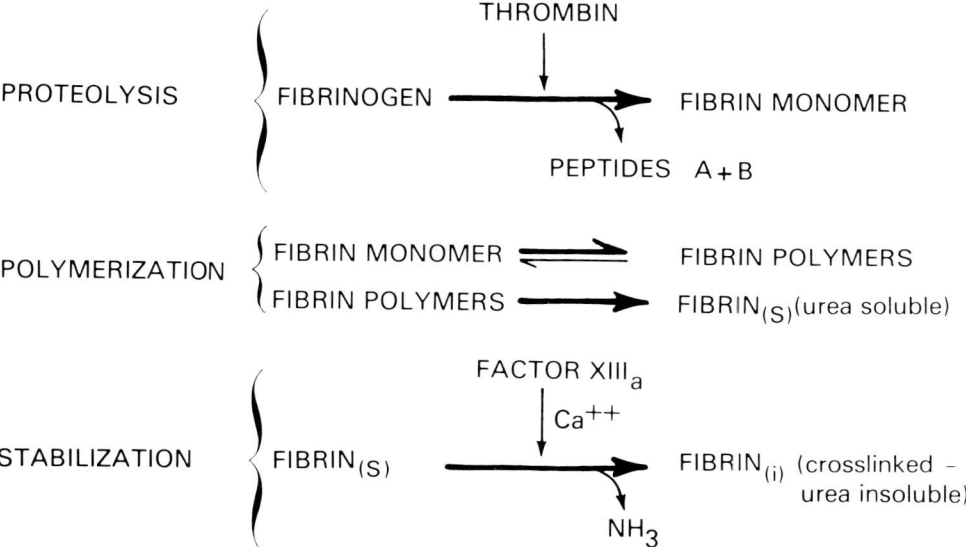

FIGURE 2. Structure of γ-carboxyglutamic acid.

FIGURE 3. The three phases of fibrin formation. Proteolysis—by the enzyme thrombin, polymerization—a self-assembly phenomenon, and stabilization—introduction of covalent isopeptide bonds by the cross-linking enzyme Factor XIII$_a$.

2. Polymerization Phase

The polymerization phase is best characterized as a nonenzymatic, spontaneous self-assembly process, resulting in end-to-end and side-to-side aggregation of fibrin monomers, resulting in the fibrin polymer[27] designated "fibrin$_s$."* Studies performed on fibrin produced by thrombin and by the snake venom enzyme reptilase (which removes only fibrinopeptide A) indicate that the polymerization pattern differs for the two products. The molecular weight to length ratio for thrombin-induced fibrin is about 2, whereas for reptilase-induced fibrin it is about 1, indicating a predominance of end-to-end polymers for the latter.[32] Moreover, the viscosity of the two fibrins is different. Based on these observations and binding studies performed with fragment D— a terminal product of fibrinolysis (see Section III.C), it has been proposed[27,33] that there exist in fibrinogen two separate complementary sets of polymerization domains. One of these sets resides in the fragment D portion of the molecule (toward the carboxy

---

* The subscript "s" designates solubility in 5 M urea solution, suggesting that the association of monomers is promoted by noncovalent, perhaps coordinate bond formation between ionizable groups.[27]

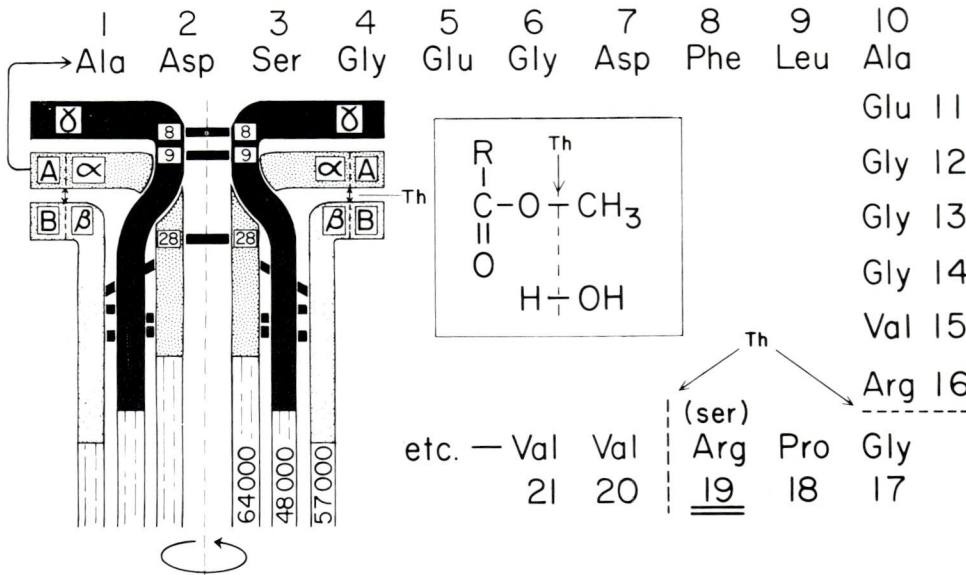

FIGURE 4. Schematic model of the amino terminal portion of the dimeric fibrinogen molecule. Disulfide bridges linking the six chains are indicated by the crossbars. The molecular size of each individual chain is indicated. Th = thrombin cleavage. The amino acid sequence of fibrinopeptide A (positions 1 to 16) plus a portion of the α chain is indicated. The serine in position 19 is found in fibrinogen Detroit. Therefore, this bond is not cleaved. The insert represents thrombin esterolytic specificity of methyl ester derivatives.

terminal region of fibrinogen). This set of domains is always exposed in the intact fibrinogen molecule. The second set of polymerization domains resides dormant (blocked) in the amino terminal area (close to the fibrinopeptides A and B) of the intact fibrinogen molecule. Upon removal of fibrinopeptide A by thrombin, the molecule undergoes a compulsory local conformational change, exposing one portion of this second (amino terminal) set of domains, which is likely complementary to the first set (carboxyterminal). This allows for end-to-end polymerization, and simultaneously permits the removal of fibrinopeptide B, which in turn uncovers the second portion of the amino terminal domain, permitting side-to-side polymerization. It has been postulated that in Fibrinogen Detroit (a well-documented dysfibrinogenemia),[27,34] although fibrinopeptide A is structurally normal and released normally by thrombin, the amino acid substitution (Arg → Ser) close to the bond split by thrombin (Figure 4) prevents or alters the conformational change necessary for exposing the first amino terminal domain and for releasing fibrinopeptide B. Consequently, clotting is abnormal.

3. Stabilization Phase

The stabilization phase of the conversion fibrinogen to fibrin is characterized by the introduction of covalent bonds within the already polymerized fibrin network. This "cross-linking" process results in fibrin$_i$*. The enzyme responsible for this ultimate series of reactions is Factor XIII$_a$ (plasma transglutaminase, fibrinoligase). It exists in plasma and in platelets as an inactive precursor (Factor XIII). The zymogen in plasma

---

* The subscript "i" designates insolubility in 5 M urea solutions. This is the kind of fibrin that forms in normal plasma.

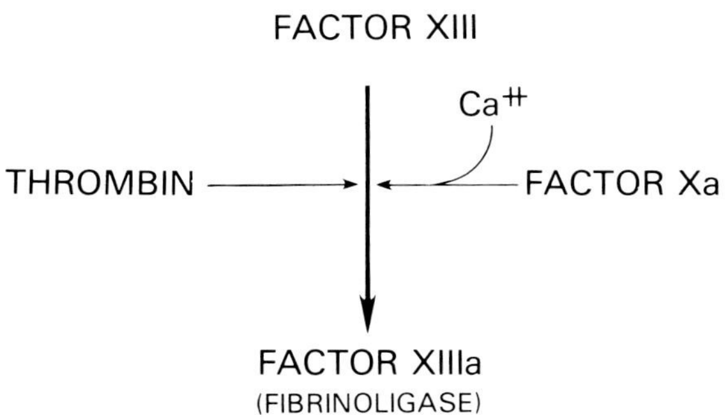

```
                    FACTOR XIII
                         |    Ca⁺⁺
                         |   ╱
THROMBIN ───────────▶    ◀──────  FACTOR Xa
                         |
                         ▼
                    FACTOR XIIIa
                    (FIBRINOLIGASE)
```

FIGURE 5. The conversion of Factor XIII to Factor XIII$_a$ (fibrinoligase) by thrombin and Factor X$_a$.

is a tetramer composed of two identical subunits termed *a* chains (molecular weight 75,000) and two identical subunits termed *b* chains (molecular weight 80,000). Its total molecular weight is about 300,000. The catalytic site resides in the *a* chains.[35] The zymogen in platelets is composed of only the two *a* chains, with a total molecular weight of 150,000.[35] The site of biosynthesis of the *a* chains has been localized to hepatocytes, megakaryocytes, spleen, and uterus, while the biosynthesis of the *b* chains is confined to the hepatocyte.[75] Factor XIII is activated to its enzymatic form by thrombin and by Factor X$_a$, the latter requiring the presence of calcium ions[36] (Figure 5). In the course of activation, a polypeptide with a molecular weight of 4000 is released from the amino terminal area of both *a* chains.[35] Factor XIII$_a$, functioning as a transpeptidase, in the presence of calcium ions, introduces isopeptide bonds between the Σ-amino groups of certain lysine residues and the γ-carboxyamide groups of certain glutamines,[37] releasing ammonia. This renders the fibrin more elastic and less amenable to lysis by fibrinolytic agents.[38] The first cross-links occur between neighboring γ chains (fast reaction), resulting in γ-γ dimers. Then, more slowly, the α chains begin and continue to be cross-linked resulting in α polymers.[39,40] Figures 6 and 7 illustrate the basic mechanism.

B. Thrombin Formation

The enzyme thrombin is derived from its inactive precursor: prothrombin (Factor II). Prothrombin is a vitamin K-dependent,[23,24] single polypeptide chain glycoprotein with a molecular weight of about 70,000 and is synthesized in the liver parenchymal cells.[13,41,42] Its concentration in plasma is about 10 mg/dl.[13,41] Thrombin has a molecular weight of about 39,000 (about one half that of prothrombin), can exist in several forms (two or more polypeptide chains),[13,43,44,46,47] and is derived from the carboxyterminal half of prothrombin.[46] In this discussion, when not otherwise stated, we refer to the two-chain thrombin (A = light chain and B = heavy chain linked by a disulfide bridge). The active center resides in the B chain. The conversion of prothrombin to thrombin occurs in several steps. The sequence varies, depending on the conditions of activation, and it is likely that, in vivo, more than one route is operative.

Two major intermediates of activation have been identified and characterized. These are known as Prethrombin 1 and Prethrombin 2.[13,44] In the process of forming these two intermediates, two activation polypeptides are released from the amino terminal portion of prothrombin. These are designated Prothrombin fragments 1 and 2, respec-

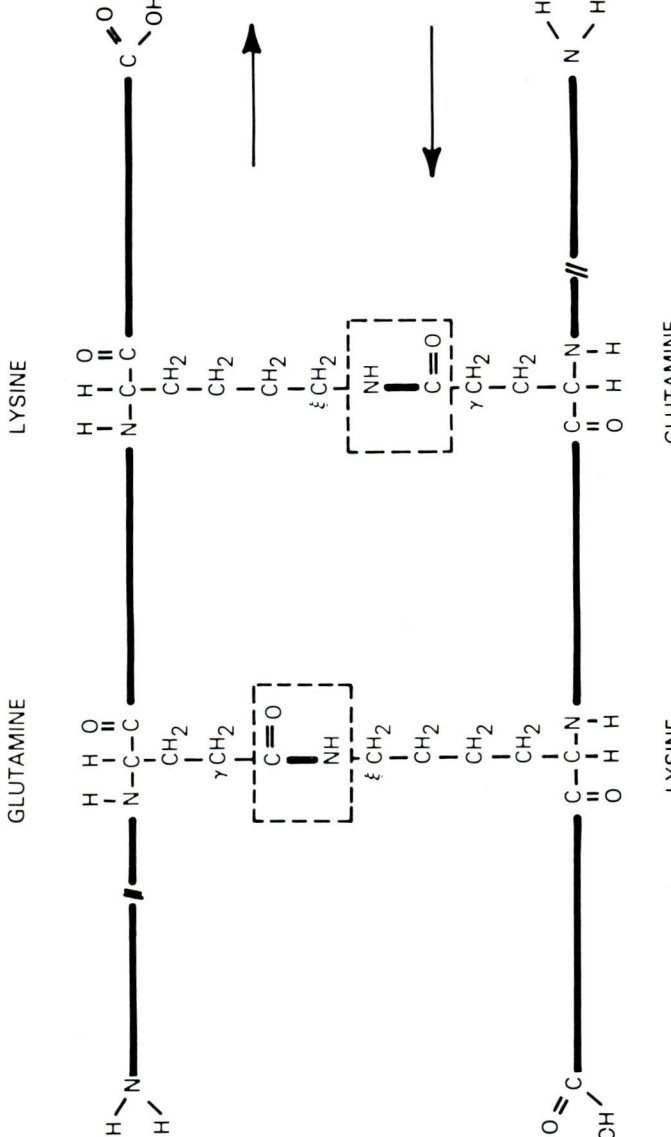

FIGURE 6. Neighboring antiparallel γ-chains isopeptide bonds between Σ-amino groups of lysine residues and γ-carboxyamide groups of glutamine residues introduced by the enzyme Factor XIII$_a$.

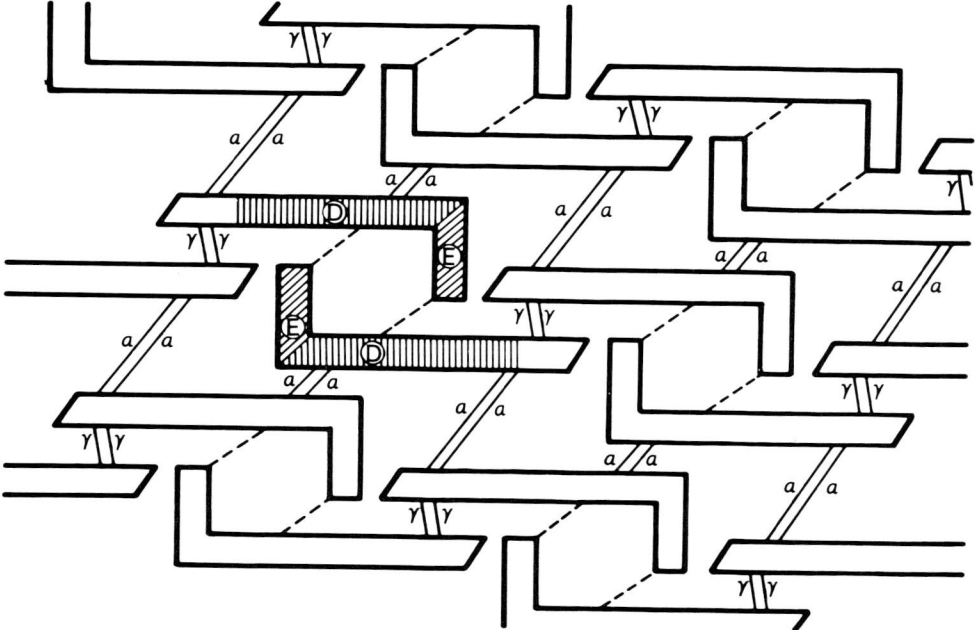

FIGURE 7. Schematic of cross-linked fibrin. γ-γ cross-links and α-α cross-links are indicated by solid lines. The complementarity of the D and E domain (center of figure) in each fibrin monomer is indicated in the center of the figure.

tively.[13,42,44,45-49]* Fragment 1 contains γ-carboxyglutamic acid residues necessary for calcium binding and contains two thirds of the carbohydrate found in prothrombin. The remainder of the carbohydrate is found in the thrombin moiety.[46,47,50] Prethrombin 1 and 2 do not possess proteolytic activity. Figure 8 illustrates in a linear fashion the various component substructures of prothrombin.

Factor X_a is the enzyme that produces thrombin from prothrombin.[51-53] However, unlike thrombin, which by itself attacks its substrate fibrinogen, Factor X_a functions optimally in association with other components, namely, Factor V, calcium ions, and phospholipids.[13,20,44] A complex constituted of all five components is formed, resulting in optimal thrombin formation (Figure 9). The phospholipids (phosphotidyl-L-serine and phosphotidylinositol) function in micellar form and are derived primarily from platelets (platelet factor 3).[13,20,54]

Since other micelles (bile salts, for example) can substitute[13] in vitro for platelet factor 3, it appears that phospholipids serve as a surface support upon which the enzyme (Factor X_a), the determiner (Factor V)**, and the substrate (prothrombin) can interact in complex mediated by calcium ions. Factor V binds to the prothrombin frag-

---

* Prethrombin 1 is a product of thrombin proteolysis.[13] Prethrombin 2 is a product of Factor X_a proteolysis.[15] Recent evidence[49] indicates that normally, in vivo, Fragments 1 and 2 are released predominantly as one (continuous) polypeptide, termed Fragment 1·2.

** The exact mode of action of Factor V is not known. It appears to serve as cofactor governing the reaction specificity between the enzyme and substrate[13,54] and/or serve (after modification by thrombin) to bind the other components of the prothrombin activation system to itself, thereby maintaining the integrity of the "complex".[44] Factor V is synthesized, at least in part, by the liver.[75] It is a single chain molecule with a molecular weight of 300,000. When fully activated by thrombin,[53] it is converted to two chains (115,000 and 73,000).

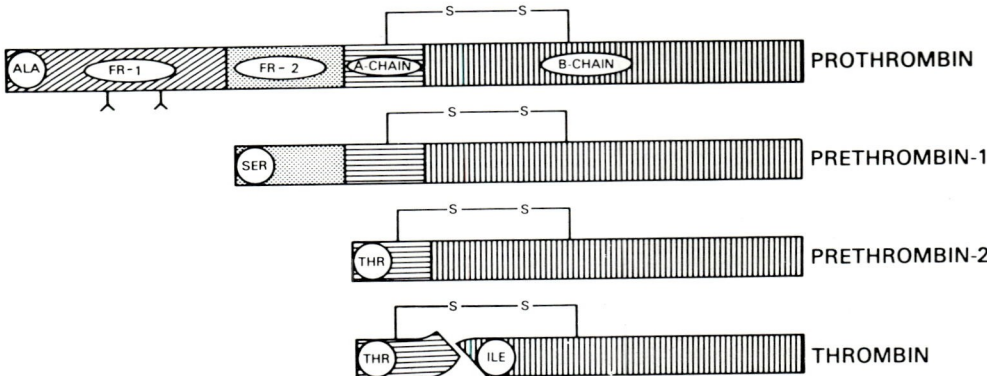

FIGURE 8.. Linear model of prothrombin, activation intermediates, and thrombin. N-Terminal amino acid residues are indicated within circles. FR-1 and FR-2 = prothrombin fragment 1 and prothrombin fragment 2, respectively. The symbol λ denotes the presence of γ-carboxyglutamic acid residues. The active site region is in the B-chain.

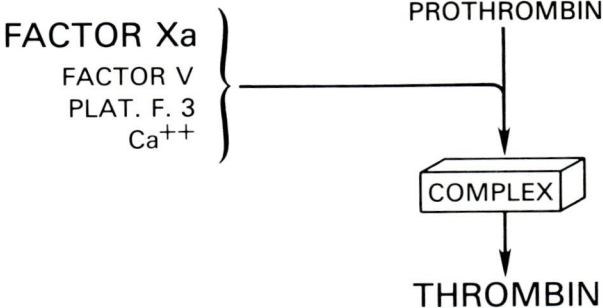

FIGURE 9. The five-component system constituting the complex necessary for optimal conversion of prothrombin to thrombin. Factor X_a = enzyme, Factor V = determiner, Ca^{++} = binder, Plat. F. 3 = platelet factor 3 — phospholipid surface, and prothrombin = substrate.

ment 2 portion of prothrombin,[55] and calcium ions bind to the prothrombin fragment 1 portion of prothrombin, which contains γ-carboxyglutamic acid residues.[13,20,24,43,44,47,48,55] Reduction in the concentration of any one of the five components composing the complex results in a paramount reduction in the rate and yield of thrombin.[13] A precise stoichiometric relationship is essential. Any perturbation of this equilibrium results in less than optimal yields of thrombin, which is reflected in delayed coagulation in vivo.[13,44,45] As already pointed out in the fibrin formation section, thrombin has a very restricted substrate specificity. This property is imparted by the structural characteristics of the substrate in the area immediately adjacent to the arginyl-glycine peptide bond cleaved by thrombin (Figure 10).

C. Factor X_a Formation

Factor X_a is the proteolytic enzyme responsible for cleaving two essential peptide bonds in prothrombin, thereby generating thrombin.[13,14,42,44,47,54,56-58] Like thrombin, Factor X_a is derived from an inactive precursor (Factor X), which is also a vitamin K-

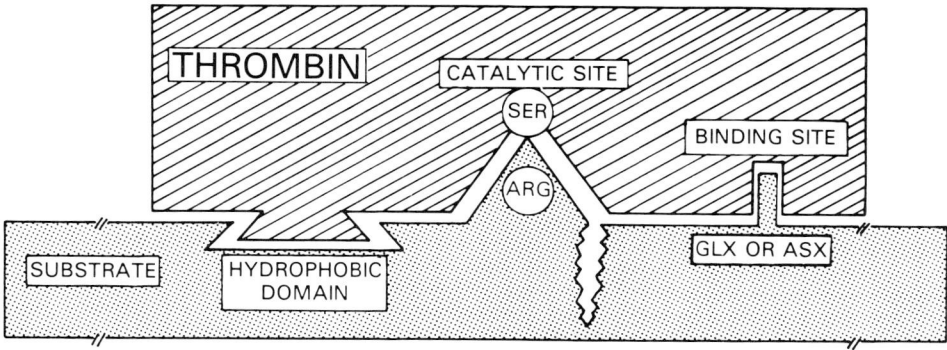

FIGURE 10. Schematic model of thrombin specificity. Note the obligatory GLX (glutamic acid or glutamine) or ASX (aspartic acid or asparagine) residues to the right, and the hydrophobic area to the left of the arginyl-X bond cleaved by thrombin. Other arginyl-X peptide bonds not conforming to this kind of arrangement are not very susceptible to cleavage by thrombin.

dependent glycoprotein containing γ-carboxyglutamic acid residues necessary for calcium binding. Its concentration in plasma is about 1 mg/dl (one tenth that of prothrombin).[14] Unlike prothrombin, which is a single polypeptide chain,[13,24,41,42,44] Factor X, as it is normally isolated from plasma, contains two polypeptide chains linked by a disulfide bridge.[14,15,44,59] The light chain has a molecular weight of about 15,000 and the heavy chain has a molecular weight of about 39,000.[14,15] It has been pointed out, however, that, theoretically, the protein should be synthesized by the liver as a single chain, as is the case with prothrombin.[59] If it is synthesized as a single chain, there must be a modification at a later time. This could occur metabolically and/or during isolation from plasma. It is of interest to note that the primary structure of the light chain of Factor X displays a great degree of homology to the structure of the N-terminal portion of prothrombin (Fragment 1).[14,15,44] This, in conjunction with the presence of γ-carboxyglutamic acid residues in the light chain,[60] is suggestive of a possible common ancestral gene for the two proteins. In contrast to prothrombin, the carbohydrate in Factor X is associated exclusively with the heavy chain (C-terminal portion of the molecule).[14]

Like in prothrombin activation, the activation of Factor X to Factor X_a involves a proteolytic process, resulting in the release of one or more polypeptide fragments. A glycopeptide (Fragment 3) with a molecular weight of 11,000 is split from the amino terminal area of the heavy (H) chain. This polypeptide contains two thirds of the carbohydrate in Factor X.[15,61,62] This reduces the molecular weight from 55,000 to 44,000 and gives rise to the active enzyme Factor $X_{a\alpha}$. A second nonobligatory cleavage can occur in either Factor $X_{a\alpha}$ or as a primary event in the zymogen, resulting in the removal of another glycopeptide (Fragment 4, molecular weight 4,000) from the carboxyterminal region of the heavy chain.[15,61,63] This latter reaction is catalyzed by thrombin and leads to the eventual formation of Factor $X_{a\beta}$. The presence or absence of this carboxyterminal polypeptide on the heavy chain does not seem to influence the biologic activity of Factor X_a.[61,63] Figure 11 illustrates the activation sequence. The active center resides in the heavy chain. It should be noted at this point that although both prothrombin and Factor X contain γ-carboxyglutamic acid residues in homologous regions, Factor X does not bind to phospholipid surfaces via calcium ions as does prothrombin. However, Factor X_a does bind.[64,65] It is possible that in Factor X the 11,000 molecular weight amino terminal glycopeptide is sterically hindering the γ-carboxyglutamic acid residues.

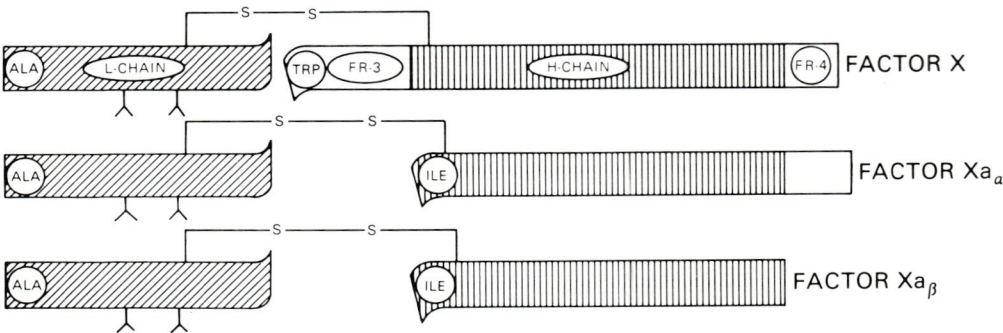

FIGURE 11. Linear model of Factor X, Factor Xa_α, and Factor Xa_β. N-Terminal amino acid residues are indicated within circles. FR-3 = Fragment 3 and FR-4 = Fragment 4. The symbol ⋏ denotes the presence of γ-carboxyglutamic acid residues. L-Chain = light chain and H-chain = heavy chain. The active site region is in the H-chain.

As in prothrombin activation to thrombin, multiple factors are involved in the activation of Factor X to Factor X_a. There are purified enzymes, venoms from various sources, and other biologic materials that activate Factor X to Factor X_a.[14,62] Our discussion will be limited to the activation of Factor X as it normally occurs in vivo. Two principal pathways of activation are operative: the "extrinsic" and the "intrinsic" pathways, and, as will be illustrated later, the two are interrelated. The term "extrinsic" denotes the requirement of substances that are not normally present in the circulation, i.e., tissue substances (thromboplastin) introduced upon injury. The term "intrinsic" denotes the participation of substances normally present in the circulation. The main distinguishing feature of the two pathways is the *rate* of Factor X_a formation.

1. Extrinsic Pathway—Rapid Formation of Factor X_a

The extrinsic pathway involves the participation of thromboplastin (tissue factor), Factor VII, and calcium ions.[19] Tissue factor is a membrane-bound protein (lipoprotein) existing in a protected state within the plasma membrane of endothelial cells.[19,66] Upon injury, it is released into the circulation, where it forms a complex with coagulation Factor VII (another vitamin K-dependent protein containing γ-carboxyglutamic acid residues) in the presence of calcium ions (Figure 12). The activity of the complex seems to be largely dependent on the concentration of tissue factor. However, the enzymatic activity responsible for the proteolytic activation of Factor X resides in the Factor VII molecule.[67]

Factor VII exists in plasma as a single chain glycoprotein, with close structural homology to prothrombin, Factor IX, and Factor X.[19] Contrary to its analogs however, Factor VII is not a zymogen in the true sense, since it has proteolytic activity, although to a limited extent.[19] In the presence of thrombin or Factor X_a and lipids and calcium ions, this activity may be increased as much as 400-fold and is accompanied by the formation of a two polypeptide chain molecule (Figure 13).[19] Upon further incubation, the two chain form of Factor VII becomes inactive, and the rate of inactivation is dependent on the concentration of Factor X_a.[67] It has been proposed that in the activation of Factor X by Factor VII, the continuing generation of Factor X_a results in a "pulse of Factor X-converting activity that can quickly disappear".[19]

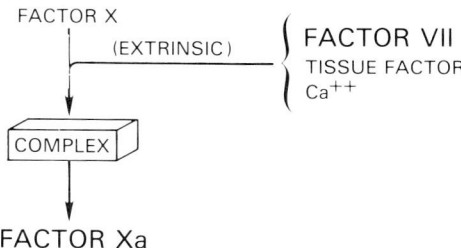

FIGURE 12. The components of the extrinsic pathway of Factor X activation. Factor X = substrate, Factor VII = enzyme, tissue factor = "activator" of Factor VII, and Ca^{++} = binder.

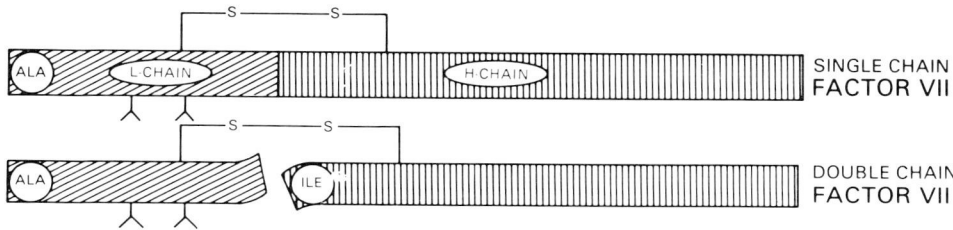

FIGURE 13. Linear model of single chain and double chain Factor VII. N-terminal amino acid residues are indicated within circles. The symbol ⋏ denotes the presence of γ-carboxyglutamic acid residues. L-Chain = light chain and H-chain = heavy chain. The active site region residues in the H-chain.

2. Intrinsic Pathway—Slow Formation of Factor X_a

The intrinsic pathway involves the participation of phospholipids, Factor VIII (antihemophilic factor), Factor IX_a, and calcium ions. These factors form a complex (much in the likeness of the prothrombin-activating complex), and it is this complex that converts Factor X to Factor X_a.[15] Under physiologic conditions, the platelets provide the phospholipids (phosphotidyl choline and phosphotidyl ethanolamine as platelet factor 3) for this reaction. Factor VIII plays the role of a regulatory protein (in the likeness of Factor V), and Factor IX_a is the enzyme. Indeed, Factor IX_a alone will convert Factor X to Factor X_a; however, the reaction is accelerated several thousand-fold in the presence of the other components. Similarly to Factor V, it appears that Factor VIII requires a modification (interaction with) thrombin or Factor X_a before it can function in the complex.[15,68-70] The nature of this modification is not known.

Factor VIII is a glycoprotein with a molecular weight exceeding one million.[68-70] Its subunit structure constitutes components with a molecular weight of about 200,000.[68-70] Three major properties of Factor VIII have been defined: (1) shortening of the clotting time (Factor $VII_{Coag.}$), (2) precipitin reaction with rabbit antibody (VIII_{Agn}), and (3) correction of defective platelet aggregation in von Willebrand's disease in the presence of the antibiotic ristocetin (VIII_{vWF}).[70,71] The coagulant activity can be separated in the laboratory from the other two activities, and it is associated with one of the low molecular weight subcomponents.[70-74] More specifically, the portion involved in the formation of the complex responsible for Factor X activation, is the Factor VIII_{Coag}. The role of Factor VIII_{vWF} is discussed in Chapters 6 and 7.

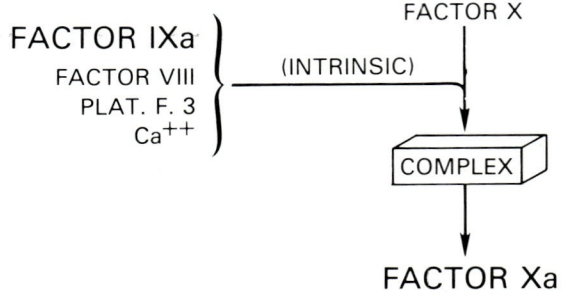

FIGURE 14. The five-component system of the intrinsic pathway of Factor X activation. Factor IX_a = enzyme, Factor VIII = determiner, Ca^{++} = binder, Plat. F.3 = platelet factor 3 — phospholipid surface, and Factor X = substrate.

The precise site of synthesis of Factor VIII is not clear. There is evidence indicating that endothelial cells[75] (primarily hepatic[76]) are the site of synthesis. Figure 14 outlines the reactions involving the intrinsic activation of Factor X to Factor X_a.

It is of interest to note that in the intrinsic and extrinsic pathway, each one of the molecular pairs that accelerate the *rate* of Factor X_a formation (and thrombin formation) is derived from separate anatomic compartments: platelets and plasma, or tissue and plasma. Injury brings them together.

D. Factor IX_a Formation

Factor IX_a is the proteolytic enzyme responsible for the intrinsic activation of Factor X to Factor X_a. Like thrombin and Factor X_a, Factor IX_a is derived from a zymogen (Factor IX) that is also a vitamin K-dependent glycoprotein containing γ-carboxyglutamic acid residues. In plasma, Factor IX exists as a single chain glycoprotein, with a molecular weight of about 55,000.[77] As in prothrombin and Factor X activation, the formation of Factor IX_a involves a proteolytic process (two steps) resulting in the release of a polypeptide(s).[77] In the first step (slow reaction), Factor IX is cleaved by hydrolysis of an internal peptide bond, giving rise to a two chain (molecular weights about 16,000 and 38,000) intermediate linked by disulfide bridges. This intermediate is not active. In the second step (fast reaction), a glycopeptide with a molecular weight of about 10,000 is released from the amino terminal portion of the heavy chain, resulting in the formation of Factor IX_a, with a molecular weight of about 45,000 (Figure 15). The heavy chain of Factor IX_a is homologous with the heavy chain of thrombin and Factor X_a and contains the active site.[15,77,79] Furthermore, the heavy chain of all three enzymes is homologous with trypsin and other serine proteases, indicating a similar biochemical mechanism for their function.[15]

Two routes of activation for Factor IX are known. One of these involves the enzyme Factor XI_a (*not* a vitamin K-dependent protein) and calcium ions.[15,77] Another pathway involves the extrinsic system activation complex (Factor VII, tissue factor, and calcium ions).[78] Figure 16 outlines the activation sequence.

E. The Early Steps in Coagulation

The exact sequence of chemical events occurring in the formation of Factor XI_a are not completely clear. Several factors are involved in this early series of reactions: surfaces, prekallikrein (Fletcher factor), high molecular weight (HMW) kininogen (Fitzgerald or Flaujeac or Williams factor), and Factor XII (Hageman factor). Although

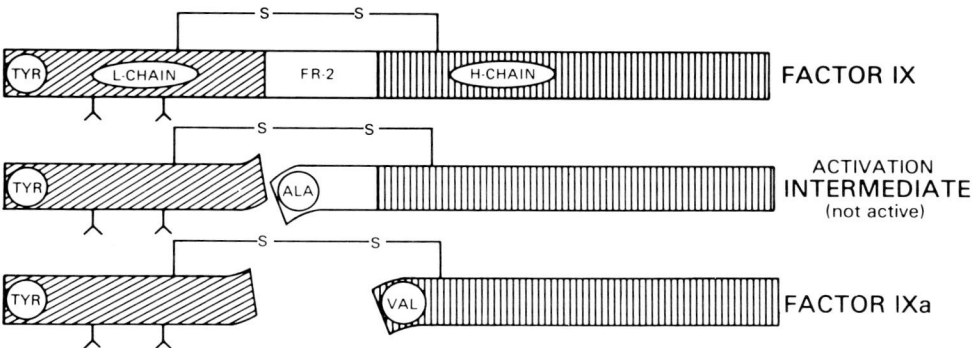

FIGURE 15. Linear model of Factor XI, activation intermediate, and Factor XI$_a$. N-Terminal amino acid residues are indicated within circles. The symbol ⊥ denotes the presence of γ-carboxyglutamic acid residues. FR-2 = Fragment 2, L-chain = light chain, and H-chain = heavy chain. The active site region resides in the H-chain.

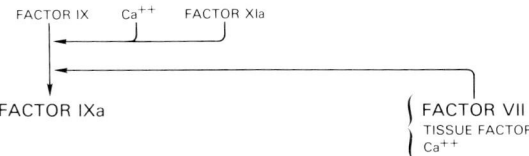

FIGURE 16. The two pathways of activation of Factor XI. The enzyme Factor XI$_a$, in the presence of Ca^{++}, directly activates Factor XI. The extrinsic system complex, i.e., Factor VII in the presence of tissue factor and Ca^{++} also activates Factor XI.

no direct evidence is available, it is likely that the biosynthesis of these factors occurs in the liver. Basically, Factor XI is activated by limited proteolysis to Factor XI$_a$ by Factor XII$_a$. Factor XI$_a$, in turn, can feedback (positive) and activate more Factor XII to XII$_a$.[80] Other enzymes (plasmin, kallikrein, and tissue proteases) can also activate Factor XII.

Factor XI is a glycoprotein with a molecular weight of 160,000, composed of two apparently similar/identical polypeptide chains linked by disulfide bridges.[15,81] The activation process consists of cleaving internal peptide bonds in the two chains, resulting in two subunits (heavy chains) with a molecular weight of 50,000 each and two subunits (light chains) with a molecular weight of 33,000 each.[81] The active site region is located in the light chains[15] (Figure 17).

In the initial step of the intrinsic coagulation sequence, Factor XII (a surface-sensitive single polypeptide chain protein with a molecular weight of about 80,000) is converted to Factor XII$_a$ by cleavage of one (or more) internal peptide bonds, resulting in two chains linked by disulfide bridge(s).[82] The heavy (amino terminal) chain contains surface-binding sites. The light (carboxyterminal) chain contains the active (proteolytic) site (Figure 18).[82] Factor XII can be "activated" in several ways.[82-87] Collagen or vascular basement membranes (exposed upon injury), phospholipids (from platelets), or washed, activated platelets themselves can serve as a surface. Factor XII, once bound to a negatively charged surface, has minimal ability to activate prekallikrein (see Section IV. Kinin Generation) and coagulation Factor XI. This activity is enhanced by HMW kininogen. The small quantities of kallikrein that are formed in this

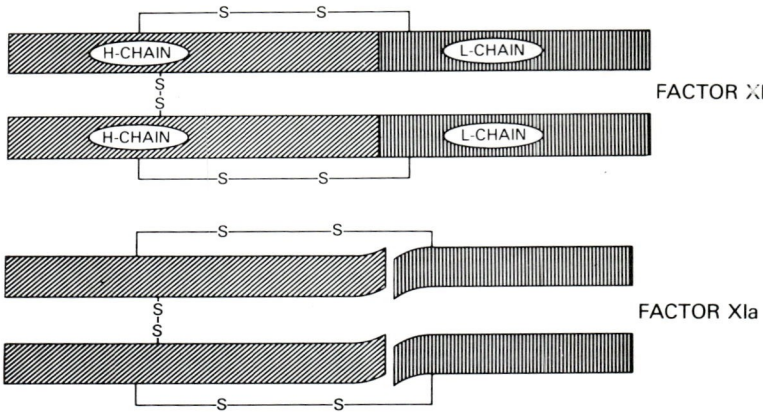

FIGURE 17. Linear model of Factor XI and Factor XI$_a$. H-Chain = heavy chain and L-Chain = light chain. The active site region is located in the L-chain.

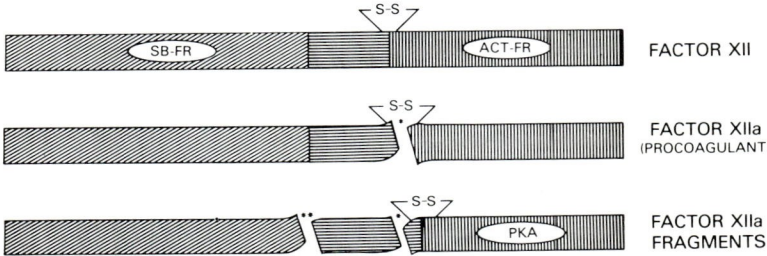

FIGURE 18. Linear model of Factor XII, Factor XII$_a$, and Factor XII fragments. SB-FR = surface-binding fragment and ACT-FR = active fragment. SB-FR is necessary for the procoagulant activity of Factor XII$_a$. PKA = prekallikrein activator. The surface-binding portion is apparently not required for this activity. The symbol * indicates that the exact location of these cleavage points is not clear. They may occur either within and/or on either side of the disulfide bridge. The symbol ** indicates cleavage occurring after prolonged incubation.

fashion then serve to enzymatically convert more Factor XII to the active form.[82,88] This latter reaction is also enhanced by HMW kininogen and constitutes a positive feedback mechanism. Furthermore, Factor XII$_a$ and/or fragments thereof[82] formed by extensive acitvation, will further activate more prekallikrein to kallikrein in the presence of HMW kininogen. It appears that HMW kininogen serves not only as the precursor of "kinins", but also as a linkage for Factor XI and prekallikrein to the exposed surface, where they are activated by surface-bound Factor XII$_a$. Once activated, Factor XI$_a$ remains localized at the site of activation, whereas kallikrein circulates free in plasma[88] (Figures 19 and 20). Similarly to the prothrombin, Factor X, and Factor IX activation complex, the "surface" seems to function as a stage upon which all of the components can interact.[17,88-93] Most likely, several pathways of activation are operative in this early (intrinsic) phase of coagulation, and the qualitative and quantitative aspects of the reactions are undoubtedly reflected in the mode and degree of activation. Figure 21 summarizes the coagulation sequence.

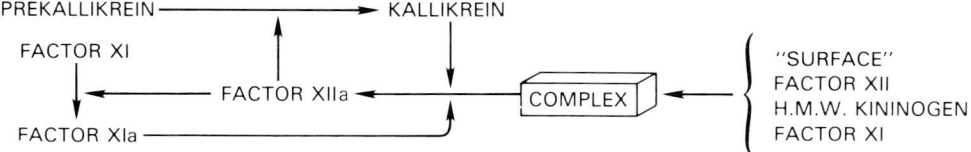

FIGURE 19. Pathways of activation in the early surface-dependent coagulation sequence. The complex constituted by: surface, Factor XII, HMW kininogen, and Factor XI generates (probably minimal) quantities of Factor XII$_a$. In turn, Factor XII$_a$ activates Factor XI to Factor XI$_a$ and prekallikrein to kallikrein. The latter enzymes then serve to further "amplify" the activation process.

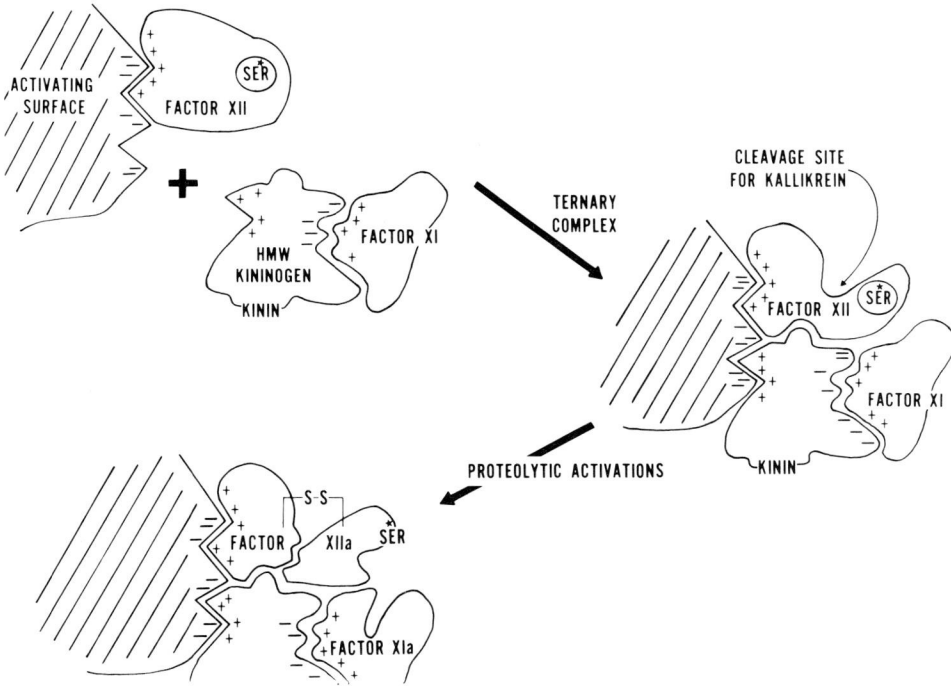

FIGURE 20. Schematic illustration of the interactions proposed in Figure 19. In this model, surface-bound Factor XII becomes "activated" by kallikrein. Factor XII$_a$, in turn "activates" surface-bound (via HMW kininogen) Factor XI. (Courtesy of Dr. John Griffin, Scripps Clinic, La Jolla, California).

F. Inhibitory Mechanisms

Like other physiologic processes, the blood coagulation mechanism is governed by a number of inhibitory devices designed to limit the extent of the various biochemical reactions and the possible dissemination of the process, resulting in pathology. To this extent, the regulation is effected by a number of negative feedback mechanisms, the involvement of specific inhibitors, and the compartmentalization of function restricting clotting to a localized process.

1. Nonproteolytic Activation of Factors XII and VII

Although blood coagulation is the result of a proteolytic sequence, it is noteworthy that the initiating step in both the intrinsic and extrinsic pathway, upon injury, is the "nonproteolytic activation" of Factor XII and Factor VII by collagen and tissue fac-

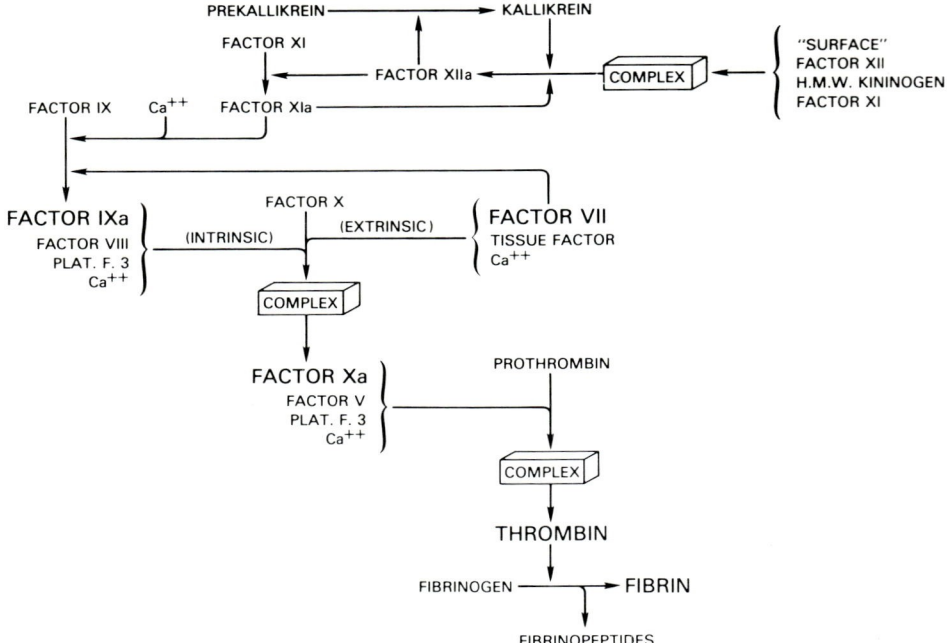

FIGURE 21. The coagulation sequence summarized.

tor, respectively, both of which appear to be totally inert toward other clotting proteins and thus can be widely distributed without risk of nonspecific "activation" of other proteins.[19]

2. Factor X_a as an Inhibitor

Once activated, the extrinsic pathway is still under control by the "pulse activation" mechanism discussed earlier,[19] i.e., the product of the reaction, Factor X_a, first activates Factor VII and subsequently destroys its activity, thereby limiting its own formation.

3. Thrombin as an Inhibitor

The enzyme thrombin, in addition to its ability to convert fibrinogen to fibrin and activate Factor XIII, has the ability to temporarily enhance the activity of Factors V and VIII, followed by immediate destruction of their activity.[13,19] Furthermore, thrombin hydrolyses prothrombin to form Prethrombin 1 (which is resistant to activation since it is lacking calcium-binding sites) and prothrombin fragment 1, which interferes with the activation process.[13] (Prothrombin fragment 2, produced by Factor X_a, inhibits fibrin formation.[13])

4. Generation of Activated Protein-C

Thrombin converts the newly discovered vitamin K-dependent factor (Protein-C) to an active protease which inhibits coagulation by degrading Factor V, and also participates in the activation of endogenous fibrinolysis.[13,22]

5. Stoichiometric Requirements

The formation of the various "complexes" is dependent upon a precise stoichiometry, requiring optimal concentration of each component for optimal function.[13,54] Reduction in the concentration of any of the components results in less than optimal activation.

6. Antithrombin III

The activity of the various enzymes (serine proteases) involved in the coagulation sequence (thrombin, Factor X_a, Factor IX_a, Factor XI_a, Factor XII_a, and kallikrein) is controlled (although to a variable extent) primarily by a plasma protein generally known as antithrombin III (heparin cofactor). Antithrombin III may in effect constitute a family of proteins (two or more) each with similar chemical properties, but varying affinities for the various enzymes.[13,94-96] This inhibitor, which is synthesized by the liver[75] and exists in plasma at a concentration of approximately 13 mg/dl, inactivates the enzymes by forming an irreversible complex, thereby blocking the active center. A mutual depletion system is involved.[13] The function of antithrombin III is optimized in the presence of heparin.[95] Although little is known about the availability of heparin at sites of vessel damage, sulfated mucopolysaccharides of heparin type have been detected on some cell surfaces.[97]

The exact mechanism of action of heparin is not clear. It has been proposed that heparin modifies (allosterically) either the enzyme molecule[94] or the antithrombin III molecule[95] in such a way as to facilitate complex formation. Most recent information[96] indicates that heparin acts catalytically by mediating complexing of antithrombin III with thrombin (and other serine proteases), forming a ternary complex. In this respect, the role of heparin may be visualized in a fashion analogous to that of phospholipid surfaces in forming complexes in the coagulation sequence (Figure 22). Heparin therapy is essentially ineffective in the absence of antithrombin III. Other inhibitors, such as α_1-antitrypsin and α_2-macroglobulin, also neutralize the activity of proteolytic enzymes, but do not seem to play a major role in thrombin modulation. α_2-Macroglobulin and C1 esterase inhibitor ($\overline{C1}$ INH), however, do play a major function in regulating the early steps in the contact phase of coagulation (see Section III).

7. Fibrin(ogen) as an Inhibitor

The fibrin matrix has a strong affinity for thrombin and, in that respect, could be considered as having an antithrombin effect.[98]

8. Fibrin(ogen) Degradation Products

The products of fibrino(geno)lysis (see Section III) function as inhibitors by interfering with fibrinogen to fibrin conversion, fibrin polymerization,[33] and perhaps interfere with platelet function.[99]

From this brief discussion, it is evident that the clotting sequence is highly regulated by a series of inhibitory forces, resulting in a perfectly modulated response limited to the site of vascular injury. In that sense, the participation of the various negative feedback loops (Table 2) allows for considerations alluding to biocybernetic principles.

III. FIBRINO(GENO)LYSIS

Fibrin deposition plays a role not only in hemostasis, but also in the inflammatory response[100] defense mechanisms against bacterial invasion[101] and wound healing.[102] For this mechanism that is perpetually ready to spring into action, the body pays the price of the potential accumulation of fibrin microdeposits, which constitute a potential hazard—thrombosis. Counterbalancing this potential danger is the fibrinolytic system that destroys fibrin deposits. In this respect, fibrin deposition may be considered a fundamental mechanism of injured tissue repair and fibrinolysis its physiologic antithesis.

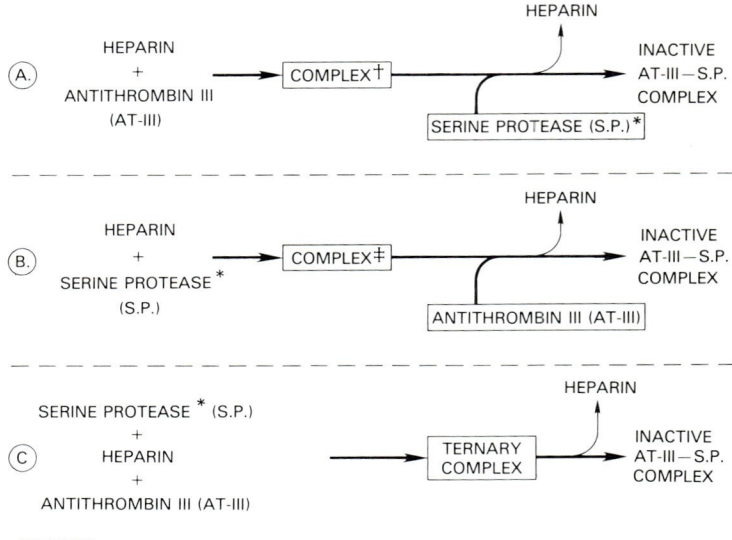

* THROMBIN, KALLIKREIN, PLASMIN, FACTORS IXa, Xa, XIa, XIIa
† STERICALLY MODIFIED AT-III
‡ STERICALLY MODIFIED S.P.

FIGURE 22. Proposed models (A, B, and C) for the inhibition of serine proteases by antithrombin III in the presence of heparin. Most likely, in vivo, mechanism C is operative.

TABLE 2

Summary of Inhibitory Mechanisms in Coagulation

1. Inactivation of Factor VII by Factor X_a.
2. Inactivation of Factors V and VIII by thrombin
3. Inhibition of prothrombin activation and fibrin formation by prothrombin fragments
4. Inhibition of Factor X_a activity through degradation of Factor V by thrombin-modified protein-C
5. Inhibition of thrombin formation with less than optimal concentration of "complex" components
6. Inhibition of proteases: thrombin, Factor XI_a, Factor X_a, Factor XI_a, Factor XII_a, and kallikrein by antithrombin-III
7. Inhibition of thrombin by adsorbing to fibrin
8. Inhibition of fibrin polymerization and platelet function by FDP

The phenomenon of fibrinolysis was recognized as early as 1700 in postmortem fluidity of blood; in 1800 in autodigestibility of fibrin, and in 1900 in streptococcal lysis. In the field of obstetrics, in early 1900, low plasma fibrinogen with rapid lysis was associated with hemorrhage. Later, enhanced fibrinolytic activity was recognized in most traumatic injuries, major surgery, liver cirrhosis, lymphomas, and other states.[103] In the late 19th century, fibrinolysis was shown to be due to proteolytic degradation of fibrin.[104] Later, in the 1940s, the enzyme responsible for this degradation was denoted plasmin (fibrinolysin), and it was established that, in plasma, it exists as a zymogen—plasminogen (profibrinolysin).[105-107]

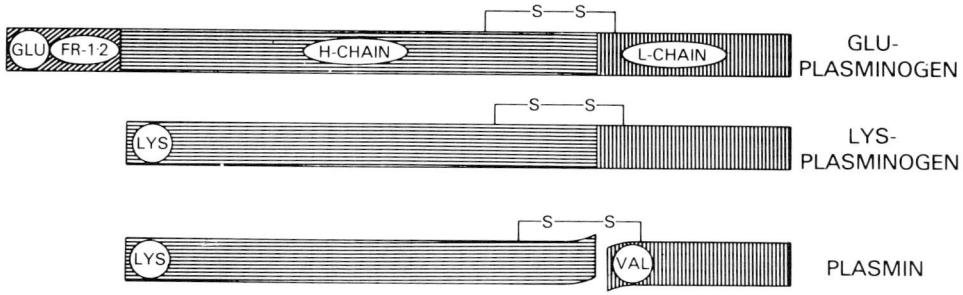

FIGURE 23. Linear model of plasminogen. N-Terminal amino acid residues are indicated within circles. GLU-Plasminogen is the native zymogen. LYS-Plasminogen is an activation intermediate with no proteolytic activity. FR-1·2 = fragment released in the conversion of GLU-plasminogen to LYS-plasminogen. H-Chain = heavy chain and L-Chain = light chain. The active site region is located in the L-chain.

A. Plasmin Formation

The enzyme responsible for lysis is plasmin. It is derived from the inactive precursor plasminogen. The latter is a single polypeptide chain protein with a molecular weight of about 90,000.[108,109] The precise tissue site of plasminogen synthesis is not clear, although there is evidence that eosinophilic leukocytes play a role in synthesis and/or transport.[110]

Plasminogen can be activated to the enzyme plasmin by a proteolytic process by several different activators. The conversion occurs in several steps, and, depending on the conditions for activation, the sequence varies. In general, the activation process involves the cleavage of peptide bonds, resulting in a molecule with two polypeptide chains with molecular weights of about 25,000 (light chain) and 48,000 (heavy chain), linked by disulfide bridges.[108,109] The active site region is located in the light chain (Figure 23). Plasmin is a general broad spectrum endopeptidase (proteolytic enzyme) similar to other serine proteases.[108,109,111,112] Its specificity is directed at lysyl residues. It has a strong affinity for fibrinogen and fibrin. However, it also hydrolyzes other clotting factors, including active Hageman factor (Factor XII_a),[89,113] activates certain components of the complement system,[114,115] and liberates kinins from kininogen.[116,117]

Of the several activators of plasminogen, the best known are (1) urokinase, a proteolytic enzyme synthesized by the kidney and found in normal urine; (2) activators from various tissues, (3) streptokinase (produced by β-hemolytic streptococci), and (4) staphylokinase (from staphylococci). Purified urokinase directly converts plasminogen to plasmin by proteolysis.[109,118] Streptokinase, a nonproteolytic enzyme, first forms a complex with the substrate (plasminogen) or the enzyme (plasmin) itself.[109,118] This results in an "activator" that converts plasminogen to plasmin. Staphylokinase converts plasminogen to plasmin by a mechanism similar to that of streptokinase.[119] Other activators are produced locally, some arising from the vascular endothelium[120,121] in response to a variety of stimuli such as injury, ischemia, exercise, pyrogens, epinephrine, electroshock, etc.[118] It is not clear whether endothelial cell activator activates plasminogen directly or through a proactivator. Activated Protein-C may be involved in this system.

Another pathway of plasminogen activation is via the intrinsic system involving Factor XII_a. This pathway of plasmin formation involves the interaction of Factor XII_a, or fragments thereof (Figure 24), with a plasma cofactor (plasminogen proactivator). This interaction results in the formation of an active component—activator—which in

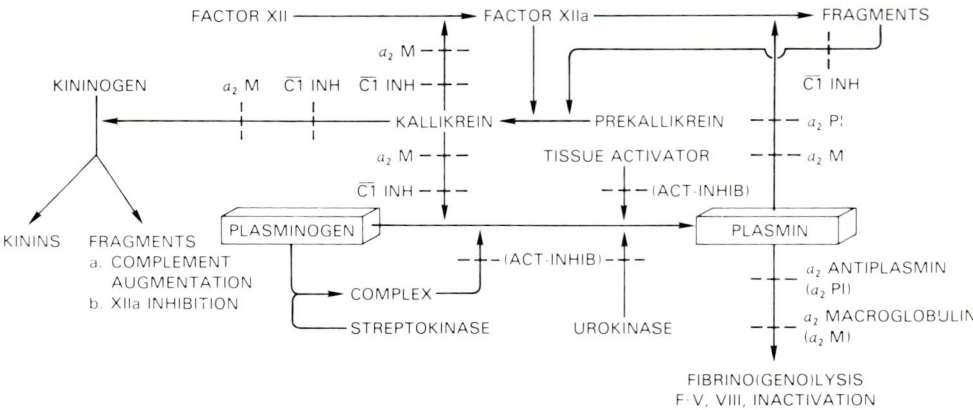

FIGURE 24. The activation of plasminogen to plasmin by urokinase, streptokinase, tissue activator, and kallikrein. The figure also illustrates the interrelationships of reciprocal activating sequences and the generation of kinins from kininogen. The control of the various reactions by the inhibitors α_2-macroglobulin (α_2M), α_2-antiplasmin (α_2-PI), C1 esterase inhibitor ($\overline{C1}$ INH), and activator inhibitor (ACT-INHIB) is indicated by dashed lines.

turn converts plasminogen to plasmin. Recent evidence[123] indicates that plasminogen proactivator (Hageman factor-cofactor) is, in fact, the same as plasma prekallikrein (Fletcher factor).* This implies that kallikrein directly activates plasminogen. Moreover, Factor XII$_a$ and, to a lesser extent, fragments thereof can directly convert plasminogen to plasmin.[124] It should be noted, however, that Factor XII and prekallikrein deficiencies do not appear to result in significant impairment of fibrinolytic nor of clotting activity in vivo, indicating that, normally, this may not be a pathway of major physiologic significance. As a matter of fact, individuals with "Fletcher trait" (prekallikrein deficiency) and "Hageman trait" (Factor XII deficiency) are generally healthy, although it has been documented that these individuals may well have a predisposition to thromboembolism[125,126] — an observation supporting the biocybernetic view.

The fibrinolytic portion of the Factor XII-dependent sequence has been found to be regulated primarily by two specific plasma inhibitors: (1) the inhibitor of the activated first component of complement ($\overline{C1}$ INH) and α_2-macroglobulin (α_2-M).[96,127-129] The two inhibitors function at various stages of the sequence and with variable efficacy.[128,130] Another plasma inhibitor that increases in activity in parallel to (intrinsic) clotting has been demonstrated (ACT-INHIB), but no characterized. This labile factor displays maximal activity in fresh serum and reacts competitively to inhibit the activation of plasminogen to plasmin, but has no direct antiplasmin nor antiplasminogen activity.[131,132] It apparently inhibits "plasminogen activator", regardless of its source.

More recently, a potent inhibitor of plasmin (α_2-antiplasmin**) has been discovered and characterized.[133,134] Its concentration in plasma is about 6 mg/dl, and its molecular weight is about 67,000. Although it contributes only about 3% of the total antiplasmin activity in plasma (on a molar basis), its extraordinary affinity for plasmin—resulting in an irreversible covalent complex—makes it a candidate for the major regulator of fibrinolytic activity in vivo. Figure 24 outlines the activation sequence.

---

* Prekallikrein and Factor XII most likely constitute a reciprocal proenzyme activating system.[17]

** A congenital deficiency of α_2 antiplasmin (Miyasato Disease), characterized by rather severe hemorrhage, has recently been documented.[134]

B. Mechanism of Fibrin Dissolution

The observation that the quantity of circulating plasminogen decreases proportionally with an increase in the amount of fibrin deposited, has led to the hypothesis that clot lysis occurs primarily from within the clot. In fact, experimentally it has been demonstrated that the more plasminogen is entrapped in the clot, and the more "activator" in the medium, the faster the clot lysis.[135] Another hypothesis proposes that a small quantity of plasmin is always being formed physiologically—not inconsistent with a continuous coagulation/lysis equilibrium—and it is stored as an inactive complex with inhibitors. Upon contact with fibrin, the plasmin inhibitor complex is dissociated and plasmin is free to hydrolyze fibrin.[136] Most likely in vivo both systems are operative.

C. Chemistry and Function of Fibrin(ogen) Degradation Products (FDP)

The precise sequence of chemical events occurring during the proteolysis of fibrinogen and fibrin by plasmin has not been established. It is clear, however, that the Aα chain of fibrinogen—more precisely, the carboxy-terminal portion—is destroyed first by plasmin. The process then continues by destruction of the Bβ chain as a second order of preference, and, finally, the γ chain is hydrolyzed.[27] This process of sequential hydrolysis is responsible for the formation of four major degradation products: X, Y, D, and E (Figure 25). During intravascular lysis, whether primary, secondary, or therapeutically induced, the titer of these degradation products is substantially increased, because their rate of formation exceeds the capacity of the reticuloendothelial system to clear them from the circulation, and can be used to assess the extent of lysis.

As mentioned earlier, these products exert various anticoagulant effects. The X, earliest degradation product, consists of a family of derivatives. Their molecular weight ranges between 260,000 and 300,000, depending on the amount of peptide material removed from the carboxyterminal portion of the Aα chains and whether or not peptides have been hydrolysed from the amino terminal portion of the Bβ chains. By itself, fragment X exerts an antithrombin action by still being clottable by thrombin, but more slowly than intact fibrinogen.[137,138] The Y product (molecular weight about 155,000) is derived from X, and, most likely, is a very short-lived intermediate of digestion. The formation of this derivative involves plasmic cleavage of peptides (molecular weight about 6000) from the amino terminal portion of Bβ chains, followed by asymmetrical splitting of three chains at one side of the partly degraded dimer (the latter three chain fragment, monomeric, is fragment D). The Y derivative, like the X derivative, also prolongs the thrombin time when added to fibrinogen.[137,138] Both X and Y form soluble complexes[137] with fibrin monomer* (SFM). This may be explained on the basis that, in the formation of the Y derivative from X, one fragment D moiety is released. Since one of the polymerization domains is located in the D area (others are located in the amino terminal portion of fibrinogen—the E area), it is understandable that in its absence polymerization would be abnormal.[27,33]

Further proteolysis of the Y fragment gives rise to a second D fragment (monomeric) and one E fragment (dimeric). Fragment D (molecular weight 90,000) interferes with the polymerization process[139] for reasons already presented. The anticoagulant function of E (molecular weight about 50,000) has not been ascertained. However, since it is derived from the amino terminal portion of fibrinogen,[140] and it too contains polymerization domains,[27] it most likely interferes with thrombin activity directly, and with polymerization as well. Figure 26 illustrates the X, Y, D, and E structures within the fibrinogen molecule.

---

* The soluble fibrin monomer (SFM) constitutes the basis for the ethanol gelation and the protamine sulfate paracoagulation tests (see Chapter 8).

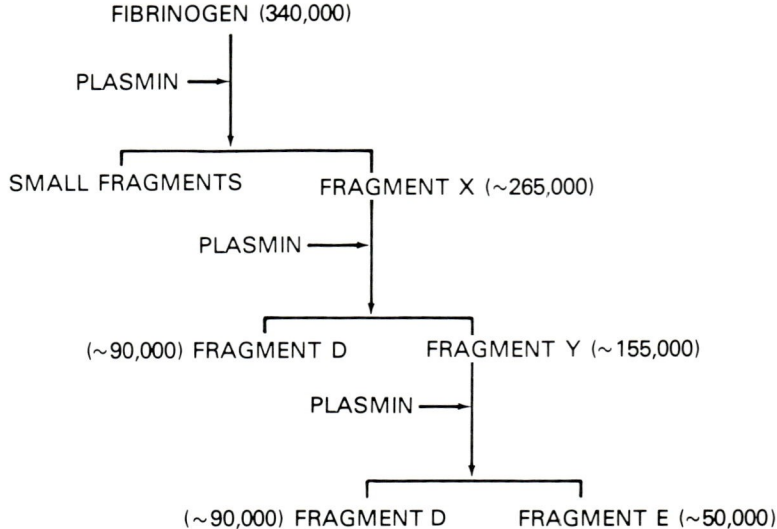

FIGURE 25. The sequential degradation of fibrin(ogen) by the enzyme plasmin. The approximate molecular size of each fragment is indicated within parentheses.

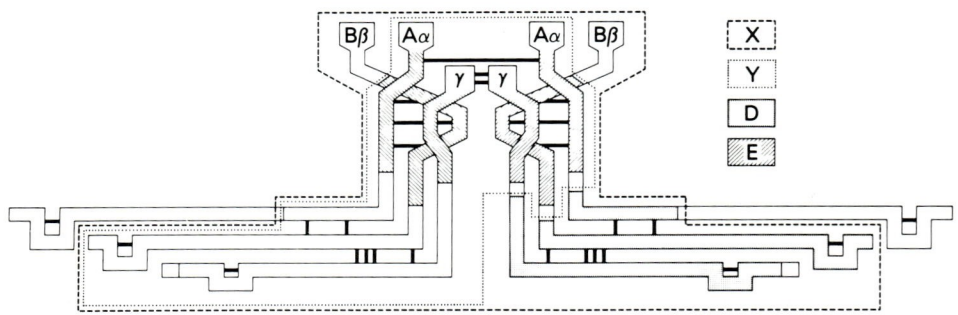

FIGURE 26. A model of fibrinogen indicating the location of fragments, X, Y, D, and E within the molecule. Note that fragment E is a dimeric structure constituting the amino terminal portion of the molecule. Fragment D is a monomeric structure (two moieties are present in each fibrinogen molecule) constituting the carboxy terminal portions of each monomer in fibrinogen.

IV. KININ GENERATION

So far we have observed the involvement of Factor XII (Hageman factor) in the clotting and lytic systems. A third role of Factor XII is the induction of substances responsible for inflammatory states and pain.[89,141-144]

There exist in human plasma multiple forms of an alpha globulin known as kininogen. Two major classes have been identified and are termed: low molecular weight (LMW) kininogen and high molecular weight (HMW) kininogen.[145-147] The latter is "Fitzgerald or Flaujeac, or Williams factor". Its molecular weight is about 120,000, and it functions in the activation of Factor XII.[89,90,148-151] The proteolytic enzyme kallikrein (which exists in plasma as an inactive precursor—prekallikrein), with a molecular weight of about 85,000 daltons, has the property of splitting off biologically active polypeptide fragments, preferentially from HMW kininogen.[117,129,148] These fragments, known generically as kinins[129,143,144] (among them the nonapeptide bradykinin), enhance vascular permeability, dilate certain blood vessels—resulting in hypotension, contract certain smooth muscles, and, perhaps, bring about the migration of leukocytes in extravascular space.[129,148,152] In addition, as pointed out earlier, kallikrein also activates Factor XII.[17,88,89] Once again, we return to Factor XII.

The initiating event in the generation of kinins in human plasma is the activation of Factor XII. Evidence has accumulated indicating that Factor XII$_a$ and/or fragments thereof[32] resulting from plasmin digestion,[89,113] directly activate prekallikrein to kallikrein, thus diverting the reaction sequence from coagulation to kinin generation.[89,129] Activation of the kinin-generating system is associated with the production of several other fragments, one of which participates in augmenting the complement pathway directly (see Section V), and one that inhibits the activation of Factor XII.[148,153,154] As expected, this portion of the activation cycle is also regulated by $\overline{C1}$ INH and α_2-M.[96,127-130] Figure 24 outlines the sequence.

It is evident from our discussion so far that enzymes may have multiple substrates and that what we consider a discrete system is really an integral portion of a physiologic continuum. In order to lend further support to this thesis, let us examine the relationship of the three systems we have discussed with immunologic defense mechanisms. For this, we turn to "complement".

V. COMPLEMENT ACTIVATION

A. Classic Mechanisms

The complement system is a multimolecular, self-assembling system constituting the primary humoral mediator of inflammation and tissue damage. In this respect, it achieves its classic effect by recognizing the presence of antigen-antibody (Ag-Ab) complex, activating, in turn, the biologically important effector proteins, eventually resulting in cell lysis or the destruction of pathogens by phagocytes (opsonization).[155-159] The complement proteins, in general, follow a specific pattern of activation. They circulate as inactive precursors throughout the extracellular compartment until they are activated sequentially by highly specific biochemical reactions.[158,159] In many instances, this involves limited proteolysis, with the formation of two fragments of unequal size. The minor fragment often contributes to the development of inflammation.[158-160] The larger fragment continues the activation sequence—much in the likeness of the coagulation sequence. To produce their immunopathologic effect, these proteins must interact in a precise sequence.[158-164] The classical route of activation follows the sequence C1, C4, C2, C3, C5 → 9. The stimulus for this response is the presense of antibodies (IgM, IgG1, IgG2, and IgG3) on the cell surface.[165-172]

Briefly, the first component in this series, C1 is a complex constituted by three subcomponents C1q,* C1r, and C1s.[158,159] When Ag-Ab complexes or the lipid A region of bacterial lipopolysaccharides (LPS)[173] interact with the C1q portion, a proteolytic enzyme (C1 esterase) is generated from the C1s component. This enzyme, in turn, can generate a second enzyme—C3 convertase—by interacting with the C4 and C2 components. C3 convertase ($\overline{C4bC2a}$), in turn, activates C3, a key component in the series—and so on.[158,159]

An alternate route of complement activation (the alternative pathway) involves properdin and other components leading to direct C3 activation.[158,159,174,175] Some of the initiators of this pathway are F(ab)$'_2$ fragment of IgG, IgE, IgA, bacterial lipopolysac-

---

* Monomeric C1q, which has structural similarities to collagen, inhibits collagen induced platelet aggregation. Polymeric C1q mimicks the effect of collagen on platelets.[200]

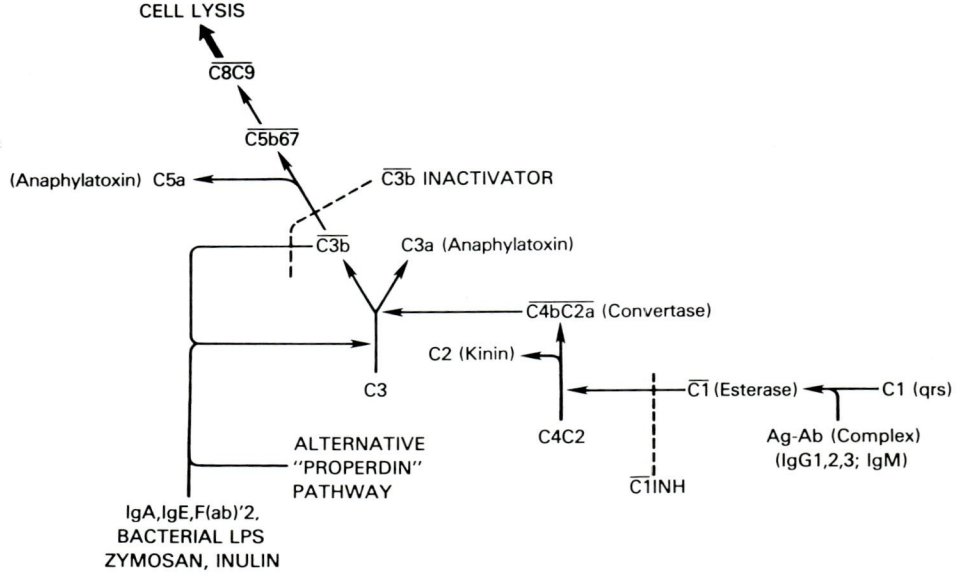

FIGURE 27. The complement sequence. Some of the components of the alternative "properdin" pathway are omitted. The inhibition of C1 esterase by the inhibitor ($\overline{C1}$ INH) and the inhibition of C3b by the inactivator is indicated by dashed lines.

charides, inulin, and zymosan.[158,159, 176-182] A potent inhibitor of $\overline{C1}$ esterase (C1 INH), an alpha-2-globulin, controls the activity of this enzyme on C4 and C2 substrates.[183] A second inhibitor (C3b Inactivator) controls the activity of C3b.[184] Figure 27 summarizes the interrelationships of the two pathways of activation. En route, various effects—chemotaxis of neutrophils into the area of immunologic reaction, enhancement of phagocytosis, elaboration of anaphylatoxin, histamine release, etc.—are mediated.[159]* Tables 3 and 4 summarize the activities of the various components.

B. The Hageman (Factor XII) Connection

The relationship of blood clotting processes with the immunologic fibrinolytic and kinin generating system has been noted for many years.[152,186-189] The first direct evidence associating clotting and other hemostatic mechanisms with immunological events was derived from the observation that the enzyme plasmin (generated by Factor XII activation in the absence of immune complexes) can initiate the classical pathway of complement activation by activating C1s to C1 esterase[115] and by cleavage of C3[114] to yield anaphylatoxin (C3a), which is chemotactic for polymorphonuclear neutrophils and releases histamine from mast cells, resulting in increased vascular permeability (Figure 28).[152,158,159,190]

It is of interest to note at this point that a vasoactive peptide distinguishable from bradykinin is generated in patients suffering from hereditary angioneurotic edema.[191,192] These patients do not synthesize adequate amounts of $\overline{C1}$ INH. Therefore, especially under conditions of stress, which have been shown to accelerate plasmin formation,[118,121] the activity of the enzyme C1 esterase is uncontrolled. It is likely then, that this accelerated activity results in a high titer of a fragment, probably C2

---

* The inflammatory response and opsonization of particles by phagocytic cells are probably more important than cell lysis per se. A C6-deficient patient cannot lyse bacteria nor sensitized sheep erythrocytes, yet the patient has never had an incidence of infection.[185]

TABLE 3

Biologic Activities of Some Complement Components

Complement component	Activity
C1	Enhances association of Ag-Ab complexes
C4b	Involved in virus neutralization; adheres (via receptor) to lymphocytes and phagocytic cells
C2	Fragment C2 kinin (present in angioneurotic edema?)
C3b	Adheres (via receptor) to lymphocytes and phagocytic cells—opsonin; participates in activation of alternative pathway; triggers production of mediators from B lymphocytes; triggers release of leukocytes from bone marrow; triggers release of Ag-Ab complexes from leukocyte surface; triggers rapid division of tumor cells
C3a	Anaphylatoxin, chemotactic factor
C5a	Anaphylatoxin
C5b67	May attack unsensitized cell, chemotactic factor
C8	Damages cell membranes (slow)
C9	Damages cell membranes (rapid)

From Frank, M. M., *Complement—Current Concepts,* The Upjohn Company, Kalamazoo, Mich., 1975. With permission.

TABLE 4

Biologic Activities Resulting from Activation of the Alternative Pathway of Complement

1. Cobra venom mediated lysis of unsensitized erythrocytes
2. Erythrocyte lysis in paroxysmal noctural hemoglobinuria
3. Bactericidal activity
4. Phagocytosis
5. Anaphylatoxin production
6. Leukotaxis
7. Mediation of arthus vasculitis
8. Proteinuria in experimentally induced glomerulonephritis
9. Renal damage of hypocomplementemic glomerulonephritis
10. Immune adherence
11. Histamine release from platelets, lysis, and enhancement of blood clotting

From Frank, M. M., *Complement—Current Concepts,* The Upjohn Company, Kalamazoo, Mich., 1975. With permission.

(Figure 27), which has been associated with the kinin activity observed in the disease—edematous lesions.[192]

Another observation of interest[154] is that concomitant with the generation of bradykinin, a kininogen fragment is generated that augments the biologic activity of C1 esterase, thereby accelerating the formation of C3 convertase (Figure 24).

Close examination of Figure 28 reveals a cycle. To further amplify the perspective of interrelationships, let us briefly reexamine some of the functional aspects of the

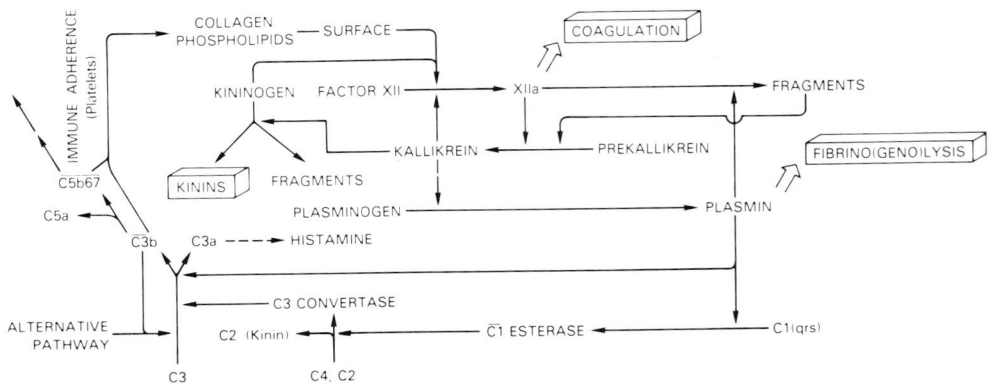

FIGURE 28. Summary of the interrelationship of coagulation, fibrino(geno)lysis, kinin generation, and complement activation. Note that the figure is cyclical. Depending on the nature (quantitative and qualitative) of the stimulus, the reaction sequence may be shifted in any direction, eliciting the appropriate responses. The modulation of these responses is under the control of inhibitors (see text).

later components of complement, especially C3. The C3b component exhibits many functions (Table 3). Its presence on the cell membrane permits binding to specific receptors on polymorphonuclear leukocytes, erythrocytes, and platelets in the immune adherence phenomenon,[155] leading to the release of lysosomal enzymes that can produce C5a (anaphylatoxin) from C5 and can fragment basement membranes, thereby possibly contributing to Factor XII activation. The involvement of the platelets naturally may result in thrombocytopenia and, with their disruption, the release of phospholipids, serotonin, ADP, etc., all of which serve to accelerate the clotting process.[193] In this respect it should be mentioned that in drug-sensitivity reactions, the drug, probably in haptenic combination with a carrier protein, reacts with a circulating antibody—elicited upon repeated exposure—to form immune complexes.[194] In the presence of complement, these adhere to platelets (though not always), precipitating accelerated platelet sequestration by reticuloendothelial organs. The observation that acquired C3 deficiency results in delayed clot lysis[195] suggests that this component or fragments thereof mediates plasmin formation in vivo either directly or perhaps through a humoral pathway independent of Factor XII.

The complex constituted of C5, C6, and C7 has been shown to be chemotactic for polymorphonuclear leukocytes.[196] How this portion of the sequence relates to clotting is not clear. It is known that activation of the alternative pathway of complement by inulin and lipopolysaccharides (LPS) causes thrombocytopenia and shortens the clotting time of blood in rabbits (and in guinea pigs upon injection of endotoxin).[155,159] This does *not* occur in C6-deficient rabbits and guinea pigs, indicating the involvement of these late components in clot promotion.[197] Interestingly, this also does not occur in C4-deficient animals.[198] Therefore, the activation of the alternative pathway may not efficiently mediate platelet damage, and, consequently, does not shorten the clotting time. Apparently the immune adherence reaction with resulting membrane damage ensues only with classical pathway activation, produced by the complex of natural antibody and platelet-bound endotoxin—in this case, the antigen.[159]

In considering these mechanisms as they relate to hyperacute rejections[199] and endotoxic shock, it appears that the clot-promoting effects of phospholipids from disrupted platelets are major contributing factors. It is possible, however, that antigen-antibody complexes, in certain circumstances, may directly damage the vascular endothelium[201] and that the platelet damage ensues as a consequence. Regardless of the precise sequence of events, it is apparent that the "contact phase" of coagulation (Factor XII activation) plays a major role in the pathophysiology of many syndromes.

VI. CONCLUDING REMARKS

Summarizing this litany of admiration for the apparent holistic nature of physiology, it is clear that further elucidation of the basic biochemical interrelationships of the systems described (and undoubtedly others, as yet elusive) will allow for a better understanding of associated pathologies and afford an opportunity for the preparation of more stable, and safer, plasma concentrates, thereby permitting more efficient applications of therapy.

In the spirit of the distinguished physiologist Claude Bernard, who hoped that someday poets, philosophers, and physiologists would speak the same language, this author indulges in encouraging the "specialist"—be he or she an immunologist, oncologist, coagulationist, pharmaceutical chemist, or technologist—to deploy his or her diagnostic and therapeutic resources with a perspective of "wholeness" in physiology.

REFERENCES

1. Morawitz, P., Beitrage zur kenntnis der blutgerinnung, *Dtsch. Arch. Klin. Med.,* 79, 1, 1904.
2. Brinkhous, K. M., A study of the clotting defect in hemophilia, the delayed formation of thrombin, *Am. J. Med. Sci.,* 198, 509, 1939.
3. Owren, P. A., Coagulation of blood; investigation on new clotting factors, *Acta Med. Scand.,* 128 (Suppl. 194), 1, 1947.
4. Alexander, B., Devries, A., Goldstein, R., and Landwehr, G., A prothrombin conversion accelerator in serum, *Science,* 109, 545, 1949.
5. Pavlovsky, A., Contribution to the pathogenesis of hemophilia, *Blood,* 2, 185, 1947.
6. Telfer, T. P., Denson, K. W., and Wright, D. R., A "new" coagulation defect, *Br. J. Haematol.,* 2, 308, 1956.
7. Rosenthal, R. L., Dreskin, O. H., and Rosenthal, N., New hemophilia-like disease caused by deficiency of a third plasma thromboplastin factor, *Proc. Soc. Exp. Biol. Med.,* 82, 171, 1953.
8. Ratnoff, O. D. and Colopy, J. E., A familial hemorrhagic trait associated with a deficiency of a clot-promoting fraction of plasma, *J. Clin. Invest.,* 34, 602, 1955.
9. Duckert, F., Jung, E., and Schmerling, D. H., A hitherto undescribed congenital haemorrhagic diathesis probably due to fibrin stabilizing factor deficiency, *Thromb. Dieth. Haemorr.,* 5, 179, 1960.
10. MacFarlane, R. G., An enzyme cascade in blood clotting mechanisms and its function as a biochemical amplifier, *Nature (London),* 202, 498, 1964.
11. Davie, E. W. and Ratnoff, O. D., Waterfall sequence for intrinsic blood clotting, *Science,* 145, 1310, 1964.
12. Mammen, E. F., Physiology and biochemistry of blood coagulation, in *Thrombosis and Bleeding Disorders,* Bang, N. U., Beller, F. K., Deutsch, E., and Mammen, E. F., Eds., Academic Press, New York, 1971, 1.
13. Seegers, W. H., Hassouna, H. I., Hewett-Emmett, D., Walz, D. A., and Andary, T. J., Prothrombin and thrombin. Selected aspects of thrombin formation, properties, inhibition and immunology, *Semin. Thromb. Hemost.,* 1, 211, 1975.
14. Henriksen, R. A. and Jackson, C. J., The chemistry and enzymology of bovine factor X, *Semin. Thromb. Hemost.,* 1, 284, 1975.
15. Davie, W. E., Fujikawa, K., Legaz, M. E., and Kato, H., Role of proteases in blood coagulation, in *Proteases and Biological Control,* Reich, E., Rifkin, D. B., and Shaw, E., Eds., Cold Spring Harbor Laboratory, Cold Spring Harbor, N.Y., 1975, 65.
16. Lorand, L., Controls in the clotting of fibrinogen, in *Proteases and Biological Control,* Reich, E., Rifkin, D. B., and Shaw, E., Eds., Cold Spring Harbor Laboratory, Cold Spring Harbor, N.Y., 1975, 79.

17. Ulevitch, R. J., Cochrane, C. G., Revak, S. K., Morrison, D. C., and Johnson, A. R., The structural and enzymatic properties of the components of Hageman factor-activated pathways, in *Proteases and Biological Control,* Reich, E., Rifkin, D. B., and Shaw, E., Eds., Cold Spring Harbor Laboratory, Cold Spring Harbor, N.Y., 1975, 85.
18. Triantaphyllopoulos, E. and Triantaphyllopoulos, D. C., Selected topics on blood coagulation, in *Critical Reviews in Biochemistry,* 1, 305, 1973.
19. Jesty, J., Maynard, J. R., Radcliffe, R. D., Silverberg, S. A., Pitlick, F. A., and Nemerson, Y., Initiation and control of the extrinsic pathway of blood coagulation, in *Proteases and Biological Control,* Reich, E., Rifkin, D. B., and Shaw, E., Eds., Cold Spring Harbor Laboratory, Cold Spring Harbor, N.Y., 1975, 171.
20. Hemker, K. C., Lindhout, M. F., and Vermeer, C., Blood coagulation factors at phospholipid surfaces, *Ann. N.Y. Acad. Sci.,* 283, 104, 1977.
21. Prydz, H., Vitamin K-dependent clotting factors, *Semin. Thromb. Hemost.,* 4, 1, 1977.
22. Walker, F. J., Sexton, P. W., and Esmon, C. T., The inhibition of blood coagulation by activated protein C through the selective inactivation of activated Factor V, *Biochim. Biophys. Acta,* in press.
23. Shah, D. V. and Suttie, J. W., Mechanism of action vitamin K, Evidence for the conversion of a precursor protein to prothrombin in the rat, *Proc. Natl. Acad. Sci. U.S.A.,* 68, 1653, 1971.
24. Magnusson, S., Sottrup-Jensen, L., Petersen, T. E., Morris, H. R., and Dell, A., Primary structure of the Vitamin K dependent part of prothrombin, *FEBS Lett.,* 44, 189, 1974.
25. Barnhart, M. I. and Anderson, G. F., Intracellular localization of fibrinogens, *Proc. Soc. Exp. Biol. Med.,* 110, 734, 1962.
26. Alving, B., Murano, G., and Walz, D., Partial chemical characterization of S-carboxymethylated chains of rabbit fibrin(ogen). Evidence for separate chain biosynthesis, Abstr., 6th Int. Congr. Thromb. Hemost., *Thromb. Hemost.,* 38, 26, 1977.
27. Murano, G., The molecular structure fibrinogen, *Semin. Thromb. Hemost.,* 1, 1, 1974.
28. Gardlund, B., Hessel, B., Marguerie, G., Murano, G., and Blomback, B., Primary structure of human fibrinogen. Characterization of disulfide containing cyanogen bromide fragments, *Eur. J. Biochem.,* 77, 595, 1977.
29. Lundblad, R. L., Fenton, J. W., and Mann, K. G., Eds., *Chemistry and Biology of Thrombin,* Ann Arbor Science, Ann Arbor, Mich., 1977.
30. Huseby, R. M., Conformational structure of the fibrinopeptides released during fibrinogen to fibrin conversion, *Physiol. Chem. Phys.,* 5, 1, 1973.
31. Walz, D. A., Seegers, W. H., Reuterby, J., and McCoy, L. E., Proteolytic specificity of thrombin, *Thromb. Res.,* 4, 713, 1974.
32. Laurent, T. C. and Blomback, B., On the significance of the release of two different peptides from fibrinogen during clotting, *Acta Chem. Scand.,* 12, 1875, 1958.
33. Kudryk, B., Collen, D., Woods, K. R., and Blomback, B., Evidence for localization of polymerization sites in fibrinogen, *J. Biol. Chem.,* 249, 3322, 1974.
34. Blomback, M., Blomback, B., Mammen, E. F., and Prasad, A. S., Fibrinogen Detroit—a molecular defect in the N-terminal disulfide knot of human fibrinogen, *Nature (London),* 218, 134, 1968.
35. Folk, J. E. and Chung, S. I. I., Blood coagulation Factor XIII. Relationship of some biological properties to subunit structure, in *Proteases and Biological Control,* Reich, E., Rifkin, D. B., and Shaw, E., Eds., Cold Spring Harbor Laboratory, Cold Spring Harbor, N.Y., 1975, 157.
36. McDonagh, J. and McDonagh, R. P., Alternative pathways for the activation of Factor XIII, *Br. J. Haematol.,* 30, 465, 1975.
37. Doolittle, R. F., Gassman, K. G., Chen, R., Sharp, J. J., and Wooding, G. L., Correlation of the mode of fibrin polymerization with the pattern of crosslinking, *Ann. N.Y. Acad. Sci.,* 202, 114, 1972.
38. McDonagh, R. P., McDonagh, J., and Duckert, F., The influence of fibrin crosslinking on the kinetics of urokinase induced clot lysis, *Br. J. Haematol.,* 21, 323, 1971.
39. McDonagh, R. P., McDonagh, J., and Blomback, J., Polypeptide chains of human fibrin. Molecular organization in crosslinking, *Ann. N.Y. Acad. Sci.,* 202, 335, 1972.
40. Finlayson, J. S., Crosslinking of fibrin, *Sem. Thromb. Hemost.,* 1, 33, 1974.
41. Seegers, W. H., *Prothrombin,* Harvard University Press, Cambridge, 1972.
42. Hemker, J. C. and Veltkamp, J. J., Eds., *Prothrombin and Related Coagulation Factors,* Boerhave series postgraduate medical education #10, Leiden University Press, The Netherlands, 1975.
43. Fenton, J. W., Fasco, M. J., Stackrow, A. B., Aronson, D. L., Young, A. M., and Finlayson, J. S., Human Thrombins, production, evaluation, and properties of α-thrombin, *J. Biol. Chem.,* 252, 3587, 1977.
44. Jackson, C. M., The biochemistry of prothrombin activation, in *Heparin Chemistry and Clinical Usage,* Kakkar, V. V. and Thomas, D. P., Eds., Academic Press, New York, 1976, 61.

45. Walz, D. A., Hewett-Emmet, D., and Seegers, W. H., Amino acid sequence of human prothrombin fragments 1 and 2, *Proc. Natl. Acad. Sci. U.S.A.*, 74, 1969, 1977.
46. Magnusson, S., Petersen, T. E., Sottrup-Jensen, L., and Claeys, H., Complete primary structure of prothrombin: isolation, structure and reactivity of thrombin, in *Proteases and Biological Control*, Reich, E., Rifkin, D. B., and Shaw, E., Eds., Cold Spring Harbor Laboratory, Cold Spring Harbor, N.Y., 1975, 123.
47. Owen, W. G., Esmon, C. T., and Jackson, C. M., The conversion of prothrombin to thrombin. I. Characterization of the reaction product formed during activation of bovine prothrombin, *J. Biol. Chem.*, 249, 594, 1974.
48. Gitel, S. N., Owen, W. G., Esmon, C. T., and Jackson, C. M., A polypeptide region of bovine prothrombin specific for binding to phospholipids, *Proc. Natl. Acad. Sci. U.S.A.*, 70, 1344, 1973.
49. Aronson, D. L., Stevan, L., Ball, A., Franza, R., and Finlayson, J. S., Generation of the combined prothrombin activation peptide (F 1·2) during the clotting of blood and plasma, *J. Clin. Invest.*, 60, 1410, 1977.
50. Morita, T., Nishihi, H., Iwanga, S., and Suzuki, J., Studies on the activation of bovine prothrombin, *J. Biochem.*, 76, 1031, 1974.
51. Milstone, J. H., TAMe esterase activity of blood thrombokinase after repeated electrophoretic fractionations, *Proc. Soc. Exp. Biol. Med.*, 103, 361, 1960.
52. Milstone, J. H. and Oulianoff, N., Removal from bovine prothrombin of the substrate for Russell's viper venom, *Thromb. Diath. Haemorrh.*, 21, 203, 1969.
53. Esmon, C. T., The subunit structure of thrombin-activated Factor V: isolation of activated Factor V, separation of subunits, and reconstitution of biological activity, *J. Biol. Chem.*, 154, 964, 1979.
54. Seegers, W. H., Sakuragawa, N., McCoy, L. E., Sedensky, J. A., and Dombrose, F. A., Prothrombin activation: Ac-Globulin, lipid, platelet membrane, and autoprothrombin C (Factor Xa) requirements, *Thromb. Res.*, 1, 293, 1972.
55. Esmon, C. T. and Jackson, C. M., The conversion of prothrombin to thrombin IV. The function of the fragment 2 region during activation in the presence of Factor V, *J. Biol. Chem.*, 249, 7791, 1974.
56. Aronson, D. L. and Menache, D., Action of human thrombokinase on human prothrombin and p-Tosyl-L-arginine methyl ester, *Biochem. Biophys. Acta*, 167, 378, 1968.
57. Esmon, C. T. and Jackson, C. M., The conversion of prothrombin to thrombin. III. The Factor Xa catalyzed activation of prothrombin, *J. Biol. Chem.*, 249, 7782, 1974.
58. Stenn, K. S. and Blout, E. R., Mechanism of bovine prothrombin activation by an insoluble preparation of bovine Factor Xa (thrombokinase), *Biochemistry*, 11, 4502, 1972.
59. McCoy, L. E., Walz, D. A., Agrawal, B. B. L., and Seegers, W. H., Isolation of L-chain polypeptide of autoprothrombin III (Factor X), Homology with prothrombin indicated, *Thromb. Res.*, 2, 293, 1973.
60. Howard, J. B. and Nelsestuen, G. L., Isolation and characterization of vitamin K-dependent region of bovine blood clotting factor X, *Proc. Natl. Acad. Sci. U.S.A.*, 72, 1281, 1975.
61. Fujikawa, K., Coan, M. H., Legaz, M. E., and Davie, E. W., The mechanism of activation of bovine Factor X (Stuart Factor) by intrinsic and extrinsic pathways, *Biochemistry*, 13, 5290, 1974.
62. Furie, B. C., Furie, B., Gottlieb, A J., and Williams, W. J., Activation of bovine Factor X by the venom coagulation protein of *Vipera Russelli*, *Biochem. Biophys. Acta*, 365, 121, 1974.
63. Jesty, J., Spencer, A. K., and Nemerson, Y., The mechanism of activation of Factor X, *J. Biol. Chem.*, 249, 5614, 1974.
64. Papahadjopoulos, D., Hougie, C., and Hanahan, D. J., Purification and properties of bovine Factor V: a change of molecular size during blood coagulation, *Biochemistry*, 3, 264, 1964.
65. Papahadjopoulos, D. and Hanahan, D. J., Observation on the interaction of phospholipids and certain clotting factors in prothrombin activator formation, *Biochem. Biophys. Acta*, 90, 436, 1964.
66. Stemerman, M. B. and Pitlick, F. A., Tissue factor antigen and blood vessels, *Thromb. Diath. Haemorrh.*, 60, 71, 1974.
67. Silvergerg, A. S., Nemerson, Y., and Zur, M., Kinetics of the activation of bovine Factor X by components of the extrinsic pathway, *J. Biol. Chem.*, 252, 8481, 1977.
68. Legaz, M. E., Weinstein, M. J., Heldebrandt, C. M., and Davie, E. W., Isolation, structure and proteolytic modification of bovine factor VIII, *Ann. N.Y. Acad. Sci.*, 240, 43, 1975.
69. Shapiro, G. A., Anderson, J. C., Pizzo, S. V., and McKee, P. A., The subunit structure of normal and hemophilic Factor VIII, *J. Clin. Invest.*, 52, 2198, 1973.
70. Irwin, J. F., Factor VIII in von Willebrand's disease, *Sem. Thromb. Hemost.*, 2, 85, 1975.
71. Hougie, C., Sargeaut, R. B., Brown, J. E., and Bouch, R. F., Evidence that Factor VIII and ristocetin aggregating factor (VIII Rist) are separate molecular entities, *Proc. Soc. Exp. Biol. Med.*, 147, 58, 1974.
72. Benson, R. E. and Dodds, W. J., Physical relationship between canine Factor VIII coagulant activity and Factor VIII related antigen, *Proc. Soc. Exp. Biol. Med.*, 153, 339, 1976.

73. **Poon, M. C. and Ratnoff, O. D.**, Evidence that functional subunits of antihemophilic factor (Factor VIII) are linked by noncovalent bonds, *Blood,* 48, 87, 1976.
74. **Lian, E. C. and Deykin, D.**, In vivo dissociation of factor VIII (AHF) activity and Factor VIII related antigen in von Willebrand's disease, *Am. J. Hematol.,* 1, 71, 1976.
75. **Workman, E. F. and Lundblad, R. L.**, The role of the liver in biosynthesis of the non-Vitamin K-dependent clotting factors, *Sem. Thromb. Hemost.,* 4, 15, 1977.
76. **Webster, W. P., Mandel, S. R., Strike, L. E., Penick, G. D., Riggs, T. R., and Brinkhous, K. M.**, Factor VIII synthesis: hepatic and renal allografts in swine with von Willebrand's disease, *Am. J. Physiol.,* 230, 1342, 1976.
77. **Lindquist, P. A., Fujikawa, K., and Davie, E. W.**, Activation of bovine Factor IX (Christmas Factor) by Factor XI$_a$ (activated plasma thromboplastin antecedent) and a protease from Russell's viper venom, *J. Biol. Chem.,* 253, 1902, 1978.
78. **Osterud, B. and Rapaport, S. I.**, A bypass mechanism for activating human Factor IX with human Factor VII and thromboplastin, Abstracts, 6th Int. Congr. Thrombosis and Hemostasis, *Thrombos. Hemost.,* 38, 179, 1977.
79. **Enfield, D. L., Ericson, L. H., Fujikawa, K., Titanis, K., Walsh, K. A., and Neurath, H.**, Bovine Factor IX (Christmas Factor). Further evidence of homology with Factor X (Stuart Factor) and prothrombin, *FEBS Lett.,* 47, 1, 1974.
80. **Neier, H. L., Thompson, R. E., and Kaplan, A. P.**, Activation of Hageman Factor by Factor XIa—HMW-Kininogen, Abstr., 6th Int. Congr. Thromb., Hemost., *Thrombos. Hemost.,* 38, 14, 1977.
81. **Bouma, B. N. and Griffin, J. H.**, Human Blood coagulation Factor XI. Purification, properties, and mechanism of activation by activated Factor XII, *J. Biol. Chem.,* 252, 6432, 1977.
82. **Griffin, J. H. and Cochrane, C. G.**, Recent advances in the understanding of contact activation reactions, *Semin. Thromb. Hemost.,* 5, 254, 1979.
83. **Hubbard, D. and Lucas, G. L.**, Ionic charges of glass surfaces and other materials and their possible role in the coagulation of blood, *J. Appl. Physiol.,* 15, 265, 1960.
84. **Niewiarowski, S., Bankowski, E., and Rogowicka, I.** Studies on the adsorption and activation of Hageman factor (Factor XII) by collagen and elastin, *Thromb. Diath. Haemorrh.,* 14, 387, 1965.
85. **Wilner, G. D., Nossel, H. C., and LeRoy, E. C.**, Activation of Hageman factor by collagen, *J. Clin. Invest.,* 47, 2608, 1968.
86. **Ratnoff, O. D. and Saito, H.**, Coagulation factors and the role of surface in their activation, *Ann. N.Y. Acad. Sci.,* 283, 88, 1977.
87. **Meier, J. L., Scott, C. F., Mandel, R., Webster, M. E., Pierce, J. V., Colman, R. W., and Kaplan, A. P.**, Requirements for contact activation of human Hageman factor, *Ann. N.Y. Acad. Sci.,* 283, 93, 1977.
88. **Wiggins, R. C., Bouma, B. N., Cochrane, C. G., and Griffin, J. H.**, Role of high molecular weight kininogen in surface-binding and activation of coagulation Factor XI and prekallikrein, *Proc. Natl. Acad. Sci. U.S.A.,* 74, 4636, 1977.
89. **Kaplan, A. P., Meier, H. L., and Mandle, R.**, The Hageman factor dependent pathways of coagulation, fibrinolysis, and kinin generation, *Semin. Thromb. Hemost.,* 3, 1, 1976.
90. **Donaldson, V. H., Glueck, H. I., Miller, M. A., Movat, H., and Habal, F.**, Kininogen deficiency in Fitzgerald trait: role of high molecular weight kininogen in clotting and fibrinolysis, *J. Lab. Clin. Med.,* 87, 327, 1976.
91. **Webster, M. E., Guimaraes, J. A., Kaplan, A. P., Colman, R. W. and Pierce, J. V.**, Activation of surface-bound Hageman factor: pre-eminent role of high molecular weight kininogen and evidence for a new factor, *Adv. Exp. Med. Biol.,* 70, 285, 1976.
92. **Liu, C. Y., Scott, C. F., Bagdasarian, A., Pierce, J., Kaplan, A., and Colman, R. W.**, Potentiation of the function of Hageman factor fragments by high molecular weight kininogen, *J. Clin. Invest.,* 60, 7, 1977.
93. **Meyer, K. L., Pierce, J. V., Colman, R. W., and Kaplan, A.**, Activation and function of human Hageman factor, *J. Clin. Invest.,* 60, 18, 1977.
94. **Hatton, M. W. C. and Regoeczi, E.**, The inactivation of thrombin and plasmin by antithrombin III in the presence of sepharose-heparin, *Thromb. Res.,* 10, 645, 1977.
95. **Rosenberg, R. D.**, Biologic actions of heparin, *Semin. Hematol.,* 14, 427, 1977.
96. **Pomerantz, M. W. and Owen, W. G.**, A catalytic role for heparin. Evidence for a ternary complex of heparin cofactor, thrombin, and heparin, *Biochim. Biophys. Acta,* 535, 66, 1978.
97. **Kraemer, P. M.**, Heparan sulfates of cultured cells, *Biochemistry,* 10, 1437, 1971.
98. **Fell, C., Ivanovic, N., Johnson, S. A., and Seegers, W. H.**, Differentiation of plasma antithrombin activities, *Proc. Soc. Exp. Biol. Med.,* 85, 199, 1954.
99. **Niewiarowski, S., Gurewich, V., Senyi, A. F., and Mustard, J. F.**, The effect of fibrinolysis on platelet function, *Thromb. Diath. Haemorrh.,* Suppl. 47, 99, 1971.

100. **Barnhart, M. I., Sulisz, L., and Bluhm, G. B.,** Role of fibrinogen and its derivatives in acute inflammation, in *Immunopathology of Inflammation*, Forscher, B. K. and Honck, J. C., Eds., Excerpta Medica, Amsterdam, 1971, 59.
101. **Hawiger, J., Hammond, D. K., and Timmons, S.,** Human fibrinogen possesses binding sites for staphylococci on Aα and Bβ polypeptide chains, *Nature (London)*, 258, 643, 1975.
102. **Duckert, F. and Beck, E. A.,** Clinical disorders due to the deficiency of Factor XIII (fibrin stabilizing factor, fibrinase), *Semin. Hematol.*, 5, 83, 1968.
103. **von Kaulla, K. N.,** *Chemistry of Thrombolysis: Human Fibrinolytic Enzymes*, Charles C Thomas, Springfield, Ill., 1963, 9.
104. **Dastre, A.,** Fibrinolyse dans le sang, *Arch. Physiol. Norm. Pathol.*, 5, 661, 1893.
105. **Kaplan, M. H.,** Nature and role of the lytic factor in hemolytic streptococcal fibrinolysis, *Proc. Soc. Exp. Biol. Med.*, 57, 40, 1944.
106. **Christensen, L. R.,** Streptococcal fibrinolysis: a proteolytic reaction due to a serum enzyme activated by streptococcal fibrinolysin, *J. Gen. Physiol.*, 28, 559, 1945.
108. **Wallen, P. and Wiman, B.,** On the generation of intermediate plasminogen and its significance for activation, in *Proteases and Biological Control*, Reich, E., Rifkin, D. B., and Shaw, E., Eds., Cold Spring Harbor Laboratory, Cold Spring Harbor, N.Y., 1975, 291.
109. **Robbins, K. C., Summaria, L., and Barlow, G. H.,** Activation of plasminogen, in *Proteases and Biological Control*, Reich, E., Rifkin, D. B., and Shaw, E., Eds., Cold Spring Harbor Laboratory, Cold Spring Harbor, N.Y., 1975, 305.
110. **Barnhart, M. I. and Riddle, J. M.,** Cellular localization of profibrinolysin (plasminogen), *Blood*, 21, 306, 1963.
111. **Mosesson, M. W.,** Fibrinogen catabolic pathways, *Semin. Thromb. Hemost.*, 1, 63, 1974.
112. **Groskopf, W. R., Hsieh, B., Summaria, L., and Robbins, K. C.,** Studies on the active center of human plasmin, *J. Biol. Chem.*, 244, 359, 1969.
113. **Kaplan, A. P. and Austen, K. F.,** A prealbumin activator of prekallikrein. II. Derivation of activators of prekallikrein from active Hageman factor by digestion with plasmin, *J. Exp. Med.*, 133, 696, 1971.
114. **Taylor, F. B. and Ward, P. A.,** Generation of chemotactic activity in rabbit serum by plasminogen—streptokinase mixtures, *J. Exp. Med.*, 126, 149, 1967.
115. **Ratnoff, O. D. and Naff, G. B.,** The conversion of C'1s to C'1 esterase by plasmin and trypsin, *J. Exp. Med.*, 125, 337, 1967.
116. **Gapanhuk, E. and Henriques, O. B.,** Kinins released from horse heat-acid denatured plasma by plasmin, plasma kallikrein, trypsin, and bothrops kininogenase, *Biochem. Pharmacol.*, 19, 2091, 1970.
117. **Habal, F. M., Burrowes, C. E., and Movat, H. Z.,** Generation of kinin, kallikrein, and plasmin and the effect of α1-antitrypsin and antithrombin III on the kininogenases, *Adv. Exp. Med. Biol.*, 70, 23, 1976.
118. **Bang, N. U.,** Physiology and biochemistry of fibrinolysis, in *Thrombosis and Bleeding Disorders*, Bang, N.U., Beller, K. F., Deutsch, E., and Mammen, E. F., Eds., Academic Press, New York, 1971, 292.
119. **Kowalska-Loth, B. and Zakrewski, K.,** The activation by staphlokinase of human plasminogen, *Acta Biochem. Polonica*, 22, 327, 1975.
120. **Aoki, N. and von Kaulla, K.,** Dissimilarity of human vascular plasminogen activator and human urokinase, *J. Lab. Clin. Invest.*, 78, 354, 1971.
121. **Radcliffe, R. and Heinze, T.,** Isolation of plasminogen activator from human plasma by chromatography on lysine-Sepharose, *Arch. Biochem. Biophys.*, 189, 185, 1978.
122. **Kaplan, A. and Austen, F.,** The fibrinolytic pathway of human plasma. Isolation and characterization of the plasminogen proactivator, *J. Exp. Med.*, 135, 1378, 1972.
123. **Vennerod, A. M. and Laake, K.,** Prekallikrein and plasminogen proactivator. Absence of plasminogen proactivator in Fletcher factor deficient plasma, *Thromb. Res.*, 8, 519, 1976.
124. **Goldsmith, G. H., Saito, H., and Ratnoff, O. D.,** The activation of plasminogen by Hageman Factor (Factor XII) and Hageman Factor fragments, *J. Clin. Invest.*, 21, 54, 1978.
125. **Glueck, H. I. and Roehill, W.,** Myocardial infarction in patient with Hageman (Factor XII) defect, *Ann. Intern. Med.*, 64, 390, 1966.
126. **Currimbhoy, Z., Vinciguerra, V., Palakavongs, P., Kuslanski, P., and Degnan, T. J.,** Fletcher factor deficiency and myocardial infarction, *Am. J. Clin. Pathol.*, 65, 970, 1975.
127. **Harpel, P. C., Mosesson, M. W., and Cooper, N. R.,** Studies on the structure and function of α_2 macroglobulin and C1 inactivator, in *Proteases and Biological Control*, Reich, E., Rifkin, D. B., and Shaw, E., Eds., Cold Spring Harbor Laboratory, Cold Spring Harbor, N.Y., 1975, 387.
128. **Schreiber, A. D.,** Plasma inhibitors of the Hageman factor dependent pathways, *Semin. Thromb. Hemost.*, 3, 43, 1976.

129. Pisano, J. J., Chemistry and Biology of the kallikrein-kinin system, in *Proteases and Biological Control*, Reich, E., Rifkin, D. B., and Shaw, E., Eds., Cold Spring Harbor Laboratory, Cold Spring Harbor, N.Y., 1975, 199.
130. Ratnoff, O. D., Pensky, J., Ogsten, D., and Naff, G. B., The inhibition of plasmin, plasma kallikrein, plasma permeability factor, and the C1s subcomponent of the first component by serum C1 esterase inhibitor, *J. Exp. Med.*, 129, 315, 1969.
131. Bennet, N., Further studies on an inhibitor of plasminogen activation in human serum, *Thromb. Diath. Haemorrh.*, 23, 553, 1970.
132. Nilson, I. and Hedner, U., Partial purification of an activator inhibitor in serum, *J. Clin. Pathol.*, 25, 621, 1972.
133. Aoki, N., Moroi, M., Matsuda, M., and Tachiya, K., The behavior of α_2-plasmin inhibitor in fibrinolytic states, *J. Clin. Invest.*, 60, 361, 1977.
134. Koie, K., Ogata, K., Kamiya, T., Takamatzu, J., and Kohakura, M., α_2 plasmin inhibitor disease (Miyasato Disease), *Lancet*, 2, 1334, 1978.
135. Alkjaersig, N., Fletcher, A. P., and Sherry, S., The mechanism of clot dissolution by plasmin, *J. Clin. Invest.*, 38, 1086, 1959.
136. Ambrus, C. M. and Marcus, G., Plasmin-antiplasmin complex as a reservoir of fibrinolytic enzyme, *Am. J. Physiol.*, 199, 491. 1960.
137. Bang, N. U. and Chang, M. L., Soluble fibrin complexes, *Semin. Thromb. Hemost.*, 2, 91, 1974.
138. Marder, V., Matchett, M., and Sherry, S., Detection of serum fibrinogen and fibrin degradation products, *Am. J. Med.*, 51, 71, 1971.
139. Gardlund, B., Kowalska-Loth, B., Grondahl, N. J., and Blomback, B., Plasmin degradation products of human fibrinogen. I. Isolation and characterization of fragments E and D and their relationship to "disulfide knots", *Thromb. Res.*, 1, 371, 1972.
140. Kowalska-Loth, B., Gardlund, B., Egberg, N., and Blomback, B., Plasmic degradation products of human fibrinogen. II. Chemical and Immunological relation between fragment E and N-DSK, *Thromb. Res.*, 2, 423, 1973.
141. Margolis, J., Activation of plasma by contact with glass, evidence for a common reaction which releases plasma kinin and initiates coagulation, *J. Physiol. (London)*, 144, 1, 1958.
142. Kaplan, A. P. and Austen, K. F., A prealbumin activator of prekallikrein, *J. Immunol.*, 105, 802, 1970.
143. Sicuteri, F., Back, N., and Haberland, G. E., Eds., *Kinins, Pharmacodynamics and Biological Roles*, Plenum Press, New York, 1976, 70.
144. Pisano, J. J. and Austen, K. F., Eds., *Chemistry and Biology of the Kallikrein Kinin System in Health and Disease*, Fogerty Int. Center Proc. No. 27, DHEW Publication No. (NIH) 76-791, Department of Health, Education and Welfare, Washington, D.C., 1974.
145. Eisen, V., Kinin forming enzymes and substrates in human plasma, *J. Physiol. (London)*, 186, 133, 1966.
146. Jacobsen, S. and Kriz, M., Some data on two purified kininogens from human plasma, *Br. J. Pharmacol.*, 29, 25, 1967.
147. Seidel, G., Two functionally different kininogens in human plasma, *Agents Actions*, 3, 12, 1973.
148. Habal, F. M. and Movat, H. Z., Kininogens of human plasma, *Semin. Thromb. Hemost.*, 3, 27, 1976.
149. Colman, R. W., Bagdasarian, A., Talamo, R. C., Scott, C. F., Seaven, M., Guimaraes, J. A., Pierce, J. V., and Kaplan, A. P., Williams trait: human kininogen deficiency with diminished levels of plasminogen proactivator and prekallikrein associated with abnormalities of the Hageman factor dependent pathway, *J. Clin. Invest.*, 56, 1650, 1975.
150. Saito, H., Ratnoff, O. D., Waldmann, R., and Abraham, J., Fitzgerald trait: deficiency of a hitherto unrecognized agent, Fitzgerald factor, participating in surface-mediated reactions of clotting, fibrinolysis, generation of kinins, and the property of diluted plasma enhancing vascular permeability (Pf/dil), *J. Clin. Invest.*, 55, 1082, 1975.
151. Wuepper, K. D., Miller, D. R., and Lacombe, M. J., Flaujeac trait: deficiency of human plasma kininogen, *J. Clin. Invest.*, 56, 1663, 1975.
152. Ratnoff, O. D., The interrelationship of clotting and immunologic mechanism, in *Immunobiology*, Good, R. A. and Fisher, D. W., Eds., Sinauer, Stanford, Conn., 1971, 135.
153. Han, Y. N., Komiya, M., Iwanaga, S., and Suzuki, T., Studies on the primary structure of bovine high molecular weight kininogen, *J. Biochem. (Tokyo)*, 77, 55, 1975.
154. Gigli, I., Kaplan, A. P., and Austen, K. F., Modulation of function of the activated first component of complement by a fragment derived from serum. I. Effect on early components of complement, *J. Exp. Med.*, 134, 1466, 1971.
155. Ruddy, S., Gigli, I., and Austen, K. F., The complement system of man, *N. Engl. J. Med.*, 287, 489, 1972.

156. **Muller-Eberhard, H. H.**, Initiation of membrane attack by complement: assembly and control of C3 and C5 convertase, in *Proteases and Biological Control*, Reich, E., Rifkin, D. B., and Shaw, E., Eds., Cold Spring Harbor Laboratory, Cold Spring Harbor, N.Y., 1975, 229.
157. **Kinsky, S. C. and Six, H. R.**, A model for the lytic action of complement, in *Proteases and Biological Control*, Reich, E., Rifkin, D. B., and Shaw, E., Eds., Cold Spring Harbor Laboratory, Cold Spring Harbor, N.Y., 1975, 243.
158. **Muller-Eberhard, H. J.**, Complement, *Annu. Rev. Biochem.*, 44, 697, 1975.
159. **Frank, M. M.**, *Complement—Current Concepts*, Upjohn, Kalamazoo, Mich., 1975.
160. **Hugli, T. E.**, Serum anaphylotoxins, formation, characterization and control, in *Proteases and Biological Control*, Reich, E., Rifkin, D. B., and Shaw, E., Eds., Cold Spring Harbor Laboratory, Cold Spring Harbor, N.Y., 1975, 273.
161. **Rapp. H. G. and Borsos, T.**, *Molecular Basis of Complement Action*, Appleton-Century-Crofts, New York, 1970.
162. **Mayer, M. M.**, Complement and complement fixation, in *Experimental Immunochemistry*, 2nd ed., Kabat, E. A., Ed., Charles C Thomas, Springfield, Ill., 1961, 133.
163. **Mayer, M. M.**, The complement system, *Sci. Am.*, 229, 54, 1973.
164. **Forssman, J.**, Die herstellung hochwertiger spezifischer schafhamolysine ohne verwendung von schafblut. Ein beitrag zur lehre von heterologer antikorpbildung, *Biochem. Z.*, 37, 78, 1911.
165. **Borsos, T. and Rapp, H. J.**, Complement fixation on cell surfaces by 19S and 7S antibodies, *Science*, 150, 505, 1965.
166. **Borsos, T.**, Immunoglobulin classes and complement fixing, in *Progress in Immunology*, Academic Press, New York, 1971, 841.
167. **Ishizaka, T. K., Borsos, T., and Rapp, H. J.**, C'1 fixation by human isoagglutinins, Fixation of C'1 by G and M but not A antibody, *J. Immunol.*, 97, 716, 1966.
168. **Fauci, A. S., Frank, M. M., and Johnson, J. S.**, The relationship between antibody affinity and the efficiency of complement fixation, *J. Immunol.*, 105, 215, 1970.
169. **Frank, M. M. and Gaither, T. A.**, Complement fixation by a single molecule of γG hemolysin, *J. Immunol.*, 104, 1458, 1970.
170. **Humphrey, J. H. and Dourmashkin, R. R.**, Electron microscope studies of immune cell lysis, in *Ciba Foundation Symposium on Complement*, J. London and A. Churchill, London, 1965, 175.
171. **Rosse, W. R.**, Fixation of the first component of complement (C'1a) by human antibodies, *J. Clin. Invest.*, 47, 2430, 1968.
172. **Leddy, J. P. and Swisher, S. N.**, Acquired immune hemolytic disorders, in *Immunological Diseases*, 2nd ed., Samter, M., Ed., Little, Brown, Boston, 1971, 1094.
173. **Cooper, N. R. and Morrison, D. C.**, Binding and activation of the first component of human complement by the lipid-A region of lipopolysaccharides, *J. Immunol.*, 120, 1862, 1978.
174. **Gotze, O.**, Proteases of the properdin system, in *Proteases and Biological Control*, Reich, E., Rifkin, D. B., and Shaw, E., Eds., Cold Spring Harbor Laboratory, Cold Spring Harbor, N.Y., 1975, 255.
175. **Pillimer, L., Blum, L., and Lepow, I. H.**, The properdin system and immunity. I. Demonstration and isolation of a new serum protein, properdin, and its role in immune phenomena, *Science*, 120, 279, 1954.
176. **Schur, P. H. and Becker, E. L.**, Pepsin digestion of rabbit and sheep antibodies. The effect on complement fixation, *J. Exp. Med.*, 118, 891, 1963.
177. **Sandberg, A. L., Oliveira, B., and Osler, A. G.**, Two complement interaction sites in guinea pig immunoglobulins, *J. Immunol.*, 106, 282, 1971.
178. **Block, K. J., Kourilsky, F. M., Ovary, Z., and Benacerraf, B.**, Properties of guinea pig 7S antibodies. III. Identification of antibodies involved in complement fixation and hemolysis, *J. Exp. Med.*, 117, 965, 1963.
179. **Gewurz, H., Shin, H. S., and Mergenhagen, S. E.**, Interactions of the complement system with endotoxic lipolysaccharide, Consumption of each of the six terminal complement components, *J. Exp. Med.*, 128, 1049, 1968.
180. **Marcus, R. L., Shin, H. S., and Mayer, M. M.**, An alternate complement pathway: C3 cleaving activity, not due to C4 2a, on endotoxic lipopolysaccharide after treatment with guinea pig serum: relation to properdin (complement components), *Proc. Natl. Acad. Sci. U.S.A.*, 68, 1351, 1971.
181. **Ellman, L., Gren, I., and Frank, M. M.**, Genetically controlled total deficiency of the fourth component of complement in the guinea pig, *Science*, 170, 74, 1970.
182. **Frank, M. M., May, J. E., Gaither, T., and Ellman, L.**, In vitro studies of complement functions in sera of C4 deficient guinea pigs, *J. Exp. Med.*, 134, 176, 1971.
183. **Pensky, I., Levy, L. R., and Lepow, I. H.**, Partial purification of a serum inhibitor of C'1 esterase, *J. Biol. Chem.*, 236, 1674, 1961.
184. **Ruddy, S. and Austen, K. F.**, C3b inactivator of man. II. Fragments produced by C3b inactivator cleavage of cell-bound or fluid phase C3b, *J. Immunol.*, 197, 742, 1971.

185. Leddy, J. P., Frank, M. M., Gaither, T., Baum, J., and Klemperer, M. R., Hereditary deficiency of the sixth component of complement in man. I. Immunochemical, biologic and family studies, *J. Clin. Invest.*, 53, 544, 1974.
186. Rocha e Silva, M. and Grana, R., Anaphylaxis-like reactions produced by *Ascaris* extracts, *Arch. Surg. (Chicago)*, 52, 523, 1946.
187. Guest, M. ., Murphy, R. C., Bodnar, S. R., Ware, A. G., and Seegers, W. H., Physiological effects of a plasma protein: blood pressure, leukocyte concentration, smooth and cardiac muscle activity, *Am. J. Physiol.*, 150, 471, 1947.
188. Rocha e Silva, M., Beraldo, W. T., and Rosenfeld, G., Bradykinin, a hypotensive and smooth muscle stimulating factor released from plasma globulin by snake venoms and trypsin, *Am. J. Physiol.*, 156, 261, 1949.
189. Schreiber, A. D. and Austen, F., Interrelationships of the fibrinolytic, coagulation, kinin generating and complement system, *Ser. Haematol.*, 6, 593, 1973.
190. Dias de Silva, W., Eisele, J. W., and Lepow, I. H., Complement as a mediator of inflammation. III. Purification of the activity with anaphylatoxin properties generated by interaction of the first four components of complement and its identification as a cleavage product of C'3, *J. Exp. Med.*, 125, 1027, 1967.
191. Alper, C. A. and Rosen, F. S., Genetic aspects of the complement system, *Adv. Immunol.*, 14, 251, 1971.
192. Rosen, R. H., Apler, C. A., Pensley, J., Klemperer, M. R., and Donaldson, V. H., Genetically determined heterogeneity of the C1 esterase inhibitor in patients with hereditary angioneurotic edema, *J. Clin. Invest.*, 50, 2143, 1971.
193. Ulutin, O. N., *The Platelets, Fundamentals and Clinical Applications,* Kagit Ve Basim Isleri, A. S., Istanbul, Turkey, 1976.
194. Shulman, N. R., Analysis of drug antibodies with autoimmune implications, in *Laboratory Diagnosis of Immunologic Disorders,* Vyas, G. M., Steitz, D. P., and Brecke, G., Eds., Grune & Stratton, New York, 1975, 31.
195. Schreiber, A. D. and Austen, K. F., Hageman factor — independent fibrinolytic pathway, *Clin. Exp. Immunol.*, 17, 587, 1974.
196. Ward, P. A., Cochrane, C. G., and Muller-Eberhard, H. F., The role of serum complement in chemotaxis of leukocytes in vitro, *J. Exp. Med.*, 122, 326, 1965.
197. Zimmerman, T. S. and Muller-Eberhard, H. F., Blood coagulation initiation by a complement mediated pathway, *J. Exp. Med.*, 134, 1601, 1971.
198. Kane, M. A., May, J. E., and Frank, M. M., Interactions of the classical and alternate complement pathway with endotoxin lipopolysaccharide—effect on platelets and blood coagulation, *J. Clin. Invest.*, 52, 370, 1973.
199. Rosenberg, J. C., Hawkins, E., and Rector, F., Mechanism of immunological injury during antibody-mediated hyperacute rejection of renal heterografts, *Transplantation,* 11, 151, 1971.
200. Cazenave, J. P., Assimeh, S. N., Painter, R. H., Packman, M. A., and Mustard, J. F., C1q inhibition of the interaction of collagen with human platelets, *J. Immunol.*, 116, 162, 1976.
201. Gaynor, E., Bouvier, C., and Spaet, T. H., Vascular lesions. Possible pathogenetic basis of the generalized Shwartzman reaction, *Science,* 170, 986, 1970.

Clinical Disorders of Hemostasis

Chapter 4

A SYSTEMATIC APPROACH TO THE DIAGNOSIS OF BLEEDING DISORDERS

Rodger L. Bick

TABLE OF CONTENTS

I. Introduction 82

II. Laboratory Screening Tests 84

III. Summary 86

References 87

I. INTRODUCTION

Disorders of hemostasis are numerous and penetrate into all areas of pathophysiology and clinical medicine. Many disorders of hemostasis are straightforward and simple; however, many are multifaceted and extremely complex in pathophysiology, as well as in diagnosis and in management. Disorders of hemostasis can be conveniently compartmentalized into hereditary and acquired, with acquired defects being much more common than hereditary defects. All acquired and hereditary defects can be further compartmentalized into defects of the vasculature defects of the platelets or defects of coagulation proteins.[1] In general, the inherited defects of hemostasis tend to be simple, confined to one hemostatic compartment and, usually, to one coagulation protein in the case of a coagulation protein disorder. By contrast, the acquired disorders of hemostasis tend to be multifaceted in etiology, as well as in pathophysiology, to involve more than one coagulation factor and, in many instances, may involve two or all three of the hemostatic compartments. Table 1 compartmentalizes and classifies a systematic approach to the diagnosis of bleeding disorders.

When approaching a patient with a bleeding disorder or a bleeding history, a systematic and logical approach to diagnosis is imperative. A simple and workable approach is to always think of the hemostasis system as being comprised of the three hemostatic compartments: *the vascular tree, the platelets,* and *the coagulation proteins.* Generally, for normal hemostasis to occur all three of these compartments must be intact. Platelets must be normal in both number and function and coagulation proteins must be quantitatively as well as qualitatively normal. Often a defect in only one hemostatic compartment can be corrected by overcompensation of the other two compartments and clinically significant bleeding may not ensue. For example, disruption of the vascular tree as in minor trauma or surgery may not lead to pathological bleeding if platelet number and function and coagulation proteins are intact and function to overcome this insult. Commonly, abnormalities in two of the three hemostatic systems must be present for pathological bleeding to occur. Hemophiliacs often do not bleed (coagulation protein abnormality) unless another of the hemostatic compartments is disrupted; for example, if the vasculature is disrupted by surgery or trauma. Once one can discern which compartment or combination of compartments contains a defect, a thorough evaluation of this compartment can then be carried out from both the clinical and laboratory standpoint. In most instances, clinical evaluation of the patient, as well as a careful history, will compartmentalize a defect of hemostasis. If the patient has petechiae and purpura, one can assume that the vasculature or the platelets (either number or function) are at fault. Petechiae and purpura never arise from coagulation protein disorders alone. By contrast, the noting of intra-articular, deep intramuscular, or intracerebral bleeding is most often a manifestation of single or multiple coagulation protein abnormalities. A careful history should pinpoint a family history of bleeding, a past history of bleeding, and the type of bleeding occurring. Obviously, patients should be carefully questioned about drugs for detection of drug-induced platelet dysfunction, drug-induced thrombocytopenia, or drug-induced vascular defects.

Probably no area of laboratory medicine is more confusing to the clinician than the field of hemostasis. The superfluity in terminology, the potpourri of techniques purported to measure the same factors, and the mystique of reagents used, such as "thromboplastin" (brain or lung derivative) and "activators" (kaolin, celite, or ellagic acid), may account for this state of affairs. Up to the present, there is still no global agreement on even such a routine procedure as the prothrombin time, in spite of more than a decade of international committee meetings. This discussion classifies the bleeding disorders according to pathogenic mechanisms and outlines laboratory procedures that will permit a systematic approach to the diagnosis of most bleeding disorders.

TABLE 1
A Systematic Approach to the Diagnosis of Bleeding Disorders

Classification	Initial screening	Definitive tests	Adjunctive tests	Clinical hints
Vascular Hereditary Acquired	TBT or Tourniquet test	ATT	Collagen work-up Tissue biopsy Autoimmune work-up Endocrine studies Paraprotein studies	Petechiae Purpura Mucosal Membrane Bleeding Telangiectasia
Platelet abnormalities Quantitative Qualitative Hereditary Acquired	Drug history Platelet count Platelet morphology Platelet adhesion TBT	Marrow exam Aggregation	Creatinine Coombs Paraproteins FDPs	Petechiae Purpura Splenomegaly Gingival bleeding
Coagulation protein disorders Hereditary Acquired	PT PTT	Factor assays Inhibitor assays Fibrinogen tests	Liver enzymes Hemotherapy trials	Family history Hemarthroses Sex Heptamegaly Surgery Postpartum
Multiple hemostatic compartment defects DIC Primary fibrino(geno)lysis	PT PTT FDP TT Platelet count	AT-III PSO_4 test Fibrinopeptide-A	Paraproteins Blood cultures Complement levels	Postoperative Postpartum Ecchymoses Petechiae Purpura Shock

A bleeding diathesis can rarely be completely defined without the aid of laboratory tests, but the selection and interpretation of these tests should be predicted on the basis of major clinical data. A careful history is therefore paramount, with particular emphasis on the family history. Drug administration, obvious or surreptitious, must be carefully considered. Detailed discussions of drugs affecting hemostasis are found in Chapters 5, 6, and 7. A history of obstetrical and surgical events associated with unusual bleeding require a search for defects in hemostasis. Vascular or platelet abnormalities usually manifest as easy and spontaneous bruisability, petechiae or purpura, commonly dependent, and bleeding from the mucous membranes, although the hereditary disorders may present primarily as gastrointestinal bleeding. Conversely, the hemophilias rarely, if ever, cause petechiae or purpura, but joint bleeding is a hallmark. In an age of social awareness, a note of caution seems warranted concerning the "battered child syndrome". Idiopathic thrombocytopenic purpura, a disease most commonly seen in children, may simulate this condition because of the painful associated hematomas. The presence of blue sclerae, hyperelasticity of the skin, and hyperextensible joints suggest a hereditary connective tissue disorder. Telangiectasia of buccal mucosal membranes or subungual areas is a classic finding in Osler-Weber-Rendu disease. Splenic enlargement most often suggest thrombocytopenia, usually secondary.

Connective tissue and vascular diseases are not commonly thought of as causes of abnormal bleeding. The rather uncommon hereditary diseases include osteogenesis imperfecta, Marfan's syndrome, pseudoxanthoma elasticum, Ehler-Danlos syndrome, and familial telangiectasia (Osler-Weber-Rendu disease). Acquired abnormalities occur in lupus erythematosus, Cushing's syndrome, scurvy, allergic purpura (Henoch-Schonlein), and the vasculidities, e.g., periateritis nodosa. These are discussed in detail in Chapter 5.

Thrombocytopenias, hereditary or acquired, may be due to (1) bone marrow failure (aplastic anemias, leukemia, myelofibrosis, myelosuppression, etc.), (2) maturation defects (megaloblastic anemias), and (3) peripheral loss (idiopathic thrombocytopenia purpura, disseminated intravascular coagulation, hypersplenism, and large angiomata).

Bleeding may also be due to platelet dysfunction, i.e., Glanzmann's thrombasthemia, uremia, and the dysproteinemias. von Willebrand's disease is clearly a plasma protein defect, but this disorder presents with bleeding suggestive of a vascular or platelet function defect.[2] Coagulation protein abnormalities, whether hereditary or acquired, may result from absent, decreased, or abnormal synthesis of a clotting factor, or the development of antibodies against these factors (circulating inhibitors or anticoagulants).

II. LABORATORY SCREENING TESTS

The initial screening of a bleeding disorder includes:

1. A blood smear and count for estimation of platelet number
2. A template bleeding time (TBT) and aspirin tolerance test (ATT) for evaluation of platelet and vascular integrity
3. A prothrombin time (PT)
4. A partial thromboplastin time (PTT)

Table 2 depicts the use of these tests in compartmentalizing a defect of hemostasis.

If a vascular or platelet defect is present, the TBT may be prolonged; the finding of a prolonged TBT or ATT in the face of a normal platelet count suggests platelet or vascular dysfunction. The ATT will help distinguish the meaning of a questionable or

TABLE 2

Screening Test Result vs. Compartment at Fault

	Compartment			
	Vascular	Quant. platelet	Qual. platelet	Coagulation Factors
Platelets	N[a]	ABN[b]	N	N
Rumpel-Leede	ABN	ABN	ABN	N
Bleeding time (template)	ABN	ABN	ABN	N
PT	N	N	N	N/ABN[c]
PTT	N	N	N	N/ABN[c]

[a] N = normal.
[b] ABN = abnormal
[c] Either the prothrombin time (PT), partial thromboplastin time (PTT), or both will be abnormal, depending upon which factor(s) is involved.

borderline TBT.[3] In addition, careful examination of the blood smear may reveal findings suggestive of an associated dyscrasia (e.g., leukemia) or the leukocytosis, shistocytosis, and reticulocytosis seen in disseminated intravascular coagulation (DIC) or thrombotic thrombocytopenia purpura (TTP). If a coagulation protein abnormality is present, either the PT, PTT, or both will be prolonged. In DIC with secondary hyperfibrinolysis, there will be a prolonged PT, PTT, and TBT, and usually a low platelet count. Primary fibrinolysis will present the same findings, except that platelets may be normal in number. More sophisticated techniques for rendering a differential diagnosis are found in appropriate chapters.

Bleeding due to a vascular defect requires careful clinical and laboratory evaluation to uncover an underlying primary disease such as Cushing's syndrome, scurvy, or Henoch-Schonlein purpura. If no primary disease can be found, the TBT, in association with an ATT and platelet function studies, will help to define the vascular nature of the disorder. The TBT should *not* be performed in the face of overt bleeding or obvious thrombocytopenia. Since the TBT and ATT are abnormal in other bleeding disorders, further studies are necessary to establish the diagnosis.

When initial screening suggests a platelet disorder, a platelet count should be done. If low, the bone marrow should be examined. If normal, the TBT, ATT, platelet aggregation and adhesiveness tests help to define qualitative abnormalities of platelets (see Chapter 6).

Coagulation factor abnormalities can frequently be diagnosed from the initial PT and PTT. The ability to perform these tests by semiautomated instruments utilizing premeasured reagents has greatly enhanced their accuracy and convenience for use by physicians in private practice with ambulatory patients requiring anticoagulant therapy. Reagents, however, should be carefully chosen. Several recent comparative studies have shown that some commercial reagents do not perform adequately.[4-8]

An abnormal PT with an abnormal PTT most commonly suggests a defect in the prothrombin complex factors (II, VII, IX, and X) and Factor V, resulting from liver disease, coumarin compounds therapy, vitamin K deficiency, or DIC. A prolonged PTT with a normal PT is highly suggestive of Factor VIII, IX, or XI deficiency, which represent the hemophilias. However, these same findings, in the face of a *negative* bleeding history, suggest Factor XI, XII, Fletcher, or Fitzgerald factor deficiency.

If the hemophilias are a strong possibility, a differential PTT, will pinpoint the specific factor deficiency. Since 85% of all hemophiliacs are Factor VIII deficient ("classical hemophilia") a Factor VIII assay may be the only other test required. Factor IX deficiency represents 10 to 15% of hemophiliacs. The remaining hereditary factor deficiencies are rare and can be diagnosed by exclusion and special laboratory procedures.

In liver disease or in suspected drug-induced bleeding (particularly antibiotics), a therapeutic trial of vitamin K may prove useful. In life-threatening situations, hemotherapeutic agents (prothrombin complex concentrate, etc.) may be necessary to establish the diagnosis and management of hemorrhage.[9]

The recognition of inhibitors (antibodies) to specific clotting factors has increased considerably in recent years. These develop in 5 to 10% of hemophiliacs, but also occur postpartum, in systemic lupus erythematosus and other diseases, and spontaneously with no obvious associated condition. The majority of these antibodies are against Factor VIII (antihemophilic factor, AHF). The diagnosis can be suspected when the PTT is prolonged and the specific factor assay demonstrates low activity. The diagnosis is confirmed when specific inhibitor tests (neutralization assays) are performed.[10] However, since most laboratories are not prepared to carry out these procedures and since some inhibitors are too low to be accurately measured, a "therapeutic test" utilizing a commercial concentrate (Factor VIII or IX) may be necessary. Failure to correct a markedly prolonged PTT or Lee-White clotting time 2 to 4 hr after infusion of enough specific concentrate to "normalize" a patient is evidence of an inhibitor, the infused material having been "neutralized" by it. Inhibitors are discussed in Chapters 7 and 10.

Afibrinogenemia and hypofibrinogenemia are suggested by finding an abnormal PT and PTT. Definitive tests necessary for confirmation are a fibrinogen level most easily estimated by the thrombin time (TT) and reptilase time (RT). If these are prolonged and immunological tests for fibrinogen are normal, a dysfibrinogemia may be present. Both DIC and primary hyperfibrinolysis will lead to multiple coagulation factor abnormalities, as previously described. With the introduction of a standardized fibrin plate technique, it is now a simple matter to demonstrate the presence of active plasmin[11,12] (fibrinolysin), either as a primary disorder or associated with a secondary disease or coagulation abnormality. This method is quantitative and far more sensitive than the euglobin lysis time and should therefore replace this latter procedure.

The mechanism of bleeding due to the hyperglobulinemias is not entirely understood, but multiple clotting defects may be demonstrated. Thus, in addition to a low platelet count, which may be seen in multiple myeloma, malfunction of platelets may be demonstrated (as described above) and prolongation of the clotting time tests may be seen. The mechanisms for this are detailed in Chapter 10. By quantitating serum protein levels, the diagnosis of one of these disorders may be made.

In an age of polypharmacy, iatrogenic bleeding must be considered, the classic example being aspirin therapy. However, a host of other drugs alone or in combination may induce bleeding tendencies and not always by the same mechanism. Drugs should be suspected when one or more clotting defects can be demonstrated, without other obvious cause, and when discontinuation of medication causes hemostasis tests to return to normal.

III. SUMMARY

1. A simple screening battery consists of a blood smear examination, TBT, PT, and PTT.
2. Petechial or purpuric bleeding is highly suggestive of vascular or platelet dysfunction, while joint bleeding is classic for hemophilia.

3. A prolonged PTT with a normal PT usually means hemophilia, 85% being Factor VIII deficiency.
4. A prolonged PT with prolonged PTT suggests liver disease or other acquired defect.
5. About 50% of hemophiliacs are uncovered following an operative procedure. On the other hand, the most common cause of postoperative hemorrhage is a *severed blood vessel* (acquired silk deficiency).
6. A family history of bleeding may be the most helpful information in diagnosing hemophilia. Conversely, carefully performed coagulation tests may reveal a clotting deficiency in the absence of historical bleeding.

REFERENCES

1. **Bick, R. L. and Shanbrom, E.**, A systematic approach to the diagnosis of bleeding disorders, *Med. Counterpoint,* 4, 27, 1972.
2. **Bowie, E. J. M., Didisheim, P., Thompson, J. H., and Owen, C. A.**, The spectrum of von Willebrand's disease, *Thromb. Diath. Haemorrh.,* 18, 40, 1967.
3. **Bick, R. L., Adams, T., and Schmalhorst, W. R.**, Bleeding times, platelet adhesion, and aspirin, *Am. J. Clin. Pathol.,* 65, 69' 1976.
4. **Shapiro, G. A., Huntzinger, S. W., and Wilson, J. E.**, Variation among commercial activated partial thromboplastin time reagents in response to heparin, *Am. J. Clin. Pathol.,* 67, 477, 1977.
5. **Teiem, A. N. and Abildgaard, W.**, On the value of the activated partial thromboplastin time (APTT) in monitoring heparin therapy, *Thromb. Haemostas.,* 35, 592, 1976.
6. **Huseby, R. and Shafer, D.**, Variables and questions related to a recent comparative heparin response evaluation, *Am. J. Clin. Pathol.,* 69, 99, 1978.
7. **Triplett, D. A., Harms, C. S., and Koepke, J. A.**, The effect of heparin on the activated partial thromboplastin time, *Am. J. Clin. Pathol.,* 70, (Suppl.), 556, 1978.
8. **Harms, C. S., Triplett, D. A., and Koepke, J. A.**, Factor VIII assay results in the 1976 College of American Pathologists Survey Program, *Am. J. Clin. Pathol.,* 70, 560, 1975.
9. **Bick, R. L., Schmalhorst, W. R., and Shanbrom, E.**, Prothrombin complex concentrate: use in controlling the hemorrhagic diathesis of chronic liver disease, *Am. J. Dig. Dis.,* 20, 741, 1975.
10. **Tse, D., Fekete, L. F., and Shanbrom, E.**, A simple procedure for the accurate quantitation of Factor VIII inhibitors, *Thromb. Diath. Haemorrh.,* 23, 19' 1970.
11. **Bick, R. L., Bishop, R. C., and Shanbrom, E.**, Fibrinolytic activity in acute myocardial infarction, *Am. J. Clin. Path.,* 57, 359, 1972.
12. **Bishop, R. C., Ekert, H., Gilchrist, G., and Fekete, Lajos F.**, The preparation and evaluation of a standardized fibrin plate for the assessment of fibrinolytic activity, *Thromb. Diath. Haemorrh.,* 23, 202, 1970.

Chapter 5

VASCULAR DISORDERS

Rodger L. Bick

TABLE OF CONTENTS

I. Introduction 90

II. Hereditary Vascular Disorders 90
    A. Ehler-Danlos Syndrome 90
    B. Marfan's Syndrome 90
    C. Osteogenesis Imperfecta 91
    D. Pseudoxanthoma Elasticum 91
    E. Osler-Weber-Rendu Disease 91

III. Acquired Vascular Disorders 92

References 94

I. INTRODUCTION

Although most vascular disorders are not strictly hematological diseases, many are characterized by or accompanied by a significant hemorrhagic diathesis and often present in this manner. Thus these diseases should be considered in the differential diagnosis of bleeding disorders. Basic physiology of the vasculature is detailed in Chapter 1.

Vascular disorders are characteristically manifest by petechiae, purpura, or telangiectasia. Although these are the most common manifestations, ecchymoses, mucous membrane bleeding (epistaxis, genitourinary, and gastrointestinal bleeding), as well as hemarthroses, may also occur. Commonly found in vascular disorders is a history of gingival bleeding with toothbrushing, bleeding after tooth extraction, and a history of easy or, more significantly, spontaneous bruisability.[1]

The diagnosis for most vascular disorders commonly requires an autoimmune investigation or connective tissue biopsy. The common abnormal laboratory features of vascular disorders are an abnormal Rumpel-Leede tourniquet test, abnormal template bleeding time, abnormal aspirin tolerance test, and normal platelet function. Screening tests often fail to differentiate between a functional platelet defect and a vascular defect. An abnormal template bleeding time, aspirin tolerance test, and Rumpel-Leede tourniquet test, in conjunction with normal platelet function studies (as defined by platelet adhesion or aggregation), is strongly suggestive of a vascular disorder.

The simplest classification of vascular disorders is into hereditary and acquired, with acquired types being more common.

II. HEREDITARY VASCULAR DISORDERS

The following are the five most common hereditary vascular disorders; four of the five diseases discussed represent the well-known hereditary collagen vascular diseases.

A. Ehler-Danlos Syndrome

The Ehler-Danlos syndrome (ED syndrome) is a rare connective tissue disorder that is inherited by autosomal dominance.[2] Interestingly, one of the earliest descriptions of this syndrome concerned the violin virtuoso Paganini, and this was thought to contribute to his remarkable dexterity and talent. The disorder is characterized by extreme vascular fragility, skin fragility, hypermobile joints, and molluscoid pseudotumors of the knees and elbows. Easy and spontaneous bruisability are hallmark characteristics of the ED syndrome. Patients commonly suffer gingival bleeding with toothbrushing and bleed after dental extraction. Also, petechiae, purpura, gastrointestinal bleeding, and hemoptysis are often present. Other characteristics commonly noted are blue sclerae and angioid streaks. In addition, aortic insufficiency and the "floppy" mitral valve syndrome may occur.

The common laboratory findings are a positive Rumpel-Leede tourniquet test, prolonged template bleeding time, and, in many instances, a platelet function defect that remains poorly characterized.[3]

The basic pathology of ED syndrome is poorly understood, but appears to represent a decrease in collagen and an increase in elastic tissue. In addition, collagen from these patients contains an abnormal amino acid composition.[4]

B. Marfan's Syndrome

This syndrome is well described and is the most popularized of the hereditary collagen vascular disorders. It is inherited as an autosomal dominant trait and is characterized by skeletal defects (manifest by long extremities and arachnodactyly), cardiovascular abnormalities (ascending aortic aneurysm or dissection), and ocular defects (primarily manifest as ectopia lentis).[5,6] In addition, hyperextensible joints are present. Of all the hereditary collagen vascular disorders, Marfan's syndrome is least characterized clinically by a hemorrhagic diathesis. However, many patients have easy and spontaneous bruising, and some may demonstrate a poorly characterized functional platelet defect.

C. Osteogenesis Imperfecta

Osteogenesis imperfecta (brittle bones and blue sclerae) is one of the more common hereditary collagen vascular diseases and is inherited as an autosomal dominant trait.[6] The disorder is characterized by a patchy lack of bone matrix. However, the matrix that does exist undergoes normal calcification. Osteogenesis imperfecta is clinically manifest as deformed and brittle bones that fracture easily. In addition, skin and subcutaneous hemorrhages are characteristic. Death commonly occurs at childbirth due to intracranial hemorrhage caused by an abnormal calvarium coupled with a vascular hemorrhagic diathesis. Easy and spontaneous bruisability, hemoptysis, epistaxis, and intracranial bleeding are common in osteogenesis imperfecta. An abnormal bleeding time and a positive tourniquet test are characteristic.[7] In addition, many cases have been described with abnormal platelet function, as defined by adhesion and aggregation studies. The basic pathophysiology of osteogenesis imperfecta appears to be related to the inability of reticulin to mature into collagen. In addition, the collagen present demonstrates an abnormal amino acid composition.[4]

D. Pseudoxanthoma Elasticum

Pseudoxanthoma elasticum (PE syndrome), unlike the other hereditary collagen vascular diseases, often does not become manifest until the second or third decade in life.[8] This rare disorder is inherited as an autosomal recessive trait. It is commonly characterized by significant hemorrhage, since abnormal elastic fibers affect the entire arterial system. Hemorrhage can occur in any organ, most commonly skin, eyes, kidneys, and gastrointestinal tract. In addition, these patients have a marked tendency to easy and spontaneous bruisability and commonly develop petechiae and purpura. Clinical characteristics include relaxed, inelastic, and redundant skin in facial, neck, axillary, orbital, and inguinal areas. Hyperkeratotic plaques develop in these areas, and subcutaneous calcinosis is also common. Death is commonly caused by gastrointestinal hemorrhage. Excessive uterine bleeding and intra-articular bleeds with formation of hemarthroses are common. The basic pathology of this disorder is poorly understood.

E. Osler-Weber-Rendu Disease

Osler-Weber-Rendu disease — hereditary hemorrhagic telangiectasia (HHT) — is a relatively common disorder and is the most common hereditary vascular disorder leading to a hemorrhagic diathesis.[9-11] The disorder is inherited as an autosomal dominant trait, but only 70% have a positive family history. The homozygous state is thought to be lethal.[12] In addition, there is evidence that the gene responsible for HHT is somehow linked to blood group O. The hallmark characteristic of this disease is epistaxis, which may be profuse and usually begins in early childbirth. The classical telangiectatic lesions of HHT may not appear until later in life, commonly the second or third decade. The classic diagnostic traits of HHT are a hereditary basis, telangiectasia, and bleeding from telangiectatic lesions. Chronic blood loss, commonly from the GI tract, is often severe enough to be manifest as a significant iron deficiency anemia of unknown etiology. The telangiectatic lesions of HHT can be of three types: pinpoint, nodular, and spiderlike.[13] Unlike telangiectasia associated with chronic liver disease, those of HHT are nonpulsatile. Telangiectasia and bleeding usually increase with advancing age, although epistaxis often decreases. The bleeding of HHT may be an occult, but common, cause of gastrointestinal hemorrhage, genitourinary bleeding, hemoptysis (due to a rupture of an A-V fistula), or of heavy menstrual flow. Approximately 20% of patients develop A-V fistulae of the lung.[14] In addition, there is an inordinately high incidence of Laennec's type cirrhosis occurring in these patients. Hamartomata of the liver and spleen may be associated with HHT.[15]

The basic pathophysiology of this disorder is poorly understood. Most investigators agree that elastic fibers are missing from the vascular walls. There are few characteristic laboratory findings in HHT. The tourniquet test and template bleeding time may be normal or abnormal, depending upon the integrity of the vascular wall in the particular area where the test is performed. The diagnosis is suggested by a history of recurrent epistaxis, occult gastrointestinal bleeding, and the noting of pinpoint, nodular, or spiderlike telangiectasia, most commonly found in the skin, subungual areas, or buccal mucosal surface.

HHT appears to be closely associated with other defects in hemostasis. Abnormal platelet function is noted in many patients with HHT.[16,17] In addition, a poorly defined defect in the fibrinolytic system may occur in these patients.[18,19] Of major importance, many patients with HHT have an associated classical disseminated intravascular coagulation syndrome. This is usually present in a chronic form, but periodically may become acute. In some individuals, spontaneous hemarthroses develop. Thus HHT may be somewhat similar to the syndrome of giant cavernous hemangiomata and, indeed, a "mini" Kasabach-Merritt syndrome may develop. When this occurs, treatment should be aimed at acute or chronic DIC (see Chapter 8).

Therapy of uncomplicated HHT depends upon the particular clinical situation and the age of the patient. Localized epistaxis often can be controlled with local supportive measures and Neo-Synephrine®. However, electrocauterization may become necessary. Most instances of troublesome bleeding in HHT, such as gingival bleeding with toothbrushing, spontaneous bruising, and gastrointestinal/genitourinary bleeding, can often be controlled with Adrenosem®.[20] This agent is administered 5 to 10 mg orally every 3 to 4 hr during waking hours and is without significant toxicity.

High-dose estrogens may be used to scarify telangiectatic lesions and control bleeding. However, this should be used as a last resort, especially in younger patients.[21] Specific therapy for significant bleeding associated with congenital vascular defects, other than HHT, is generally not available and depends primarily upon supportive measures and control of the underlying disease process.

III. ACQUIRED VASCULAR DISORDERS

The acquired vascular disorders are far more common than inherited forms and should be suspected in individuals who develop a hemorrhagic diathesis manifest by petechiae and purpura and other forms of bleeding in the appropriate clinical setting.[1]

The acquired collagen diseases may all be associated with a significant vascular defect and, indeed, many may present as a hemorrhagic diathesis manifest by petechiae, purpura, or easy and spontaneous bruising. The common disorders are lupus erythematosis, dermatomyositis, scleroderma, rheumatoid arthritis, and polyarteritis nodosa.[22]

Cushing's syndrome is commonly associated with a vascular defect thought to arise from abnormal mucopolysaccharides in vascular supporting tissues. Patients with Cushing's syndrome often present with petechiae and purpura that are commonly dependent.[23]

TABLE 1

Vascular Disorders

Hereditary vascular disorders
  Ehler-Danlos syndrome
  Marfan's syndrome
  Osteogenesis imperfecta
  Pseudoxanthoma elasticum
  Hereditary hemorrhagic telangiectasia
Acquired vascular disorders
  Collagen vascular disorders
  Cushing's syndrome
  Macroglobulinemia
  Multiple myeloma
  Amyloidosis
  Allergic purpuras
  Autoerythrocytic sensitization syndrome
  Aspirin ingestion

The paraprotein disorders and amyloidosis may present as a vascular defect with petechiae and purpura.[24,25] It should be recalled that these disorders may also be associated with a significant functional platelet defect and the precise mechanism leading to petechiae, purpura, bruising, and bleeding may be difficult to define in these patients.

The so-called allergic purpuras include Henoch-Schonlein purpura, purpura simplex, purpura fulminans, and senile purpura. In these disorders, a template bleeding time and tourniquet test may be normal or abnormal.[26]

Perhaps the most common acquired vascular defect is that due to aspirin ingestion. It has been documented that aspirin interferes with platelet metabolic functions, thereby inducing a functional platelet defect that commonly leads to petechiae, purpura, and easy and spontaneous bruisability.[27] However, aspirin also interferes with vascular function. The acetyl group of ASA acts as an acetylcholine esterase inhibitor and this abolishes normal vasoconstrictive responses to microvascular injury.[28]

Autoerythrocytic sensitization syndrome presents as painful purpura, with pain often preceding appearance of purpura. The disorder is commonly seen in young females with a positive psychiatric history.[29,30] The proposed mechanism for development of purpura in these individuals is chronic subcutaneous extravasation of red cells via conscious or unconscious trauma to the skin. This is followed by sensitization to components of the patients' own red cells. A variant of this syndrome, sensitization to red cell nucleic acids, has been described. Successful therapy for autoerythrocytic sensitization has been limited to psychiatric support. Individuals with other vascular disorders and chronic extravasation of red cells can also develop a type of autoerythrocytic sensitization, presumably from the same mechanism as outlined above.

The above are the most common disorders associated with acquired vascular defects. When presented with a patient manifesting unexplained petechiae, purpura, or easy and spontaneous bruisability, the presence of one of the above primary diseases should be considered.

Table 1 summarizes the common hereditary and acquired vascular defects.

REFERENCES

1. **Bick, R. L. and Shanbrom, E.**, A systematic approach to the diagnosis of bleeding disorders, *Med. Counterpoint,* 4, 27, 1972.
2. **Johnson, S. A. and Falls, E. F.**, Ehlers-syndrome: a clinical and genetic study, *Arch. Dermatol. Suppl.,* 60 (Suppl.), 82, 1949.
3. **Roberts, H. R. and Kroncke, F. G.**, Tests of platelet activity: application to clinical diagnosis, in *The Platelet,* Brinkhous, K. W., Shermer, R. W., and Mostofi, F. K., Eds., Williams & Wilkins, Baltimore, 1971.
4. **Pinnell, S. R., Krane, S. M., Kenzora, J., and Glincher, M. J.**, A new hereditable disorder of connective tissue with hydroxylysine-deficient collagen, *N. Engl. J. Med.,* 286, 1013, 1972.
5. **Futcher, P. H. and Southworth, H.**, Arachnodactyly and its medical complications, *Arch. Intern. Med.,* 61, 693, 1938.
6. **Anderson, M. and Pratt-Thomas, R. H.**, Marfan's syndrome, *Am. Heart J.,* 46, 911, 1953.
7. **Seibel, B. M., Briedman, I. A., and Schwartz, S. O.**, Hemorrhagic disease in osteogenesis imperfecta: study of platelet function defect, *Am. J. Med.,* 22, 315, 1957.
8. **Polimer, I. J.**, Pseudoxanthoma elasticum and gastrointestinal bleeding, *J. Maine Med. Assoc.,* 58, 76, 1967.
9. **Osler, W.**, On multiple hereditary telangiectasia with recurrent hemorrhages, *Q. J. Med.,* 1, 53, 1907.
10. **Osler, W.**, On telangiectasia circumscripta universalis, *Bull. Johns Hopkins Hosp.,* 18, 401, 1907.
11. **Hans, F. M.**, Multiple hereditary telangiectasia causinghemorrhage (hereditary hemorrhagic telangiectasia), *Bull. Johns Hopkins Hosp.,* 20, 63, 1909.
12. **Harrison, D. F. N.**, Familial haemorrhagic telangiectasia, *Q. J. Med.,* 33, 25, 1964.
13. **Osler, W.**, On a family form of recurring epistaxis, associated with telangiectasia of the skin and mucous membranes, *Johns Hopkins Med. Bull.,* 12, 333, 1901.
14. **Hodgsom, C. H. and Kaye, R. L.**, Pulmonary arteriovenous fistula and hereditary hemorrhagic telangiectasia, *Dis. Chest,* 43, 449, 1963.
15. **Fitz-Hugh, T.**, Splenomegaly and hepatic enlargement in hereditary hemorrhagic telangiectasia, *Am. J. Med. Sci.,* 181, 261, 1931.
16. **Bick, R. L. and Fekete, L. F.**, Hereditary hemorrhagic telangiectasia and associated thrombohemorrhagic diseases, *Thromb. Haemostasis,* 38, 179, 1977.
17. **Quick, A. L.**, Telangiectasia, in *Hemorrhagic Diseases and Thrombosis,* Lea & Febiger, Philadelphia, 1966.
18. **McDervitt, T. J. and Toh, A. S.**, Epistaxis: management and prevention, *The Laryngoscope,* 47, 1109, 1967.
19. **Ryan, A. J.**, Control of bleeding in familial telangiectasia, *Meriden Hosp. Bull.,* 7, 1, 1958.
20. **Stich, M. H.**, Carbazochrome salicylate therapy in hereditary hemorrhagic telangiectasia, *N. Y. State J. Med.,* 59, 2725, 1959.
21. **Koch, H. J., Escher, G. L., and Lewis, J. S.**, Hormonal management of hereditary hemorrhagic telangiectasia, *JAMA,* 149, 1376, 1952.
22. **Sheps, S. C.**, Vasculitis, in *Peripheral Vascular Diseases,* Fairbairn, J. F., Juergens, J. L., and Spittel, S. A., Eds., W.B. Saunders, Philadelphia, 1972, 18.
23. **Forsham, P. H.**, The adrenal cortex, in *Textbook of Endocrinology,* Williams, R. H., Ed., W.B. Saunders, Philadelphia, 1968.
24. **Lackner, H.**, Hemostatic abnormalities associated with paraprotein abnormalities, *Semin. Hematol.,* 10, 125, 1973.
25. **Bick, R. L., Klein, C. A., Fekete, L. F., and Wilson, W. L.**, Alterations of hemostasis associated with malignant paraprotein disorders, *Trans. Am. Soc. Hematol.,* p. 167, 1976.
26. **Taylor, J. R. and Kellum, R. E.**, Anaphylactoid purpura, in *Immunological Diseases,* Vol. 2, Sempter, M., Ed., Little, Brown, Boston, 1971.
27. **Quick, A. J.**, Hemostasis and thrombosis: a new look, *Minn. Med.,* 50, 1333, 1967.
28. **Cohen, L. S.**, The clinical pharmacology of acetylsalicylic acid, in *Thrombosis, Platelets, Anticoagulation and Acetylsalicylic Acid,* Domoso, E. and Haft, J. I., Eds., Stratton Medical, New York, 1976.
29. **Gardner, F. N. and Diamond, L. K.**, Autoerthrocytic sensitization, *Blood,* 10, 675, 1955.
30. **Hersle, K. and Mobacken, H.**, Autoerthrocyte sensitization syndrome, *Br. J. Dermatol.,* 81, 574, 1969.

Chapter 6

PLATELET DISORDERS

Douglas Triplett

TABLE OF CONTENTS

Introduction 97

PART 1: Qualitative Disorders of Platelet Function — Inherited
I.   Disorders of Adhesion 99
     A.   von Willebrand's Syndrome 99
          1.   Pathophysiology 99
          2.   Clinical Features 104
          3.   Laboratory Diagnosis 105
          4.   Therapy 106
     B.   Acquired von Willebrand's Syndrome 107
     C.   Bernard-Soulier Syndrome 108
          1.   Pathophysiology 108
          2.   Clinical Features 109
          3.   Laboratory Diagnosis 109
          4.   Therapy 109
     D.   Impaired Adhesion To Collagen 109

II. Disorders of Primary Aggregation 110
     A.   Glanzmann's Thrombasthenia 110
          1.   Pathophysiology 110
          2.   Clinical Features 111
          3.   Laboratory Diagnosis 111
          4.   Therapy 111
     B.   Essential Athrombia 111

III. Disorders of Secondary Aggregation 111
     A.   Storage Pool Disease 111
          1.   Pathophysiology 112
          2.   Clinical Features 113
          3.   Laboratory Diagnosis 114
          4.   Therapy 114
     B.   "Aspirin-Like" Defect 114
          1.   Pathophysiology 115
          2.   Clinical Features 115
          3.   Laboratory Diagnosis 115
          4.   Therapy 116
     C.   Defects of Release Reaction and Factor VIII 116

IV. Platelet Factor 3 Deficiency 116

V.   Platelet Abnormalities Associated With Other Congenital Defects 116

        A. Giant Platelets Associated With Renal Dysfunction 116
        B. May-Hegglin Anomaly 117
        C. Hereditary Disorders of Connective Tissue and Mucopolysaccharidosis 117
        D. Glycogen Storage Disease 117
        E. Afibrinogenemia 117

VI. Miscellaneous 117

PART 2: Acquired Qualitative Platelet Disorders
I. Uremia 118
        A. Pathophysiology 118
        B. Clinical Features 119
        C. Laboratory Diagnosis 119
        D. Therapy 119

II. Qualitative Platelet Disorders Associated with Myeloproliferative Syndromes 119

III. Dysproteinemia 119

IV. Qualitative Platelet Defects in Patients with Antibodies to Platelets 120

V. Scurvy 120

VI. Cyanotic Congenital Heart Disease 120

VII. Cirrhosis 120

VIII. Drugs 120

PART 3: Quantitative Abnormalities of Platelets — Thrombocytopenia
I. Thrombocytopenia 122
        A. Platelet Production 122
        B. Platelet Kinetics 124
        C. Platelet Count 125
        D. Pathophysiology of Thrombocytopenia 126

II. Amegakaryocytic Thrombocytopenias 126
        A. Congenital Hypoplasia 126
        B. Acquired Hypoplasia 128
        C. Bone Marrow Infiltration 128

III. Megakaryocytic Thrombocytopenias 128
        A. Ineffective Thrombopoiesis 129
        B. Altered Distribution of Platelets 129
        C. Nonimmunologic Destructive Thrombocytopenias 129
        D. Immunologic Thrombocytopenias 130
                1. Isoimmune Thrombocytopenia 130
                2. Drug-Induced Immunologic Thrombocytopenic Purpura 130
                3. Posttransfusion Thrombocytopenia Due to Isoantibodies 131
                4. Other Immunologic Thrombocytopenias 131
                5. Idiopathic Thrombocytopenic Purpura 131

PART 4: Quantitative Disorders of Platelets — Thrombocytosis and Thrombocythemia

I. Thrombocytosis 135

II. Thrombocythemia 137

References 138

INTRODUCTION

Until recently, of the three components of hemostasis, platelet function was probably the least understood, and therapy of platelet disorders was often inadequately managed. However, the key role of the platelet in hemostasis, probably the most essential biologic defense mechanism in the higher forms of life, has made this cell the major focus of study in hemorrhagic and thrombotic diseases in recent years. As a result, a number of new laboratory procedures have been developed to evaluate the platelet's contribution to hemostasis, the inflammatory and immunologic responses, and its possible importance in the pathogenesis of atherosclerosis. Also, the subject of platelet pharmacology has become a center of intensive research in the hope of developing new drugs for the control of thrombosis and atherosclerosis.

Phylogenetically, the platelet represents the earliest component of the hemostatic system. An excellent example is the horseshoe crab *(Limulus)*, a species that has been in existence for some 300,000,000 years, in which cells analogous to platelets (amebocytes) are the only cellular elements in the blood.[1] Donne, in 1842, published the first clear description of platelets.[2] He felt that they might represent derivatives from chyle or perhaps precursors of leukocytes. Forty years later, Bizzozero identified platelets as cells distinct from erythrocytes and leukocytes.[3] The contribution of the platelet to the body's defense against vascular injury was first described in 1886 by Eberth and Schimmelbusch.[4] It was not until 1906 that the origin of platelets from the megakaryocytes of the bone marrow was recognized by Wright.[5] In the ensuing seventy years, the platelet has remained a fertile source of study for anatomists, physiologists, biochemists, and clinicians.

Disorders of platelet sunction are somewhat difficult to classify, because of the rarity of many forms and the numerous incompletely studied cases. Consequently, considerable nosologic confusion still surrounds this field. In this chapter, the inherited and acquired qualitative abnormalities of platelet function will be discussed, as well as the thrombocytopenic states and the various clinical states associated with an increased platelet count. Major emphasis will be placed upon the disorders in which a clear understanding of the pathophysiology has been elucidated. The various hereditary and acquired abnormalities of platelet function in which the underlying defects are poorly understood will be briefly reviewed.

PART 1: QUALITATIVE DISORDERS OF PLATELET FUNCTION — INHERITED

Qualitative disorders of platelets are quite common if the many acquired dysfunctional platelet states are included. A qualitative disorder of platelets should be sus-

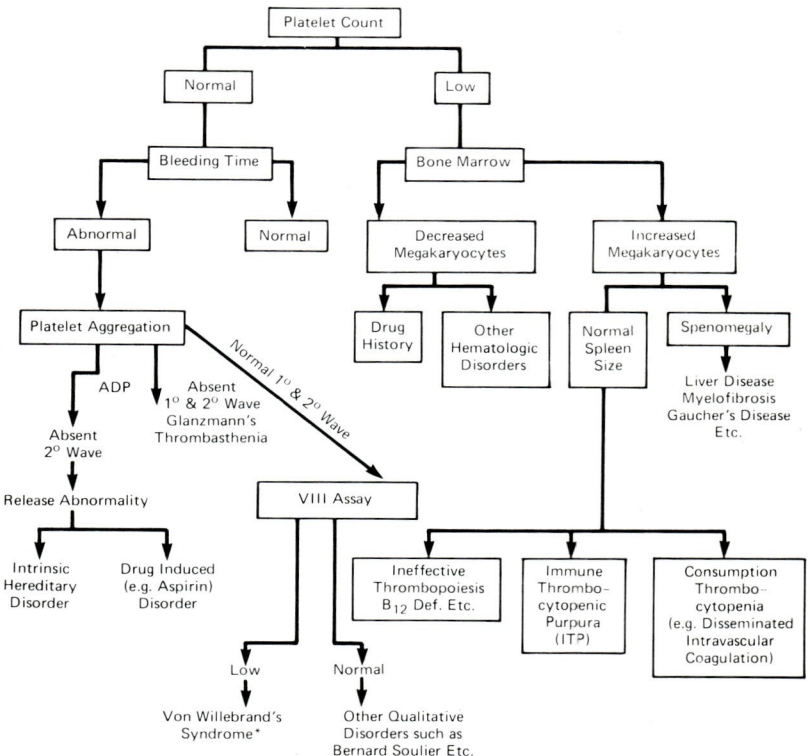

FIGURE 1. Flow diagram for diagnosis of platelet disorders. (From Triplett, D. A., *Platelet Function: Laboratory Evaluation and Clinical Application,* Triplett, D. A., Ed., American Society of Clinical Pathologists, Chicago, 1978. With permission.)

pected if there is some clinical or laboratory evidence of platelet dysfunction (i.e., laboratory evidence such as a long bleeding time or clinical evidence such as recurrent mucosal bleeding, easy bruising, menorrhagia, etc.) in the face of a *normal platelet count.* In Figure 1, a flow diagram for the diagnosis of both qualitative and quantitative abnormalities of platelet function is illustrated. A platelet count is the first step in evaluating platelet function. In the presence of a decreased platelet count, the etiology of the thrombocytopenia should be determined, and the first appropriate laboratory procedure would be a bone marrow study. In contrast, the presence of a normal platelet count together with clinical symptomatology of platelet dysfunction would indicate the performance of a bleeding time as the next procedure in the diagnostic workup. The subsequent steps in the laboratory evaluation are outlined leading to specific diagnoses.

In the past, the terms thrombocytopathia or thrombopathia (literally, an abnormal thrombus) were used in the broadest sense to identify any bleeding disorder in which a defect in platelet function was found, other than the type of defect seen in Glanzmann's disease.[6] In addition, some authors used both of these terms to refer to patients who had abnormalities in platelet factor 3 availability. As a result, a review of the older literature in the field of platelet dysfunction is rather difficult because of the poorly defined terms. The early investigators independently devised methods of studying platelet function and created new terms with which to describe their results. However, very little communication seems to have occurred among research groups, and both terminology and methodology proliferated. Most of the patients described prior to 1967 were diagnosed by demonstrating abnormalities in platelet factor 3 assays. However, with the introduction of platelet aggregation using an aggregometer and the other laboratory procedures for evaluating platelet functions, such as retention in glass-bead columns, ADP content, ristocetin-induced aggregation, etc., patients can now be more comprehensively evaluated and their qualitative abnormalities better classified.[7] Therefore, the terms thrombopathia and thrombocytopathia should be discarded because of their past association with abnormalities of platelet factor 3.

There have been a number of classifications proposed for qualitative abnormalities of platelet function. In Table 1, the various disorders are classified in two major groups: hereditary and acquired.

It will be noted that disorders of platelet function may be associated with a wide variety of disease states. Despite the recent advances in laboratory evaluation, the functional abnormality in many cases is still poorly understood. Thus much work remains to be done in identifying and classifying qualitative abnormalities of platelet function.

I. DISORDERS OF ADHESION

A. von Willebrand's Syndrome

In 1926, von Willebrand first reported a familial bleeding disorder in a group of patients studied on the Aland Islands in the Gulf of Bothnia between Finland and Sweden.[8] The first patient was a 5 year old girl with a history of severe bleeding. The family history was also strikingly positive in that four of her seven sisters had died of intractable hemorrhage. von Willebrand subsequently studied the entire family and found that 23 of 66 identified members gave a positive history for bleeding abnormalities.[9] The type of bleeding was primarily mucosal, and the affected family members were found to have prolonged bleeding times. However, their platelet counts were found to be normal; therefore, it was postulated that their platelets and blood vessels were abnormal, thus accounting for their clinical bleeding. Of the affected family members, women outnumbered men two to one and tended to have more severe clinical bleeding. Consequently, von Willebrand suggested that the abnormality was inherited as a sex-linked dominant trait. However, subsequent studies have led to the conclusion that it is inherited as an autosomal dominant trait.*

1. Pathophysiology

von Willebrand reevaluated these patients in 1933 by means of a capillary "thrombometer."[10] This test measured the duration of liquidity when whole blood was pumped back and forth in a capillary tube. Since it was normal in hemophiliac patients, and abnormal in the Aland Island patients, von Willebrand and Jurgens[10] concluded that the bleeding was a consequence of a "constitutional thrombopathy". The diagnosis for the next 20 years was based on a long bleeding time together with a normal platelet count and a normal whole blood clotting time with an autosomal pattern of inheritance. In 1953, Alexander and Goldstein noted that patients with von Willebrand's syndrome had a reduced Factor VIII activity.[11] Other investigators soon reported similar patients with low Factor VIII activity and prolonged bleeding times, and it became apparent that von Willebrand's syndrome was a relatively common bleeding disorder.[12] In the mid 1950s it was recognized that transfusion was effective in treating these patients.[11] Both the prolonged bleeding times and the low Factor VIII

---

* Recently autosomal recessive forms have been described

TABLE 1

Hereditary and Acquired Qualitative Platelet Disorders

Hereditary

I. Abnormalities of platelet adhesiveness
    A. Bernard-Soulier syndrome
    B. von Willebrand's syndrome
    C. Impaired adhesion to collagen
        1. Platelet membrane abnormality
        2. Intrinsic collagen abnormality
II. Abnormalities of primary aggregation
    A. Glanzmann's thrombasthenia
    B. Essential athrombia
III. Abnormalities of secondary aggregation
    A. Storage pool disease
        1. Wiskott-Aldrich syndrome
        2. Thrombocytopenia with absent radii
        3. Hermansky-Pudlak syndrome
        4. Chediak-Higashi syndrome
    B. "Aspirin-like" defect
        1. Cyclo-oxygenase deficiency
        2. Thromboxane synthetase deficiency
    C. Other hereditary diseases with platelet "release" abnormalities
        1. May-Hegglin anomaly
        2. Glycogen storage disease (Type 1)
        3. Ehlers-Danlos syndrome
        4. Pseudoxanthoma elasticum
        5. Marfan's syndrome
        6. Osteogenesis imperfecta
        7. Hurler's syndrome
        8. Hunter's syndrome
IV. Isolated deficiency of platelet factor 3
    A. Glucose-6 — phosphate dehydrogenase deficiency
V. Disorders of platelet function associated with plasma coagulation factor deficiency
    A. Afibrinogenemia
    B. Factor VIII deficiency
    C. Factor IX deficiency
VI. Miscellaneous
    A. Giant platelet syndrome with renal dysfunction

Acquired

I. Uremia
II. Myeloproliferative disorders
    A. Hemorrhagic thrombocythemia
    B. Myeloid metaplasia with myelofibrosis
    C. Polycythemia rubra vera
    D. Acute myelocytic leukemia
    E. Di Guglielmo's syndrome
    F. Paroxysmal nocturnal hemoglobinuria
    G. Preleukemic syndromes
    H. Sideroblastic anemias
III. Immunoproliferative disorders
    A. Waldenstrom's macroglobulinemia
    B. Plasma cell myeloma
IV. Antiplatelet antibodies
    A. Idiopathic thrombocytopenic purpura
    B. Systemic lupus erythematosus
V. Presence of fibrin(ogen) split products
    A. Cirrhosis
    B. Disseminated intravascular coagulation

TABLE 1 (continued)

Hereditary and Acquired Qualitative Platelet Disorders

Acquired

VI. Associated with anemias
    A. Pernicious anemia
    B. Iron deficiency anemia
VII. Drug-induced disorders
    A. Anti-inflammatory agents (e.g., aspirin)
    B. Antidepressants
    C. Adrenergic blocking agents
    D. Miscellaneous (e.g., papaverine and dextran)
VIII. Cyanotic congenital heart disease (?)
IX. Leukemic reticuloendotheliosis (hairy cell leukemia)
X. Scurvy

activities were corrected after the infusion of blood, plasma, or plasma fractions. The results of these experiments indicated that the impaired hemostasis in von Willebrand's syndrome was the result of a plasma factor deficiency. The Factor VIII response after transfusion in von Willebrand's disease was, however, distinctly different from that of hemophilia A. Peak Factor VIII levels were noted several hours after infusion was completed, rather than immediately, and the elevation persisted several days.[13] In 1961, Borchgrevink noted that in blood issuing from bleeding time wounds there was a failure of the platelet count to progressively decrease.[14] He proposed an abnormality in platelet adhesion as an explanation for this observation. In 1963, Salzman noted that when platelets were passed through a column of glass-beads there was reduced platelet "adhesiveness" in patients with von Willebrand's syndrome.[15] Thus in the mid 1960s the tetrad for the diagnosis of von Willebrand's syndrome was: prolonged bleeding time, decreased Factor VIII activity, decreased platelet retention in glass-bead columns, and an autosomal dominant pattern of inheritance.

With progress in purifying the Factor VIII protein, immunochemical studies became possible. Zimmerman, Ratnoff, and Powell were the first to prepare a satisfactory rabbit factor VIII antibody with good specificity.[16] Immunoprecipitation and antibody neutralization studies using this antibody demonstrated that classic hemophilia A plasmas contained normal quantities of Factor VIII-related antigen. In contrast, the Factor VIII-related antigen levels in plasmas from patients with von Willebrand's syndrome were reduced in parallel with the Factor VIII activity.[17] These observations indicated that hemophiliac patients synthesize normal amounts of a nonfunctional Factor VIII-like protein, but synthesis of Factor VIII protein is reduced in von Willebrand's syndrome.

In 1971, Howard and Firkin introduced ristocetin as another tool in the diagnosis of von Willebrand's syndrome.[18] Ristocetin is an antibiotic that was found to aggregate platelets and cause severe thrombocytopenia in vivo.[19] Ristocetin was found to induce platelet aggregation in normal patients, but not in patients with von Willebrand's syndrome. Further study established a defective or reduced plasma component in these patients, which was a necessary cofactor for ristocetin-induced aggregation. The platelets of von Willebrand's syndrome were entirely normal when this plasma component was added to platelet-rich plasma.[20] Subsequently, an assay measuring this plasma factor was reported.[21]

The rapid accumulation of information about Factor VIII has led to a number of different terminologies for components of the Factor VIII complex. Table 2 provides a summary of the various terms that have been suggested for components of the Factor VIII complex, as well as a shorthand designation for the various properties.

Recently, Baumgartner devised an in vitro system to evaluate the interaction of pla-

TABLE 2

Properties of the Factor VIII Complex

Designation	Abbreviation	Other designations
Factor VIII procoagulant activity (as measured by modified APTT)	VIII_C	Antihemophilic factor
Factor VIII — related antigen (as measured by Rocket immunoelectrophoresis)	VIII_{Ag_n}	AHF antigen von Willebrand's disease Antigen
von Willebrand's factor (plasma activity that will correct a platelet function defect in von Willebrand's disease)	VIII_{VWF}	Vascular factor
(1) Factor that supports Ristocetin-induced aggregation of washed normal platelets (in vitro) (2) Factor that corrects glass-bead retention of blood (in vitro) (3) Factor that corrects subendothelial adhesion in Baumgartner procedure (in vitro) (4) Necessary for normal bleeding time (in vivo)	VWF_R	

telets with damaged blood vessel walls.[22] The endothelial cell lining of a rabbit aorta is removed by a balloon catheter and segments of this vessel are then exposed to blood flow in in vitro chambers under conditions of controlled perfusion. Platelet adhesion and aggregation to this surface are then determined by both light and electron microscopy. Tschopp, Weiss, and Baumgartner detected a consistent decrease in platelet adhesion to the subendothelium when citrated blood of patients with von Willebrand's syndrome is tested in this system.[23] However, platelet aggregation (i.e., platelet-platelet interaction) in these patients was entirely normal. These findings suggest that the prolonged bleeding time in patients with von Willebrand's syndrome may be due to a defect in adhesion of platelets to an element of the damaged vessel wall. Normal plasma or Factor VIII concentrates were able to normalize that platelet adhesion in this in vitro test system, again indicating that the platelets were intrinsically normal, but the patients lacked a plasma factor necessary for adhesion.

Recent investigations have emphasized the importance of the endothelial cell in the biology of the Factor VIII complex. Immunofluorescence studies performed on a variety of human tissues with a monospecific rabbit antihuman Factor VIII antibody have demonstrated that, in vivo, only endothelial cells, platelets, and megakaryocytes contain Factor VIII-related antigen.[24] These results are very exciting because the site of Factor VIII antigen synthesis previously was unknown. Endothelial cell cultures have also been established, and these have been found to release Factor VIII antigen

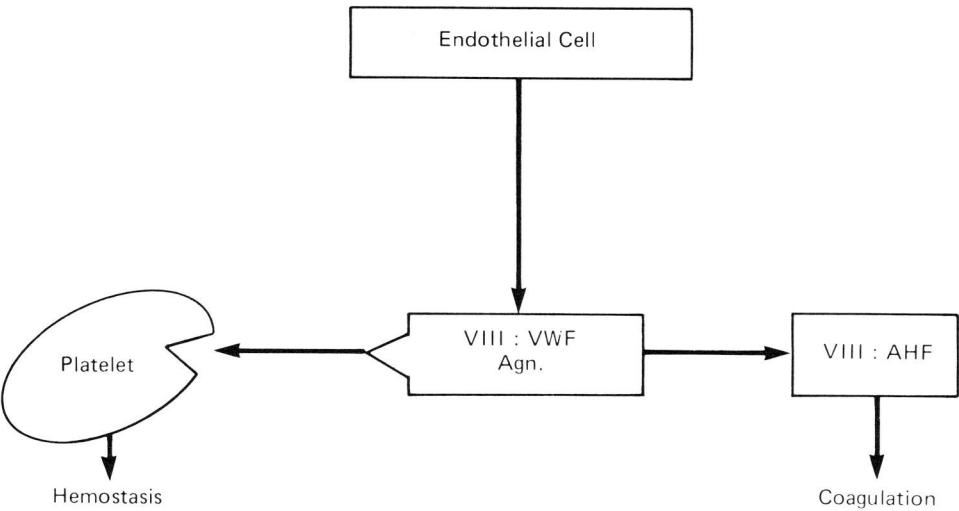

FIGURE 2. Hypothesis of the relationship of the endothelial cell to components of Factor VIII.[29] (From Jaffe, E. A., *N. Engl. J. Med.*, 296, 377, 1977. With permission.)

into the culture supernatant.[25] Further studies using Sepharose 4 B® chromatography and immunodiffusion analysis have revealed that the antigen released is identical to the normal Factor VIII antigen present in plasma.[26] Studies in patients with severe von Willebrand's syndrome have shown that these patients have very little or no Factor VIII antigen in their endothelial cells and platelets.[27] These data strongly suggest that endothelial cells are the major site of synthesis of plasma Factor VIII antigen in vivo and that classic von Willebrand's syndrome results from the failure of these cells to synthesize and release Factor VIII antigen and von Willebrand Factor. Furthermore, it has been found that the endothelial cells do not synthesize the portion of the Factor VIII molecule necessary for coagulant activity.[28] There are at least two possible explanations for the absence of the Factor VIII procoagulant activity.[29] One may be that the endothelial cells synthesize an inactive precursor molecule that contains only the antigen and von Willebrand Factor and that a conversion is necessary to produce the procoagulant activity at a second site. The second hypothesis suggests that the endothelial cells synthesize a molecule that contains the antigen and the von Willebrand Factor, and this acts as a carrier for a different molecule that contains the Factor VIII procoagulant activity. The proposed relationship of the endothelial cells to components of the Factor VIII complex is illustrated in Figure 2.[29]

Over the past several years a number of variants of von Willebrand's syndrome have been reported and reviewed (Table 3).[30] In these variants, there may be selective and sometimes discordant decreases in the various components of Factor VIII complex. For example, in some patients the antigen is present in normal amounts; however, the von Willebrand Factor is decreased. Electrophoresis with sodium dodecyl sulfate gels have shown that the Factor VIII antigen migrated normally, but lacked carbohydrate; these patients also had decreased von Willebrand Factor.[31] Other abnormalities in the Factor VIII antigen have been demonstrated by crossed immunoelectrophoresis.[32] Thus these variant syndromes may be caused by an alteration in the type or quantity of carbohydrate or perhaps amino acid substitution in the Factor VIII molecule, rather than an absence of the Factor VIII protein. The severity and type of clinical defect would depend on the degree of deficiency or abnormality in the Factor VIII complex (antigen and von Willebrand Factor).[33]

TABLE 3

Variants of von Willebrand's Syndrome

Laboratory characteristics	Type 1	Type 2	Type 3	Type 4	Type 5	Type 6
Factor VIII$_c$	Decreased	Variable decreased to normal	Normal	Decreased	Decreased	Decreased
Factor VIII-related antigen	Decreased	Normal	Decreased	Normal	Normal	Decreased
von Willebrand factor	Decreased	Decreased	Decreased	Decreased	Decreased	Normal
Ristocetin-induced aggregation	Decreased	Decreased	Usually normal	Normal	Normal	Variable decreased to normal
Miscellaneous	Largest group; classical von Willebrand			? Sex linked		

Recent evidence indicates that in persons heterozygous for von Willebrand's syndrome, the Factor VIII procoagulant activity levels may be proportionately increased over the Factor VIII antigen concentrations.[34] This finding would be analogous to the situation in carriers of hemophilia in whom antigen levels exceed procoagulant activity measurements. These observations again confirm that the Factor VIII antigen and Factor VIII procoagulant activity are under independent genetic control. If these observations prove to be consistent, one would then be able to more thoroughly investigate the genetics of this syndrome.

2. Clinical Features

von Willebrand's syndrome represents a heterogenous group of patients — genetically, pathophysiologically, and clinically.[35] Following von Willebrand's original description, it quickly became apparent that the frequency of this disorder was greater than that of classic hemophilia A. The clinical picture is dominated by cutaneous and mucosal bleeding, although in the severely affected patients hemarthroses and dissecting intramuscular hematomas may develop.[36] Serious hemorrhages due to traumatic injuries or following surgical procedures represent a significant hazard in many patients.[37] Early in life, epistaxis is the most common symptom. Bleeding from the gums is also prominent, and shedding of deciduous teeth is often accompanied by troublesome bleeding. Menorrhagia occurs regularly and occasionally patients may have severe post partum hemorrhage, which may be fatal. Gastrointestinal bleeding and hematuria have also been described. Recently, an association between von Willebrand's syndrome and hereditary hemorrhagic telangiectasia has been emphasized.[38] In these patients, gastrointestinal hemorrhage is a prominent clinical feature.

Common symptoms of von Willebrand's syndrome: easy bruising, epistaxis, and menorrhagia may occur in patients who have no other apparent abnormality of hemostasis. It is therefore important for the clinician to suspect the disease in patients with mild bleeding problems and to evaluate their clinical and family history carefully. In the past, many male patients have been misdiagnosed as having mild hemophilia A, when in fact they suffered from von Willebrand's syndrome.

Many investigators have noted that the disease may decrease in severity with advancing age.[37] This is particularly true with respect to epistaxis. Also, during pregnancy, when the Factor VIII level rises significantly, the bleeding symptoms may become milder.[39]

3. Laboratory Diagnosis

Because of the many variants of von Willebrand's syndrome, the laboratory diagnosis may be extremely difficult and require a number of specialized procedures that are not available in the routine coagulation laboratory. Of the routine tests, both the bleeding time and the activated partial thromboplastin time (APTT) may be abnormal. The abnormality in the APTT reflects the slight to moderate reduction in the Factor VIII procoagulant activity. Plasma Factor VIII procoagulant activity may vary greatly. In the majority of patients the activity ranges from 5 to 15% of normal; however, values of 30% are not uncommon, and, occasionally, in the severe patient, one may find levels of 1 to 2% activity.[37] It is important to emphasize that Factor VIII activity may be extremely labile. As discussed above, there is a progressive increase in the Factor VIII activity as well as the Factor VIII antigen in normal women during pregnancy. This is also seen in women with von Willebrand's syndrome.[40] Women treated with oral contraceptives may also have increased Factor VIII activity.[41] In addition, such diverse situations as acute stress, vigorous exercise, epinephrine infusion, and active bleeding may elevate the Factor VIII activity (Table 4).[42] The latter point is of particular importance. A consultation is often requested on the patient who has active gastrointestinal bleeding and in whom a hemorrhagic diathesis is suspected. In addition to the stress of acute hemorrhage, these patients may have received blood transfusions prior to the consultation and consequently the Factor VIII level may have increased in response to stress and transfusion and appear spuriously normal.

In severe cases, both the Duke and Ivy bleeding times are prolonged.[43] However, because of its insensitivity, the Duke bleeding time procedure is no longer recommended. The Ivy bleeding time and template bleeding time modification are much more sensitive than the Duke procedure and are more characteristically prolonged in patients with von Willebrand's syndrome.[44] Aspirin, which will prolong the normal bleeding time slightly, often has a pronounced effect in a patient with von Willebrand's syndrome.[45] Quick thinks that the "aspirin tolerance test" is one of the more important diagnostic criteria.[46]

Decreased platelet retention in glass-bead columns has also proved to be a valuable diagnostic tool in the von Willebrand syndrome.[47] However, there have been many difficulties in reproducibility and standardization of the glass-bead retention assays. Variables in this procedure include the choice of anticoagulant, the way the blood is handled after venipuncture, the time interval between doing the venipuncture and assay, type of glass beads used, the plastic tubing, and the blood flow rate.[48] The original Salzman method, in which blood flowed directly from the vein through a glass-bead column into a vacutainer, has fallen into disfavor primarily because of the variability of the flow rate. Currently, the modification of Bowie et al., in which an infusion pump is used is the most popular procedure.[49] With the appropriate precautions, a decrease in platelet retention has proved to be a valuable tool in the diagnosis of von Willebrand's syndrome. However, it should be emphasized that there are a number of other disorders in which decreased glass-bead retention will be found. These include thrombasthenia,[50] storage pool disease, defective nucleotide release, uremia,[51] valvular heart disease,[52] disseminated intravascular coagulation, myeloproliferative disorders, and afibrinogenemia.

Ristocetin-induced platelet aggregation is characteristically absent in patients with severe von Willebrand's syndrome. Low and normal aggregation tracings, however, have been recognized in individuals with mild disease.[53] It has also been noted that the ristocetin aggregation pattern can be corrected by adding normal platelet-poor plasma to the patient's platelet-rich plasma.

Quantitative assays for the von Willebrand factor have been developed using normal washed platelets and ristocetin-induced aggregation. In this procedure, there is a dose-

TABLE 4

Physiologic and Pathologic Causes of Increased Factor VIII Activity (VIII_c)

Transient
    Adrenaline infusion
    Exercise
    Fever
    Surgery
    Oral contraceptives
    Pregnancy
    Prednisone
    After cessation of Coumarin type anticoagulants
    Hyperthyroidism
    Cushing's syndrome
    Following pneumoencephalography
    Following hypoglycemia
Permanent
    Plasma cell myeloma
    Advancing age
    Males
    Blood Group A
    Diabetes mellitus
    Coronary artery disease
    Menopause

response pattern reflecting the amount of von Willebrand factor present in the plasma. Concentrations of the von Willebrand factor in test plasmas are compared with pooled normal plasma standards. However, washing platelets is laborious, and the procedure has not gained popularity in most diagnostic coagulation laboratories.[54] Other modifications using formaldehyde-fixed platelets in place of freshly washed platelets and the use of platelets that have undergone gel filtration have been proposed.[55]

It should also be emphasized that there are certain other situations in which one may encounter abnormal ristocetin-induced aggregation. These include: infectious mononucleosis, idiopathic thrombocytopenic purpura, acute leukemia, and the Bernard-Soulier syndrome.[56] In addition, aspirin has been reported as affecting ristocetin-induced aggregation.

The use of rabbit antibodies to Factor VIII-related antigen has aided immensely in the diagnosis of patients with von Willebrand's syndrome. As was previously discussed, these patients have a parallel decrease in the Factor VIII-related antigen together with the Factor VIII procoagulant activity, as assayed by the modified activated partial thromboplastin time.[57] This is in contrast to the classic hemophilia A patient in whom one finds a normal Factor VIII-related antigen and a decreased Factor VIII procoagulant activity (Table 5). A number of assay systems have been developed, including rocket immunoelectrophoresis, radioimmunoassays, and immunoradiometric assays (IRMA) as well as hemagglutination inhibition procedures.[58,59] Also, with the recognition of variants of the von Willebrand syndrome, crossed immunoelectrophoresis has been used.

The laboratory findings in the classical case of von Willebrand's syndrome include: decreased Factor VIII procoagulant activity, decreased platelet retention in glass-bead columns, prolonged bleeding time, decreased ristocetin-induced aggregation, and a parallel decrease in the Factor VIII-related antigen.

4. Therapy

The original investigators in the field found that the infusion of human plasma frac-

TABLE 5

Laboratory and Clinical Features of von Willebrand's Syndrome and Hemophilia A

	von Willebrand's syndrome	Hemophilia A (VIII deficiency)
Pattern of inheritance	Autosomal dominant	Sex-linked recessive
Bleeding time	Prolonged	Normal
Factor VIII_C	Decreased	Decreased
Factor VIII_{Ag^n}	Decreased	Normal
Factor VIII_{vWF}	Decreased	Normal
Platelet retention	Decreased	Normal
Clinical picture	Mucosal bleeding (epistaxis, GI bleeding, etc.); easy bruising	Intra-articular and deep muscle hemorrhages

tions corrected the abnormal bleeding time and increased the Factor VIII procoagulant activity in patients with von Willebrand's syndrome.[60] Subsequently, similar observations were made following cryoprecipitate infusions. These infusions produce a gradual and sustained rise in the coagulant Factor VIII activity of the recipient, which reaches a plateau in 6 to 20 hr and persists for 48 to 72 hr. The Factor VIII levels that are attained cannot be attributed to the Factor VIII present in the infused plasma, since comparable results may be obtained with plasma deficient in Factor VIII and even with normal serum. In 1967, Perkins demonstrated that the infusion of commercial concentrates of Factor VIII, although raising the Factor VIII procoagulant levels, failed to correct the prolonged bleeding time of patients with von Willebrand's syndrome.[61] Recent investigators have examined not only the Factor VIII procoagulant and Factor VIII antigen responses, but also the response of the Factor VIII-ristocetin cofactor.[62] The results of these studies have indicated that there is frequently a disassociation between the Factor VIII procoagulant activity, Factor VIII-ristocetin cofactor activity, and Factor VIII antigen. Although one may see a sustained increase in the Factor VIII procoagulant activity, there is a more rapid disappearance of the Factor VIII-related antigen and an even quicker disappearance of the Factor VIII-ristocetin cofactor. The Factor VIII-ristocetin cofactor has a half disappearance time of approximately 18 hr, in contrast to the Factor VIII procoagulant activity of 48 hr and the Factor VIII-related antigen of 30 to 37 hr (Figure 3). Although Factor VIII concentrates will increase the Factor VIII procoagulant activity, they fail to correct the bleeding time and the Factor VIII-ristocetin cofactor activity.

Based on these observations, the current recommendation for therapy is cryoprecipitate, which should be given every 15 to 20 hr. The amount of cryoprecipitate needed must be adjusted to the individual patient and clinical situation. The most effective means of following the therapy is the bleeding time correction noted after infusion of cryoprecipitate.

B. Acquired von Willebrand's Syndrome

A number of patients have been described who have acquired von Willebrand's syndrome.[13,60,63-70] These patients are characterized by a long bleeding time and low Factor VIII procoagulant activity, together with a low Factor VIII-related antigen. Abnormal ristocetin-induced aggregation and decreased platelet retention in glass-bead columns have also been reported. However, the response to transfusion has been minimal, with

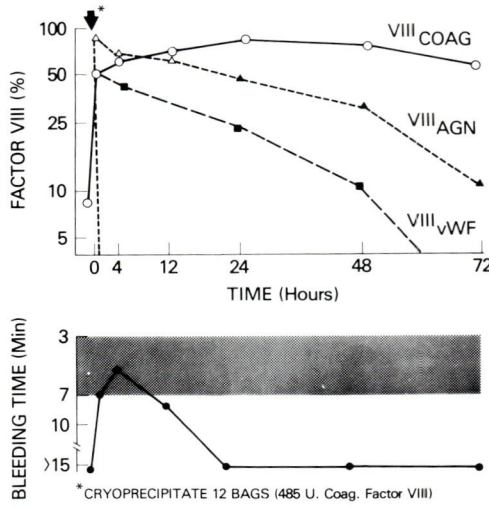

FIGURE 3. Response of patient to infusion of cryoprecipitate. Shaded part of graph indicates normal bleeding time. (From Chediak, J. R., Telfer, M. C., and Green, D., *Am. J. Med.*, 62, 369, 1977. With permission.)

a small increase in Factor VIII activity as measured in the modified activated partial thromboplastin time. There has also been no late rise in Factor VIII activity, thus distinguishing the transfusion response from that seen in hereditary von Willebrand's syndrome.[60] Systemic lupus erythematosus has been associated with acquired von Willebrand's syndrome in two instances, and in three patients a monoclonal immunoglobulin spike has been found. Also, in one additional patient an inhibitor was found that was directed against that part of the Factor VIII molecule necessary for normal platelet retention and ristocetin-induced aggregation.[71] In that particular patient, the patient's serum did not inactivate the Factor VIII procoagulant activity.

C. Bernard-Soulier Syndrome

Bernard and Soulier were the first to describe a hereditary bleeding disorder characterized by a long bleeding time, a mild thrombocytopenia, and "giant" morphologically atypical-appearing platelets.[72] This disorder is inherited as an incomplete autosomal recessive trait, and laboratory abnormalities may be demonstrable in clinically unaffected heterozygotes.

1. Pathophysiology

The fact that the bleeding time was disproportionately long in these patients when correlated with their level of thrombocytopenia led to additional studies of platelet function. The prothrombin consumption time was found to be abnormal.[73] Platelet factor 3 activity as measured by kaolin-induced activation of platelet-rich plasma, however, yielded normal results.[74] Bernard-Soulier platelets aggregate normally with ADP, collagen, epinephrine, and thrombin. Bithell et al. reported two distinct findings in these patients, the first being a lack of platelet shape change in response to ADP, and the second being a significantly more rapid degree of aggregation in response to collagen and ADP.[73] Bernard-Soulier platelets are not aggregated by bovine fibrinogen* or

---

* This product contains Factor VIII.

the antibiotic ristocetin.[73,75,76] Unlike von Willebrand's disease, the defective ristocetin-induced aggregation is not corrected by normal plasma or purified Factor VIII preparations. However, plasma from these patients supports ristocetin-induced aggregation of platelets from patients with von Willebrand's syndrome.[75]

In view of the normal reaction of Bernard-Soulier platelets with collagen and their normal ADP mediated aggregation, Caen et al. proposed that the bleeding disorder was due to an abnormal interaction with the subendothelium.[76] Subsequently, this was confirmed by Weiss et al., using the Baumgartner technique in vitro.[75] It was, therefore, proposed that the Bernard-Soulier platelets lack a receptor for the von Willebrand factor, which is necessary for the normal reaction of platelets with ristocetin and vascular subendothelium.

The membrane abnormality in Bernard-Soulier syndrome was further studied, and it was found that there was a reduced sialic acid content in these platelets and also a reduced electrophoretic mobility.[77] Recently, a significant reduction in a membrane glycoprotein with a molecular weight of 155,000 has been found.[78] This glycoprotein deficiency is different from that found in Glanzmann's thrombasthenia. It, therefore, seems that the decreased adhesion to the subendothelium in this disorder may be the result of a specific abnormality in the platelet membrane glycoprotein content.

Recently, a patient with Bernard-Soulier syndrome was found to have an IgG antibody that agglutinated normal platelets, but not Bernard-Soulier platelets.[79] At high dilutions, this antibody also prevents ristocetin as well as bovine fibrinogen aggregation, without interferring with ADP-induced aggregation. The antibody reacted with a component found in normal platelet membranes, but not in those of Bernard-Soulier platelets. The molecular weight of the component was $150,000 \pm 10,000$. Using the Baumgartner technique, it was subsequently found that this antibody prevented the adhesion of normal platelets to the subendothelium.[80]

Recent work has also indicated that platelets from Bernard-Soulier syndrome do not bind Factor V, Factor XI,[81] and thrombin.

These giant platelets have also been found to have ultrastructural abnormalities. These have included regions of membrane complexes associated with the dense tubular system. Similar structures have also been seen in megakaryocytes of these patients.[82]

2. Clinical Features

These patients may have moderate to severe bleeding manifestations of the purpuric type, including easy bruising, epistaxis, and menorrhagia. Heterozygotes are almost invariably asymptomatic, although in an occasional patient one may find the characteristic giant platelets on peripheral smear.

3. Laboratory Diagnosis

The laboratory findings in Bernard-Soulier syndrome include: giant platelets on peripheral smear, decreased platelet retention in glass-bead columns, abnormal ristocetin-induced aggregation that is not corrected by the addition of normal platelet-poor plasma, and a prolonged bleeding time disproportionate to the mild thrombocytopenia. The remainder of the aggregation studies in these patients are characteristically normal, as are the clot retraction and platelet factor 3 assays.

4. Therapy

The treatment of choice in a bleeding patient with Bernard-Soulier syndrome would be platelet concentrates, the dosage of which would be individualized according to the patient and clinical situation.

D. Impaired Adhesion to Collagen

There have been two reports describing patients whose platelets showed impaired adhesion to collagen fibers.[83] In these cases, adhesion was initiated by stirring platelet-rich plasma with suspensions of collagen, and the degree of adhesion to collagen fibers was estimated by light microscopy. The reactivity of the patient's platelets to adenosine diphosphate was found to be normal; however, there was abnormal collagen-induced platelet aggregation. This would lead one to speculate that the abnormality was one of a receptor in the platelet membrane specific for the collagen-platelet interaction.

Caen and Legrand have described a disorder in which there is an apparent abnormality of collagen, rather than the platelet.[84] They found that in their group of patients, the platelet counts were essentially normal, as were platelet factor 3, platelet factor 4, and platelet acid phosphotase content. However, the bleeding times were strikingly prolonged. Platelet aggregation studies performed with adenosine diphosphate (ADP) and collagen were essentially normal, as were platelet retention studies. Electron microscopy of collagen taken from the connective tissue of these patients was abnormal. Acid-extractable skin collagen taken from skin biopsies in these cases was unable to induce aggregation in platelet-rich plasma from normal controls. Clinically, these patients suffered from easy bruising, spontaneous hemorrhages, and abnormal wound healing.

II. DISORDERS OF PRIMARY AGGREGATION

A. Glanzmann's Thrombasthenia

The term thrombasthenia should only be used to describe the disorder in which ADP-induced platelet aggregation is absent. In 1918, Glanzmann, a Swiss pediatrician from Bern, described a group of patients with normal or slightly decreased platelet counts and abnormal clot retraction; thus he recognized the role of platelets in clot retraction.[85] It is interesting to note that according to his original papers some of his patients actually had thrombocytopenia by modern standards, and none of them had a prolongation of the bleeding time. Fonio and Schwend added to the diagnostic criteria of the disease the prolongation of the bleeding time and the importance of the isolated appearance of the platelets on the peripheral smear.[86] Braunsteiner and Pakesch noted a speeding abnormality when the platelets were examined by electron microscopy, as well as an absence of aggregation during coagulation.[87]

1. Pathophysiology

Despite the absence of aggregation, platelets will undergo a shape change when exposed to ADP.[88] The binding of ADP to the membrane of thrombasthenic platelets is within the normal range.[89] However, neither ADP nor epinephrine will induce the release reaction.[88] Nevertheless, the release mechanism appears to be intact as collagen, kaolin, or thrombin are able to induce release.[90] The platelets will adhere to collagen in the subendothelium and respond normally to ristocetin or bovine fibrinogen.[91] Platelet factor 3 availability is decreased and, as noted above, characteristically there is an absence of clot retraction.[92]

Studies of platelet enzymes in various biochemical pathways have failed to reveal consistent abnormalities. Deficiencies of glyceraldehyde 3-phosphodehydrogenase and pyruvate kinase have been demonstrated, as has a deficiency of glutathione peroxidase.[93] Another abnormality in the glutathione pathway has also been described, a reduction of the glutathione reductase activity.[94] These findings suggest that the ability of the thrombasthenic platelet to withstand oxidative stress is deficient.

A deficiency of platelet fibrinogen has also been demonstrated, and recent studies using a rabbit human-contractile protein antibody have shown that thrombasthenic platelets contain less surface contractile protein than do normal platelets.[95] Glycoprotein II of the platelet surface membrane is absent or grossly abnormal. Perhaps this is the major membrane abnormality in thrombasthenia.[96]

All of these findings are somewhat confusing and point out the heterogeneity of the disorder. One would anticipate that in the future there will be a subclassification or multiple subclassifications of the general disorder termed thrombasthenia.

2. Clinical Features

The disease has been recognized in both sexes and appears to follow an autosomal recessive pattern of inheritance. The frequency of consanguinity among certain groups of people, particularly the gypsies of France, has been emphasized as supporting the recessive pattern.[97]

The bleeding in these patients is quite severe, and the onset is usually early in life. The characteristic pattern of bleeding is purpuric in nature, with mucosal and cutaneous bleeding often occurring spontaneously and being further aggravated by trauma. A peculiar clinical observation, somewhat similar to that of von Willebrand's syndrome, is the decrease in severity of the bleeding as the patient grows older. In addition to the characteristic pattern of bleeding described above, cases have been reported in which hemarthroses were present.

3. Laboratory Diagnosis

The typical laboratory findings include a normal platelet count and a prolonged bleeding time.[98] Platelet retention in glass-bead columns is decreased, and there is an absence of the primary wave of aggregation in response to ADP. Also, epinephrine, thrombin, and collagen fail to induce aggregation.[92] Clot retraction is either absent or markedly decreased. When using the Baumgartner technique for adhesion, these platelets are found to adhere normally, but have an absence of aggregation.

4. Therapy

Transfusion of platelet concentrates remains the only effective way of managing bleeding episodes in these patients. Therapy with steroids has not proved to be beneficial.

B. Essential Athrombia

Essential athrombia refers to a disorder that resembles thrombasthenia of Glanzmann in all respects except for the presence of detectable clot retraction.[99] The bleeding time is typically prolonged, while the clot retraction and platelet factor 3 activity are normal. Platelets will not aggregate when stimulated by diluted collagen suspensions, epinephrine, thrombin, or ADP. Ristocetin-induced aggregation is normal and the platelet count is also within the normal range.[100]

III. DISORDERS OF SECONDARY AGGREGATION

A. Storage Pool Disease

This group of disorders previously was classified in the ill-defined heterogenous clinical disorders known as thrombocytopathies or thrombopathies. For many years it was believed that the platelet factor 3 content was deficient. In 1967, Weiss[101] and Hardisty and Hutton[102] independently described groups of patients whose platelets were aggregated normally by ADP (primary wave), but not by collagen. The lack of collagen-induced aggregation was attributed to a defect in the release of the nonmetabolic pool of adenosine diphosphate. This abnormality was also manifested by a lack of the secondary phase of aggregation in response to exogenous ADP and epinephrine (Figure 4). Following these initial observations, numerous additional patients have been described with similar aggregation profiles.[103-110]

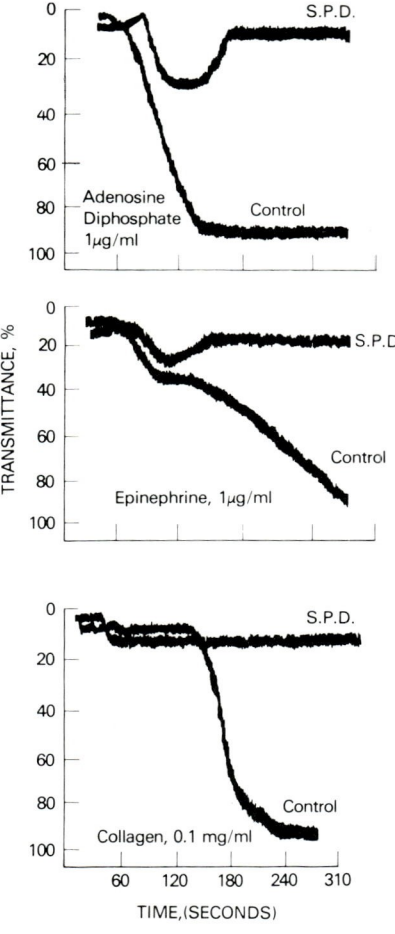

FIGURE 4. Representative aggregation tracings from a patient with storage pool disease (S.P.D.).

Two general defects may account for lack of release of the storage pool of adenosine diphosphate. In the first, the storage pool ADP is normal when assayed, but there is an apparent abnormal mechanism for the release reaction, the so-called "aspirin-like defect" or primary release defect. The characteristic finding in the second defect is a decreased amount of adenosine diphosphate in the storage pool with an intact release mechanism.

1. Pathophysiology

Storage pool disease is characterized by a deficiency of the storage ADP and ATP. In normal platelets, ADP is more selectively concentrated in the dense bodies than is ATP, and, consequently, a deficiency of storage adenine nucleotides has the overall effect of decreasing platelet ADP to a greater extent than ATP. As a result of this greater diminution of ADP, the ATP to ADP ratio is greater than in normal platelets.[107] This finding is diagnostic for storage pool disease. The decrease in the storage pool of adenine nucleotides is best demonstrated by incubation of the platelets with H^3-labeled adenine.

The deficiency of the storage pool ADP explains the abnormalities seen in the aggregation response. In addition to being deficient in ADP, the platelets of patients with storage pool disease will also have decreased amounts of serotonin and calcium.[111] By electron microscopy, the number of visible dense bodies is markedly diminished, while the number of alpha granules is within normal limits.[106] The exact nature of the defect has not been elucidated. However, an animal model has recently become available. This inbred strain of rat (the Fawn-hooded strain) has the characteristic findings of storage pool deficiency, and it has been noted that the content of the dense bodies is deficient even in young platelets that are being fragmented from the megakaryocytic cytoplasm. Thus the disorder appears to be one of an abnormal thrombopoiesis with decreased incorporation of ADP into the platelet at the time of production. One other interesting aspect of this animal model is the bizarre behavior these rats frequently exhibit.

Other findings in patients with storage deficiency include a report of one family in which there was an abnormal lipid content in the platelets.[112] These patients characteristically had small platelets and when their lipids were analyzed, they were found to have an increased lecithin and a decreased phosphatidyl ethanolamine; however, this type of defect has not been observed in other patients studied to date. This particular family had a distinctly autosomal dominant pattern of inheritance, whereas the inheritance pattern in other families has been variable.

In storage pool deficiency, the metabolic turnover of serotonin is also increased.[113] This may be due to the inability to selectively concentrate the serotonin in the dense bodies and subsequent degradation of the serotonin by mitochondrial monoamine oxidase. Recent work has indicated that the release mechanism in patients with storage pool deficiency may be abnormal as well. There are defects in both release I (dense bodies) and release II (α granules).[114] Studies using arachidonic acid-induced aggregation have shown that storage pool disease platelets can convert arachidonic acid to prostaglandin intermediates, but cannot respond to these intermediates with appropriate aggregation.[115] These findings are just the reverse of the situation in aspirin-treated platelets.[116]

2. Clinical Features

Storage pool disease represents a heterogenous group of patients.[117] A number of different clinical syndromes have been identified in which there is a deficiency of the nonmetabolic ADP content of the platelets. Included among these are patients with oculocutaneous albinism (Hermansky-Pudlak syndrome.).[105,106] The number of dense bodies in their platelets is decreased and in the single patient studied to date, the number of melanocytes was also decreased. However, the number of melanosome granules was normal, in marked contrast to the usual patients with albinism. Storage pool deficiency has also been described in patients with Wiskott-Aldrich syndrome.[118] This syndrome is a sex-linked recessive hereditary disorder, which is characterized by recurrent clinical pyogenic infections and eczema. In addition, these patients have thrombocytopenia and immunologic abnormalities. The recurrent infections are secondary to both B-cell and T-cell dysfunction. Isohemagglutinins are absent and serum IgM is reduced, while IgG and IgA are normal. An increased incidence of lymphoproliferative malignancies has also been described in these patients. The thrombocytopenia has been demonstrated to be secondary to a shortened platelet survival.[119] As a result of the shortened survival, one would logically assume that there would be an increased percentage of large platelets representing the younger more hemostatically effective platelets released from a responding bone marrow. However, abnormally small platelets are found, a feature that appears to be of unique diagnostic importance. By electron microscopy, these platelets are found to have deficiencies in the number of both alpha granules and dense bodies. Kuramoto et al. have demonstrated an interesting metabolic defect in the platelets of patients with Wiskott-Aldrich syndrome.[120] This abnormality is characterized by a deficient carbon dioxide production in the citric acid cycle following exposure of platelets to latex particles and aggregating agents.

It has been suggested that Wiskott-Aldrich syndrome may represent a broader spectrum of disease than has been recognized previously. Several kindred have been described in which thrombocytopenia has occurred as a sex-linked recessive disorder with very few or no immunologic or dermatologic manifestations.[121] In these patients, the response to splenectomy has been excellent. Thus it becomes of some diagnostic and therapeutic importance to identify these variants of the Wiskott-Aldrich syndrome. This group of patients appears to be the one subgroup of the hereditary thrombocytopenias that will respond to splenectomy.

A storage pool defect has also been described in the syndrome of thrombocytopenia with absent radius (TAR baby syndrome).[122] In these patients, there are often multiple skeletal, renal, and cardiac abnormalities, together with thrombocytopenia. Bilateral absence of the radii is the most common associated finding. Bone marrow examination is characterized by a marked decrease in the number of megakaryocytes.

Chediak-Steinbrinck Higashi anomaly has also been associated with storage pool defect.[123] This autosomal recessive disorder is characterized by partial ocular and cutaneous albinism and an increased susceptibility to pyogenic infections. In most of the granule-containing cells, one finds very large lysosome-like organelles. These abnormal granules are most readily seen in the blood and bone marrow granulocytes. Children with this disorder often exhibit pale hair, photophobia, recurrent infections, and adenopathy. Often they die at a relatively early age of a lymphoma-like illness.

The platelet dysfunction that has been described in the newborn has been attributed to a storage pool abnormality by some investigators.[124]

In addition to the specific findings noted above for the various entities associated with storage pool disease, clinically the patients may experience nild to moderate bleeding, with the predominant manifestations being muco-cutaneous hemorrhage. Hematuria and epistaxis are relatively common; however, petechiae are uncommon. In many patients the only complaint may be that of easy bruising.

3. Laboratory Diagnosis

Except in the Wiskott-Aldrich syndrome and thrombocytopenia with absent radii syndrome, one would expect to find a normal platelet count together with a prolonged bleeding time. Platelet retention in glass-bead columns is decreased, and aggregation studies will reveal a normal primary wave of aggregation in response to ADP and epinephrine, but an absent second phase of aggregation together with an absent aggregation response to collagen. However, very high concentrations of collagen can induce aggregation even in storage pool disease. Ristocetin-induced aggregation is characteristically normal. Electron microscopic studies on these platelets will show a decrease in the number of dense bodies.

4. Therapy

The treatment of choice for bleeding problems in these patients is platelet concentrates. Often, however, these patients have a very mild clinical bleeding syndrome and it may go entirely undetected.

B. "Aspirin-Like" Defect

Following the description of the storage pool disease, it became evident that there was another group of disorders that gave laboratory findings very similar to those of storage pool disease. This group of patients is characterized by a normal content of

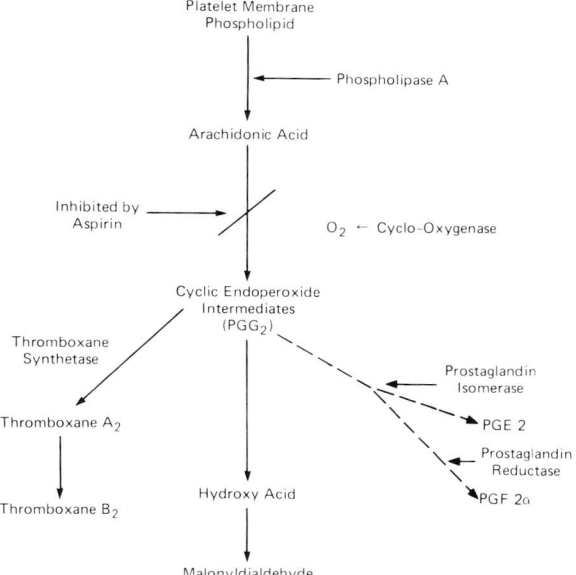

FIGURE 5. Platelet prostaglandin synthesis and metabolism.

ADP in their dense bodies, but an inability to appropriately release the contents of the granules upon proper stimulation.[125]

1. Pathophysiology

Impairment of the second phase of aggregation due to abnormalities in the release mechanism has been observed in a number of patients with idiopathic bleeding disorders. The adenosine diphosphate content in platelets of these patients is normal; however, upon stimulation with collagen and other release-inducing agents the dense body contents are not released. Because of the similarity of this defect to the acquired abnormality seen following aspirin ingestion, Weiss proposed that this abnormality in release should be referred to as "aspirin-like defect". However, recent work indicates that in some cases the defect in platelet function is different than that induced by aspirin.[125] Abnormalities in platelet factor 3 availability and decreased platelet retention have been reported in occasional patients. These abnormalities are not observed after aspirin ingestion. Malmsten et al. recently identified an enzymatic defect in patients with abnormal release reaction. They were able to demonstrate a deficiency in cyclo-oxygenase, the enzyme that converts arachidonic acid to the cyclic endoperoxides (Figure 5).[126] Weiss has also described a patient that appears to have a release abnormality based on a deficiency of the enzyme thromboxane synthetase.[127] Electron microscopic studies have also revealed striking dilatation of the surface connecting system in a single patient with aspirin-like defect.[128]

2. Clinical Features

This is a heterogenous group of disorders and the clinical picture is dominated by easy bruising and mucosal bleeding. Recurrent epistaxis and/or menorrhagia are frequent complaints. The pattern of inheritance has not been well established, although in many families it appears to be dominant.

3. Laboratory Diagnosis

The laboratory findings include: a normal platelet count, prolonged bleeding time, normal or decreased retention in glass-bead columns, normal primary wave of ADP aggregation (but absent secondary wave), absent collagen-induced aggregation, normal ristocetin-induced aggregation, and a normal primary wave of aggregation in response to epinephrine with an absent secondary wave. By electron microscopy, the number of dense bodies is normal. If one uses the Baumgartner technique for adhesion studies, there will be normal adhesion, but decreased aggregation. Clot retraction is typically normal.

4. Therapy

The treatment of choice in these patients is platelet concentrates. Some investigators, however, have pointed out that patients with both storage pool disease and aspirin-like defect may respond to steroids. Also the combination of platelet concentrates and cryoprecipitate has proved effective.

C. Defects of Release Reaction and Factor VIII

Platelet release abnormalities have been described in patients who show decreased levels of one or more of the three components of the Factor VIII complex.[129] Superficially, therefore, these patients may resemble von Willebrand's syndrome. There have been several patients reported in the literature in which a male patient had both a mild hemophilia A and also suffered from an intrinsic abnormality of platelet release or storage pool defect. Therefore, adequate treatment of this type of patient would require both the use of cryoprecipitate and platelet concentrates.

IV. PLATELET FACTOR 3 DEFICIENCY

As pointed out earlier, prior to the introduction of the more selective tests of platelet functions such as aggregation and retention, qualitative defects of platelets were attributed to a lack of platelet factor 3. Subsequently, more elaborate evaluation of these patients have, in most instances, revealed abnormalities in aggregation and other aspects of platelet function. However, an occasional patient may show an isolated defect of platelet factor 3 with normal platelet aggregation, retention, and bleeding time. This type of abnormality has been reported in patients with glucose 6-phosphate dehydrogenase deficiency (B-negative type).[130] Weiss also has reported a patient who had an excessive bleeding tendency and whose platelets were deficient in procoagulant activity (platelet factor 3), but aggregated normally to all reagents tested. In addition, this patient had a normal bleeding time.[117] There have also been other scattered reports of similar patients.[131]

V. PLATELET ABNORMALITIES ASSOCIATED WITH OTHER CONGENITAL DEFECTS

A. Giant Platelets Associated with Renal Dysfunction

Since Alport originally described the association of hereditary nephritis and deafness in 1927, a number of abnormalities have been recorded as being part of the syndrome that bears his name.[132] With the single exception of ocular defects, the other abnormalities are quite rare, and a true hereditary transmission is questionable. Recently, the association of Alport's syndrome together with thrombocytopenia and giant platelets has been reported in four kindreds.[133-135] The members of these families have a lifelong history of bleeding, usually mild epistaxis; but in at least one instance, central nervous system bleeding was fatal. In two of the four kindred, the in vitro function studies were normal; however, in the other kindred, aggregation response to collagen and epinephrine, as well as the release of platelet factor 3, was impaired.[133] It has been suggested that the giant platelets may result from a degenerative process of the megakaryocytes leading to nuclear regression and cytoplasmic fragmentation, rather than the usual lines of demarcation forming normal sized platelets.[135]

B. May-Hegglin Anomaly

In 1945, Hegglin first described the familial occurrence of thrombocytopenia associated with giant platelets and Dohle bodies in the peripheral and marrow granulocytes.[136] This abnormality is transmitted as an autosomal dominant trait. The affected patients all have giant platelets and Dohle bodies, but the thrombocytopenia may be variable. Significant clinical bleeding may be present, but most patients are asymptomatic. There have been isolated reports of platelet functional abnormalities in this disorder, but in most instances laboratory evaluation of platelet function has been within normal limits.[137] Bone marrow examination reveals an adequate number of megakaryocytes. There is some disagreement as to the platelet survival studies.[138]

C. Hereditary Disorders of Connective Tissue and Mucopolysaccharidosis

Abnormalities of the coagulation mechanism have been reported in occasional patients with genetically determined disorders of the connective tissue. This group of diseases include osteogenesis imperfecta, Marfan's syndrome, Ehlers-Danlos syndrome, pseudoxanthoma elasticum, Hurler and Hunter syndromes, and other mucopolysaccharidoses. Of these, the Ehlers-Danlos syndrome is most commonly associated with bleeding. A chance discovery of large platelets and clotting deficiencies in five members of a family with Marfan's syndrome led to these observations.[139] Frequently these patients have abnormally large platelets on peripheral smear, and there have been reports of abnormal ADP-induced aggregation.[140] The results of the aggregation studies reported to date indicate that there is an abnormality in the release reaction. This type of abnormality places these patients in the so-called "aspirin-like defect" group.[141]

D. Glycogen Storage Disease

A mild bleeding disorder has been reported in patients with glycogen storage disease type I (deficiency of glucose 6-phosphatase).[142] Laboratory evaluation of platelet function has included the following: prolonged bleeding time, deficiency in platelet factor 3 activity, and abnormalities in aggregation with both ADP and collagen suggesting a release problem. This may be an acquired disorder secondary to the abnormal glycogen metabolism, because when these patients are appropriately treated, the platelet abnormalities can be corrected.

E. Afibrinogenemia

Most deficiencies of coagulation proteins are associated with a normal bleeding time; however, afibrinogenemia is usually found to have a prolonged bleeding time. In patients with hereditary afibrinogenemia, platelet function studies in vitro are also abnormal.[143] There is a deficiency in platelet aggregation with low concentrations of ADP, and retention of platelets in glass-bead columns is decreased. Variable abnormalities in platelet factor 3 activity have also been reported.[144] The prolonged bleeding time as well as the platelet abnormalities demonstrable in the laboratory can be corrected by the addition of fibrinogen to the test system.

VI. MISCELLANEOUS

Platelet function defects have also been reported in other hereditary disorders, including glucose 6-phosphate dehydrogenase deficiency of the B-negative type, Wilson's disease, and hereditary hemorrhagic telangiectasia. In addition, platelet hyperfunction has been reported in association with homocystinuria. The survival of platelets in homocystinuric patients is decreased.

PART 2: ACQUIRED QUALITATIVE PLATELET DISORDERS

I. UREMIA

The first report of platelet dysfunction in association with uremia was by Lewis and co-workers in 1956.[145] They carefully studied the coagulation mechanism of twelve patients with uremia, and although there was significant thrombocytopenia in only three patients, seven of the twelve were found to have decreased prothrombin consumption and eight reduced "thromboplastic" function. Following this, Larrain and Langdell published observations on dogs who were made uremic by ureteral ligation.[146] In every case, serum prothrombin time decreased as uremia progressed. None of the animals developed abnormal capillary fragility, prolongation of the bleeding time, or thrombocytopenia. They concluded that impaired platelet function was the cause of the coagulation defect seen in acute uremia. Following this, in 1966, Castaldi and associates reported their observations on 19 uremic patients of whom seven were bleeding at the time of study.[147] They were able to demonstrate a number of qualitative defects including a prolonged Ivy bleeding time, diminished in vivo platelet adhesiveness by the method of Borchgrevink, and abnormal clot retraction. In addition, platelet aggregation with adenosine diphosphate and platelet factor 3 studies were abnormal. Rabiner and Hrodek found that the majority of uremic patients had a defective availability of platelet factor 3, but that a significant number had not only a decreased release of platelet factor 3, but also a diminished content.[148] They studied the effect of dialysis on platelet factor 3 and found that these abnormalities were corrected within 48 hr after dialysis. It was also found that one could maintain a normal platelet factor 3 in chronic renal failure by repeated dialysis. Subsequently, Joist and associates found abnormal spreading of platelets on siliconized slides, decreased aggregation with ADP, epinephrine, and collagen, and a decreased release of platelet factor 3 with kaolin and collagen.[149] They also found that these abnormalities in uremic patients could be corrected by dialysis.

A. Pathophysiology

There have been a number of studies performed in an effort to determine which of the metabolites or electrolytes characteristically abnormal in patients with renal failure is responsible for the qualitative platelet abnormality. Initially, urea was implicated; however, subsequent work by Somer et al. essentially ruled out urea.[150] Eknoyan et al. reported that platelet retention was decreased in normal subjects after the infusion of urea, but this reduction was only observed after 24 hr.[151] Stewart and Castaldi also found that in vivo addition of ureate, creatinine, phosphate, potassium, and magnesium similar to concentrations found in uremia had no effect on platelet aggregation or platelet factor 3.[152] Horowitz et al. in 1967 reported abnormal ADP-induced platelet factor 3 activation in 16 of 17 patients with uremia.[153] In addition, he observed that uremic platelet-poor plasma prevented ADP-induced platelet factor 3 activation of normal platelet-rich plasma following a 60 min incubation. This inhibition by uremic plasma could be overcome by the addition of small amounts of calcium. Thus the question of whether platelet aggregation by ADP or collagen is abnormal in uremia is not settled; both normal and abnormal results have been reported, and the concentration of calcium used in the test may be critical.

Guanidinosuccinic acid has been implicated as the metabolite responsible for the defective platelet function.[154] Blood levels of phenol and hydroxyphenolacetic acid have also been implicated as additional metabolites that can inhibit platelet function.[155] It is interesting to note that the aggregation abnormality produced by guanidinosuccinic acid can be demonstrated by preincubation of platelet-rich plasma with this compound for approximately 1 hr. However, the effect produced by phenolic acid requires 2 to 3 hr of preincubation.

B. Clinical Features

The bleeding one may see in uremic patients is occasionally quite severe. Ecchymoses and intractable slow gastrointestinal bleeding are common, and large hemorrhages in serous cavities and muscles may also occur.

C. Laboratory Diagnosis

As illustrated above, a number of different abnormalities in platelet function have been described in patients with uremia. At the present time, there appears to be a lack of consistency in these results from laboratory to laboratory. Consequently, a typical picture of platelet dysfunction cannot be described.

D. Therapy

Hemodialysis and/or peritoneal dialysis are of temporary therapeutic value.

II. QUALITATIVE PLATELET DISORDERS ASSOCIATED WITH MYELOPROLIFERATIVE SYNDROMES

Bleeding has long been recognized as a complication of the myeloproliferative syndromes (i.e., hemorrhagic thrombocythemia, myeloid metaplasia with myelofibrosis, polycythemia rubra vera, etc.). Often these patients may present with bleeding manifestations including ecchymoses, epistaxis, and intractable gastrointestinal bleeding. In addition to the hemorrhagic problems, they may also present with thrombotic problems. These disorders are covered later in the chapter in the discussion of the quantitative abnormalities of platelets.

III. DYSPROTEINEMIAS

Acquired circulating anticoagulants and coagulation abnormalities associated with malignant paraproteins are discused more extensively in Chapter 10.

Bleeding may complicate any of the various types of paraproteinemias, but is most frequently seen as a complication of Waldenstrom's macroglobulinemia.[156] A number of different laboratory findings have been reported in these patients, including deficient platelet factor 3 activity, reduced platelet retention in glass-bead columns, and varying abnormalities of aggregation.[157] These abnormalities in platelet function have been attributed to a coating of the platelet membrane with the abnormal protein. In addition to the interaction of the protein with the platelet, a coating of the collagen fibers by the abnormal protein has been reported.[158]

As will be discussed later, a number of abnormalities of coagulation have been described in patients with malignant paraproteinemias. However, in general, these abnormalities correlate poorly with clinical bleeding. The most consistent correlation between an abnormality in the laboratory and the clinical state of the patient have been findings of abnormal platelet function. These include a prolonged bleeding time, decreased platelet retention in glass-bead columns, and, also, an increased serum viscosity. Recently, it has also been pointed out that the presence of cryoglobulins is associated with an increased tendency toward clinical bleeding in these patients.

Plasmapheresis is the treatment of choice in these disorders, along with chemotherapy.[159]

IV. QUALITATIVE PLATELET DEFECTS IN PATIENTS WITH ANTIBODIES TO PLATELETS

Various qualitative disorders of platelet function have been described in patients with autoimmune thrombocytopenic purpura.[160] Patients with antiplatelet antibodies may have an acquired type of storage pool syndrome as a result of loss of their dense body contents following the reaction of the antibody with the platelet membrane. In addition, an acquired storage pool syndrome has also been described in patients with chronic disseminated intravascular coagulation.[161]

V. SCURVY

Abnormal platelet function has been reported in a number of cases of scurvy in man as well as animals.[162] Aggregation studies have been consistent with an abnormality in the release reaction.

VI. CYANOTIC CONGENITAL HEART DISEASE

There have been a number of platelet abnormalities described in patients with cyanotic congenital heart disease, including a deficiency of platelet factor 3 and abnormal aggregation.[163] However, other studies have demonstrated essentially normal platelet function in these patients.

VII. CIRRHOSIS

The varying changes in platelet aggregation that have been reported with liver cirrhosis probably reflect the changing hemostatic picture in the cirrhotic patient. It is known that fragment E of the fibrin degradation products will inhibit thrombin-induced aggregation, whereas fragment D will not.[228] Thus the presence of small fibrin degradation products would tend to inhibit in vitro platelet aggregation.[164,165] The presence of fibrin monomers will accelerate platelet aggregation. Thus it appears that the changing ratio of fibrin-split products to fibrin monomers is the most satisfactory explanation for the varying patterns of platelet aggregation found in cirrhotic patients.[166] This ratio will vary from patient to patient and from time to time in the same patient.

VIII. DRUGS

There are many pharmacologic compounds and drugs that will affect platelet function (Table 6). Among these drugs, aspirin is certainly the most common offender. It has long been known that small doses of acetylsalicylic acid will prolong the bleeding time in patients with inherited clotting disorders. Aspirin does not inhibit the primary phase of ADP-induced aggregation, although it does inhibit the secondary phase and release caused by ADP and epinephrine. Aspirin inhibits cyclo-oxygenase, which results in decreased production of cyclic endoperoxide intermediates, which are important in mediating the platelet release reaction. Aspirin selectively inhibits the release I reaction (i.e., dense body release), while release II occurs normally.[114]

TABLE 6

Drugs that Inhibit Platelet Function

Anti-inflammatory and analgesics
  Aspirin
  Sulfinpyrazone (Anturane®)
  Ibuprofen (Motrin®)
  Indomethacin (Indocin®)
  Phenylbutazone (Butazolidin®, weak inhibitor)
  Mefenamic acid (Ponstel®)
  Colchicine
Anticoagulants
  Heparin (?)
  Coumadin® (?)
  Dextran
Psychiatric drugs
  Phenothiazines
  Tricyclic antidepressants (e.g., Tofranil®, Triavil®, and Elavil®)
Cardiovascular drugs (i.e., vasodilators and antilipemic)
  Dipyridamole (Persantine®)
  Papaverine (Myobid®)
  Theophylline
  Clofibrate (Atromid®)
  Nicotinic acid
Anesthetics
  Cocaine (local)
  Procaine (local)
  Volatile general anesthetics
Genitourinary drugs
  Furosemide (Lasix®)
  Nitrofurantoin (Furadantin®)
Sympathetic blocking agents
  Phenoxybenzamine hydrochloride (Dibenzyline®)
  Propranolol (Inderal®)
Miscellaneous
  Glycerol guaiacolate ether (cough suppressant)
  Vinblastine sulfate (Velban®)
  Antihistamines (Benadryl®)
  Hydroxychloroquine sulfate
  Sodium nitroprusside
Antibiotics
  Penicillin G
  Carbenicillin
  Ticarcillin
  Ampicillin
  Gentamycin

These defects are seen after the ingestion of a 0.3 g tablet of aspirin, and the effects of a single dose may be demonstrable for 4 to 7 days. The use of aspirin or any of the 400 aspirin-containing preparations currently available should be avoided in patients with underlying bleeding disorders or when maximal hemostasis is desirable.

Indomethacin and phenylbutazone also inhibit release and aggregation, but the inhibitory effects of a single dose are detectable for only a few hours. Platelet aggregation and release are not inhibited by sodium salicylate, acetaminophen, propoxyphene, or codeine.[167]

Dipyridamole and sulfinpyrazone have also been found to inhibit platelet aggregation when used in high concentrations.[168] However, in the doses used clinically they are not inhibitory. The mechanism whereby they function in vivo is not clear.

Aspirin, dipyridamole, and sulfinpyrazone have been used clinically to treat transient cerebral ischemic attacks, acute myocardial infarction, glomerular disease, allograft rejection, and microangiopathic disorders, In addition, they have also been used to prevent thrombosis on prosthetic surfaces such as heart valves, shunts, catheters, and membranes.[169] Recently, some success has been recorded with the use of these drugs in treating recurrent venous thrombosis.[170] Clinical trials in these areas continue.

PART 3: QUANTITATIVE ABNORMALITIES OF PLATELETS — THROMBOCYTOPENIA

I. THROMBOCYTOPENIA

Thrombocytopenia (less than 100,000 platelets per cubic millimeter) is the most common cause of serious bleeding encountered clinically. There are many causes of thrombocytopenia, but they can be broadly divided into two large groups: decreased platelet production and increased platelet destruction or utilization. In the majority of cases one or the other of these mechanisms will be responsible; however, in some cases both may be operative. A precise etiologic diagnosis is of paramount importance for optimal treatment and prognosis.

The clinical importance of thrombocytopenia is related to the bleeding hazard, but this is variable and often is not closely correlated to the platelet count. At one end of the spectrum, patients with platelet counts as low as 20,000 and sometimes lower will have little or no bleeding or purpura. At the other end, patients with platelet counts slightly less than 100,000 per cubic millimeter may experience widespread purpura and frank bleeding. Prior to discussing the differential diagnosis and clinical evaluation of patients with thrombocytopenia, platelet production and kinetics will be briefly reviewed.

A. Platelet Production

Platelets are produced by fragmentation of giant, multinucleated cells called megakaryocytes, which constitute less than 1% of the nucleated elements of the normal human bone marrow. Megakaryocytes arise from the multipotential stem cell, which is capable of differentiating into the erythrocytic, myelocytic, and megakaryocytic series.[171] The earliest recognizable member of the megakaryocytic series is the megakaryoblast. It is characterized by deeply basophilic cytoplasm and irregular nucleus with a loose chromatin pattern and several nucleoli. Megakaryoblasts typically have a diameter of 20 to 30 μm. In contrast to other elements of the bone marrow, as the megakaryocyte matures there is nuclear division with an absence of cytoplasmic division; a process that is known as endomitosis. As a result, the nucleus becomes more lobulated and pyknotic, and the cytoplasm will increase in quantity and become more eosinophilic and granular. With each nuclear division, the ploidy doubles until the full complement is reached. In a normal marrow, approximately two thirds of the megakaryocytes are 16N (8 nuclear lobes), approximately one fourth are 32N (16 nuclear lobes), and the remainder are 8N (4 nuclear lobes). With the appropriate thrombopoietic stimulus, ploidy may reach 64 or 128N. The morphologic classification applied to the maturing megakaryocytic series includes: megakaryoblasts for the earliest recognized form, promegakaryocyte or basophilic megakaryocyte for the intermediate forms, and mature (eosinophilic or granular) megakaryocyte for the late forms.

The developing megakaryocyte contains a Golgi complex and many polyribosomes that are primarily found in the perinuclear regions.[172] As the cytoplasm matures, granular elements that are destined to become platelet organelles are elaborated in the Golgi region.[173] Tubular channels, which are destined to form the demarcation membrane of platelets will also appear in the cytoplasm.[172] These demarcation membranes, although structurally resembling smooth endoplasmic reticulum, will take up ruthenium red and horseradish peroxidase, thus indicating they are indeed invaginations of the megakaryocytic membrane.[174] In the mature platelet-producing megakaryocyte, the demarcation membrane system will tend to coalesce about cytoplasmic fragments, thus forming the margins of individual platelets. An extension of these demarcation membranes in the circulating platelet is the open canalicular system, which can be demonstrated on electron microscopy. In a normal marrow, approximately one fourth of the megakaryocytes have no apparent granulation, one fourth show a partial granulation, and the remaining 50% appear fully granulated. The amount of cytoplasm accumulated by each megakaryocyte is roughly proportional to the ploidy value of the individual cell.[175]

The time required for the complete sequence of the megakaryocytic differentiation and maturation has been calculated as approximately 3 days in the rabbit, but in man it has been estimated at approximately 4 to 5 days.[176]

Wright, in 1910, suggested that the mature megakaryocyte extended filaments of cytoplasm into the sinusoids, where they were detached and fragmented into individual platelets.[177] Microcinematographic studies of the rabbit bone marrow have confirmed his theory.[178] The mature platelets frequently seen associated with megakaryocytes in marrow aspirate preparations are probably artifactual, having come from the peripheral blood which has diluted the aspirate. Not infrequently, one may encounter bare nuclei or megakaryocytes that have totally shed their cytoplasm. These nuclei will be processed by the reticuloendothelial system.

It has been calculated that between 2000 and 7700 platelets are released by each megakaryocyte.[178] The number released may depend on the ploidy value of the individual cells.

Following thrombocytopenia, the marrow may increase platelet production as a result of three possible mechanisms: (1) an increase in the size of the individual megakaryocytes, which may be related to an increase in the average number of nuclei per cell,[175] (2) an increase in the total number of megakaryocytes as a result of an influx of cells from the stem cell pool,[175,176] and (3) a shortening of the maturation time of the megakaryocyte. It has been postulated that a hormone exists that will specifically stimulate platelet production. This "thrombopoietin" has been studied by a number of investigators and has characteristics of a glycoprotein. Evidence that such a hormone exists in man is provided by studies of a child who was severely thrombocytopenic and whose marrow contained only immature megakaryocytes. However, on the infusion of fresh, normal plasma, normal megakaryocytic maturation ensued, and there was a corresponding increase in the peripheral platelet count to a normal range.[179] As a result of these studies, it was postulated that the patient suffered from a congenital deficiency of thrombopoietin.

The maximal marrow response to thrombocytopenia has been suggested to be approximately eight times the basal level. There is approximately a 3 to 5 day lag between the onset of peripheral thrombocytopenia and evidence for acceleration of platelet production.[180] This lag probably represents the maturation time of the megakaryocytes. The platelets that are released by a reactive marrow in response to thrombocytopenia, generally, are larger in volume and metabolically more active than the circulating platelets. Evidence has been provided that these platelets may be preferentially sequestered in the spleen for several days prior to their eventual entry into the circulating blood.[181] These younger platelets, in addition to being metabolically active, are more effective in the hemostatic process. This, in part, explains the dichotomy that at times exists in patients with severe autoimmune thrombocytopenia. Although these patients may have platelet counts in the range of 10,000 per cubic millimeter, they may have very few bleeding problems, thus indicating the marked effectiveness of the platelet population. This is in marked contrast to patients who have disorders in production of platelets, such as aplastic anemia. In this situation, the circulating platelets tend to be small and not as hemostatically effective as large platelets. Therefore, at a comparable platelet count, this type of patient will experience significantly more clinical bleeding problems than will the patient suffering from a destructive thrombocytopenia with an appropriate marrow response.

B. Platelet Kinetics

The isotopes that have been used to label platelets for life span determinations have included ^{51}chromium and ^{32}phosphorus — diisopropyl fluorophosphate. The chromate ion binds to adenine nucleotides and to various platelet proteins, including thrombosthenin.[182] The radioactive diisopropyl fluorophosphate (DF ^{32}P) is bound by serine residues in platelet enzymes.[183] Chromate ion is useful in man only as an in vitro whole population label, whereas diisopropyl fluorophosphate may be used to label either a cohort or total population and can also be used in vivo and in vitro. Other compounds that have been used include ^{75}Se selenomethionine and ^{35}S sulfate.[184] Both of these compounds are incorporated into megakaryocytes and, following this, into the circulating platelet. They have been used as cohort labels in animals.

With the use of the ^{51}Cr chromate as an in vitro label, the initial in vivo recovery of labeled platelets will average approximately 65% in normal persons, but in asplenic individuals approximately 90% will be recovered.[185] Thus it appears that approximately two thirds of the total platelet mass is present in the circulation, while one third is sequestered in the spleen. These splenic platelets that are present in the sinusoids or between the cells of the red pulp are interchangeable with the circulating platelet pool and, as pointed out earlier, contain a disproportionately high percentage of young platelets.[181]

Platelet life span, as estimated by in vitro labeling with ^{51}Cr chromate, will range from 9 to 12 days in man.[186] Nearly identical values have been obtained using diisopropyl fluorophosphate — ^{32}P.[187] Similar survival times have been found in canine and bovine studies.[188] In the steady state, platelet production is balanced by platelet destruction.[176] The platelet turnover rate has been estimated at approximately 35,000 platelets per microliter per day.

There is good clinical and experimental evidence that damaged or senile platelets are sequestered principally in the spleen, where they are destroyed.[189] There has been much controversy regarding the major determinants of normal platelet survival. In the majority of the survival studies employing ^{51}Cr as a label, the survival curve has been rectilinear, thus suggesting platelet destruction is primarily due to senescence.[186] However, studies using diisopropyl fluorophosphate — ^{32}P as an in vivo platelet label in animals have suggested a curvilinear pattern of the survival curves.[190] This would thus suggest random destruction as being the prime mechanism for platelet destruction and removal. The available data suggest that platelet survival curves in man are neither rectilinear nor curvilinear, in that both random destruction and senescence determine the fate of the platelet.[191]

As discussed earlier, platelet production is thought to be controlled by a humoral substance, which has been termed thrombopoietin.[179] A number of studies have also proposed the presence of inhibitors of platelet production that are produced in the spleen. However, these studies are not convincing. There does appear to be a relationship between erythrocyte and platelet production, as witnessed in the demonstration of thrombopoietic activity in plasma from anemic animals and the association of renal polycythemia and thrombocytosis.[192,193] Also, thrombocytosis sometimes accompanies

TABLE 7

Thrombocytolytic States

1. Atherosclerosis
2. Thromboembolism
3. Carcinomatosis
4. Hodgkin's disease
5. Prosthetic cardiac valves
6. Cirrhosis
7. Gout
8. Systemic lupus erythematosus
9. Acute febrile illness
10. Smoking
11. Postoperative status
12. Animal fat ingestion
13. Some patients with idiopathic thrombocytopenic purpura in remission
14. Aortic aneurysm
15. Bypass procedures for coronary artery disease
16. Shunt procedures for renal dialysis
17. Cyanotic congenital heart disease
18. Megaloblastic anemia
19. Diabetes mellitus with retinopathy
20. Chronic disseminated intravascular coagulation
21. Homocystinuria

prolonged hypoxia and iron deficiency anemia.[194,195] Estrogens are known to produce thrombocytopenia when given in large doses.[196] This is apparently due to decreased marrow production, as the megakaryocytes may be virtually eliminated after a 2 to 3 week course of high-dose estrogen therapy. These studies, however, were performed in dogs. Variable findings have been reported in man.[197]

C. Platelet Count

The platelet count in the venous blood of normal adults averages approximately 250,000 per microliter, with a normal range of 140,000 to 440,000, as measured by phase contrast microscopy. Mean platelet count in the normal neonate is similar to that of the adult.[198] No differences have been demonstrated between normal men and women.[199] During pregnancy there is a slight decrease in the platelet count, which may fall even further during the first stage of labor and on the first or second post partum day.[200]

The administration of epinephrine produces an increase in the platelet count of 20 to 50%, which will not occur in asplenic individuals and presumably is the result of mobilization of the sequestered platelets from the splenic pool.[201] A thrombocytosis will also follow exercise, and this is thought to be due to release of platelets from megakaryocytes found in the lungs.[202] This thrombocytosis is unaffected by splenectomy.

It has recently been reported that smoking may shorten platelet survival and produce "hyperaggregability" of platelets.[176] A number of clinical situations have been identified in which there is accelerated platelet destruction with normal platelet counts (Table 7). This is referred to as a compensated thrombocytolytic state. Presumably, the marrow megakaryocyte reserve is adequate to compensate for the shortened life span of the platelet. Once the life span has shortened to such a degree that the marrow reserve is exceeded, clinical thrombocytopenia will follow.

As discussed earlier, younger platelets differ from their older cohorts.[203]

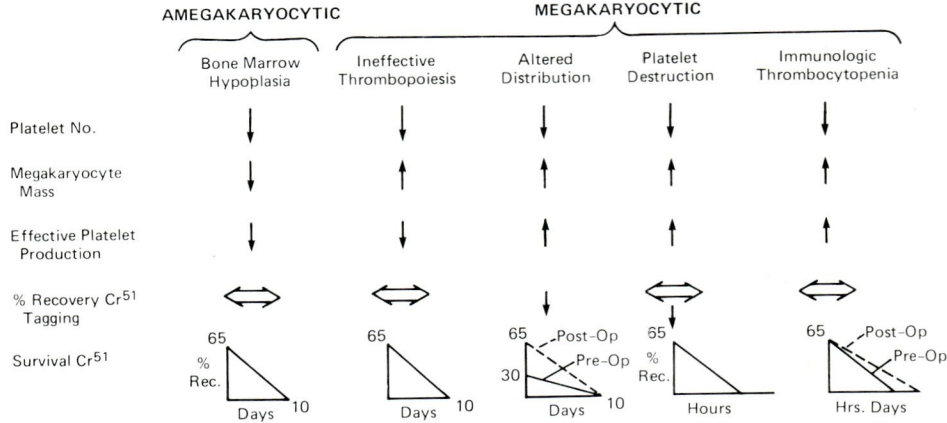

FIGURE 6. Platelet kinetics in thrombocytopenic states.

D. Pathophysiology of Thrombocytopenia

Thrombocytopenia may be defined as a subnormal number of platelets in the circulating blood. It is the most common cause of abnormal bleeding. Thrombocytopenic states are divided into two major groups: (1) the amegakaryocytic thrombocytopenias, which occur because of a loss of megakaryocytes in the bone marrow and (2) the megakaryocytic thrombocytopenias, which occur as a result of increased consumption of platelets or because of defective platelet production (Figure 6 and Table 8).

Accelerated platelet destruction may result from either intrinsic abnormalities in the platelet or extra corpuscular abnormalities. Intrinsic abnormalities are relatively rare, but have been demonstrated in certain forms of hereditary thrombocytopenia, such as the Wiskott-Aldrich syndrome.[176] In most instances, accelerated platelet destruction is due to extrinsic problems, including immunologic phenomena, destruction associated with consumption such as in intravascular coagulation and microangiopathic processes.

II. AMEGAKARYOCYTIC THROMBOCYTOPENIAS

A. Congenital Hypoplasia

Hypoplasia of the marrow megakaryocytes may be seen in a wide variety of clinical situations. The congenital thrombocytopenias include Fanconi's syndrome,[204] thrombocytopenia with absent radius (TAR baby syndrome),[205] suppression of the marrow megakaryocytes as a result of an intrauterine infection usually with a viral agent such as rubella,[206] or exposure of the fetus to drugs in the maternal circulation, such as thiazides.[207] The Fanconi's syndrome is characterized by pancytopenia, bone marrow hypoplasia, and various associated congenital anomalies. These anomalies include dwarfism, microcephaly, hypogenitalism, strabismus, anomalies of the thumbs, radial bones, and kidneys, as well as mental retardation and microophthalmia.[208] Also, atrophy of the spleen is common. Consanguinity of the parents has been reported in a number of instances, and a number of chromosomal abnormalities have been found. Not infrequently, thrombocytopenia and the complications of thrombocytopenia may be the first clinical evidence of the aplastic state of the bone marrow.

Thrombocytopenia associated with absent radii has been previously discussed in the portion of this chapter dealing with qualitative platelet abnormalities. Bone marrow examination in these patients will reveal a lack of megakaryocytes.

TABLE 8

Classification of Thrombocytopenia

Amegakaryocytic thrombocytopenia

I. Congenital hypoplasia
   A. Fanconi's syndrome (constitutional anemia)
   B. Thrombocytopenia with absent radii (TAR baby syndrome)
   C. Deficiency of thrombopoietin
   D. Rubella and other viral illnesses
   E. Neonatal thrombocytopenia resulting from maternal ingestion of thiazide diuretics
   F. Hereditary thrombocytopenias
      1. May-Hegglin anomaly
      2. Bernard-Soulier syndrome

II. Infiltrative diseases
   A. Metastatic carcinoma
   B. Leukemias
   C. Lymphomas
   D. Myelofibrosis
   E. Osteopetrosis
   F. Miliary tuberculosis
   G. Histiocytosis

III. Acquired hypoplasia
   A. Radiation and myelosuppressive drugs
   B. Drugs (thiazides, estrogens, alcohol)
   C. Tidal platelet dysgenesis
   D. Aplastic anemia

Megakaryocytic thrombocytopenia

I. Ineffective thrombopoiesis
   A. Vitamin B_{12} deficiency
   B. Folate deficiency
   C. Preleukemia
   D. Acute myelomonocytic leukemia
   E. Paroxysmal nocturnal hemoglobinuria
   F. Cyclic thrombocytopenia
   G. Di Guglielmo's syndrome
   H. Iron deficiency anemia

II. Altered distribution of platelets
   A. Splenomegaly (cirrhosis, Gaucher's disease, etc.)
   B. Hypothermia

III. Nonimmunologic destructive thrombocytopenia
   A. Disseminated intravascular coagulation
   B. Bacterial, viral, rickettsial, mycotic, and protozoal infection
   C. Acute hemolytic reactions (e.g., erythroblastosis fetalis)
   D. Thrombotic thrombocytopenic purpura
   E. Hemolytic uremic syndrome
   F. Kasabach-Merritt syndrome
   G. Infectious mononucleosis
   H. Waring blender syndrome
   I. Ristocetin induced

IV. Immunologic thrombocytopenia
   A. Isoimmune thrombocytopenia
      1. Newborns
      2. Following multiple transfusions
   B. Drug-induced thrombocytopenia
   C. Posttransfusion purpura
   D. Idiopathic thrombocytopenic purpura
      1. Acute
      2. Recurrent
      3. Chronic

TABLE 8 (continued)

Classification of Thrombocytopenia

Megakaryocytic thrombocytopenia

Loss of platelets

I. Multiple blood transfusions
II. Extracorporeal circulation

Thrombocytopenia that is seen in newborn infants infected with rubella is quite severe, with platelet counts as low as 70,000.[206]

Maternal ingestion of thiazide diuretics is associated with fetal thrombocytopenia as a result of a direct toxic effect of the thiazide on the fetal marrow megakaryocytes. Recovery will usually occur in a matter of weeks after birth.

B. Acquired Hypoplasia

In the adult population, thrombocytopenia as a result of marrow hypoplasia can be due to exposure to toxic drugs, chemicals, or various physical agents. Ionizing radiation, alkylating agents, antimetabolites, and other cytotoxic drugs will result in marrow hypoplasia and resulting thrombocytopenia. Platelets are frequently the last cell type to return to normal following recovery from bone marrow hypoplasia, and in some patients a thrombocytopenia may persist indefinitely.

In addition to the various agents that nonselectively suppress all marrow cellular elements, there are certain drugs that will selectively suppress megakaryocytes. These include chlorothiazides and its various congeners. Thiazides have been implicated in producing thrombocytopenia by at least two different mechanisms: either drug-induced platelet antibodies[209] or direct suppression of thrombopoiesis.[210] The latter is by far the most common. As many as 25% of patients taking thiazides may have a mild asymptomatic thrombocytopenia.[211] As discussed earlier, estrogenic hormones are known to affect platelet production in animals. A similar effect has been reported in man following administration of diethylstilbestrol.[212]

There is evidence that ethanol will suppress platelet production,[213] and, more recently, it has been pointed out that ethanol will also induce certain qualitative abnormalities in platelets.[214] Platelet kinetic studies have demonstrated an accelerated platelet destruction, as well as a subnormal compensatory increase in marrow thrombopoiesis.[213] The megakaryocytes are usually normal or even increased in number when the marrow is examined. Relatively large doses of ethanol are required to produce this effect. Bleeding is a relatively rare complication, and when the ethanol is withdrawn, the platelet count returns to normal or even supranormal levels within a matter of weeks.

C. Bone Marrow Infiltration

Thrombocytopenia is a relatively uncommon complication of disorders in which the marrow is replaced by abnormal cells, such as in disseminated carcinomatosis. However, in the acute leukemias, one very frequently finds a thrombocytopenia as a result of marrow replacement by malignant elements. This may also be the case in lymphomas and occasionally in patients with disseminated granulomatous disease, such as tuberculosis and histoplasmosis.

III. MEGAKARYOCYTIC THROMBOCYTOPENIAS

The megakaryocytic thrombocytopenic states can be subclassified into four groups. There may be a deficiency of platelet numbers because of: (1) ineffective synthesis, (2) altered distribution in the body, (3) increased destruction peripherally, or (4) circulating antibodies to platelets.

A. Ineffective Thrombopoiesis

Thrombocytopenia is a relatively consistent finding in patients with megaloblastic hematopoiesis. The thrombocytopenia is due to ineffective thrombopoiesis, which is characterized by diminished platelet production despite the presence of an increased marrow megakaryocytic mass.[175] The abnormality in production is presumed to be secondary to impaired DNA synthesis and a resulting limitation in the nuclear endoreduplication.[215] In the Wright's stained bone marrow, megakaryocytes will often appear hyperlobulated and platelets abnormally large. In addition to the abnormal maturation in the bone marrow, a moderate shortening of platelet survival has been described.[216] Ineffective thrombopoiesis has also been seen in DiGuglielmo's syndrome, paroxysmal nocturnal hemoglobinuria, certain forms of preleukemia, and acute myelomonocytic leukemias.

Although cyclic thrombocytopenia is an unusual clinical state, it falls within the group of ineffective thrombopoiesis.[217] In this disorder, there is alternating thrombocytosis and thrombocytopenia at regular intervals.

B. Altered Distribution of Platelets

The splenic platelet pool normally contains approximately one third of the total platelet mass.[176] When the spleen is enlarged, the splenic pool increases proportionately, and the number of platelets sequestered in the spleen also increases. Thus, depending on the degree of splenomegaly, the normal body to spleen distribution of 70 to 30% can be reversed.

For some reason, when thrombocytopenia occurs as a result of altered distribution the bone marrow does not respond with increased thrombopoiesis. In cirrhotics with portal hypertension and splenomegaly, mild thrombocytopenia of around 60 to 80,000 platelets per cubic millimeter is frequently found. It is important to emphasize that with splenomegaly some degree of hypersplenism or increased platelet destruction may coexist, with increased sequestration making the thrombocytopenia more severe.[216] Altered distribution, with increased splenic sequestration, may be seen in a number of clinical states, including sarcoidosis, Gaucher's disease, Hodgkin's disease, various lymphomas, and Felty's syndrome.

Hypothermic anesthesia has been complicated by thrombocytopenia. This is usually of no clinical consequence.[218]

C. Nonimmunologic Destructive Thrombocytopenias

Nonimmunologic destructive thrombocytopenias are varied. A classic example of this type of acquired thrombocytopenia is disseminated intravascular coagulation (DIC). The degree of thrombocytopenia encountered in DIC depends on the rate at which platelets are consumed and their production rate. In low-grade DIC states, platelet counts may not be suppressed as long as the bone marrow can keep the production rate in line with the rate of destruction. Usually, however, with acute DIC, platelet counts drop precipitously and do not return to normal until the underlying disease is treated.

With the increase in cardiac surgery and prosthetic valve replacement, as well as arterial and venous graft surgery, frequent examples of random platelet destruction through mechanical trauma have also been reported. The so-called Waring blender syndrome, which is the mechanical destruction of red cells by cardiac prosthetic valves, typifies what happens to intravascular cellular elements under these circumstances.

Thrombocytopenias may complicate a number of bacterial, viral, or rickettsial infections.[219,220] There may be a number of pathophysiologic mechanisms, including: (1) direct suppression of platelet production as is seen in certain viral infections, (2) direct interaction between platelets, viruses, and bacteria, resulting in accelerated platelet destruction, and (3) associated disseminated intravascular coagulation triggered by the infectious agent. Thrombocytopenia in a febrile patient should always alert the clinician to the possibility of bacteremia.[220] Infections that are most often complicated by thrombocytopenia include gram-negative bacteremias,[221] Rocky Mountain spotted fever, typhus, mumps, and malaria. The platelet count is also reduced in up to 50% of patients with infectious mononucleosis.[222]

Thrombotic thrombocytopenic purpura (TTP) was first described in 1925 by Moschcowitz.[223] It is characterized by a triad of hemolytic anemia with microangiopathic changes in the red blood cells, thrombocytopenia, and a fluctuating bizarre neurologic syndrome.[224] Fever and renal dysfunction are also present.[225] Typical pathologic changes are widespread hyaline occlusions of small blood vessels. The hemolytic uremic syndrome in children is somewhat similar in its clinical manifestations to thrombotic thrombocytopenic purpura.[226]

D. Immunologic Thrombocytopenias

The fourth group of megakaryocytic thrombocytopenias is related to immunologic causes. Platelets that are coated with antiplatelet antibodies will have shortened life spans, because they are removed from the circulation by the reticuloendothelial cells in the liver and spleen. Causes of the production of antiplatelet antibodies are numerous.

1. Isoimmune Thrombocytopenia

Isoimmune thrombocytopenia is the result of platelet antibodies that arise from active immunization of a patient to platelet antigens. A typical example is the immunization of a mother by fetal platelet isoantigens.[227] Immunization to four such isoantigens has been described: i.e., Pl^{A1}, Pl^{E2}, $PlGrLy^{B1}$, and $PlGrLy^{C1}$.[228] The first-born child has been affected in approximately one half of the reported cases, which is in contrast to erythroblastosis fetalis due to incompatibility in the Rh system. Affected infants may appear normal at birth, but soon develop scattered petechial and purpuric hemorrhages.[229] In the symptomatic cases, platelet levels are usually less than 30,000 per cubic millimeter and may diminish even further during the first few hours after birth. Without treatment, the thrombocytopenia will persist for 2 to 3 weeks.

Platelet isoantibodies may also occur in patients who have received multiple transfusions. Platelets and leukocytes share histocompatibility antigens and this may be of great importance in caring for patients in instances of aplastic anemia and acute leukemias, who need long-term platelet replacements with little chance of marrow remission. In these situations, it is often necessary to attempt to provide closely matched platelets to the recipient.

2. Drug-Induced Immunologic Thrombocytopenic Purpura

Quinine-induced purpura was first described by Vipan in 1865.[230] Following this, Rosenthal, in 1928, showed that thrombocytopenia could be reinduced in patients by again administering the drug after the initial recovery.[231] Drug-induced platelet antibodies are the result of an idiosyncratic reaction, which will develop in only a very small portion of the persons exposed to a given drug. An IgM antibody has been documented in some cases of thrombocytopenia due to thiazide ingestion and also in a single case associated with rifampin.[210,232] However, in the majority of cases, the responsible antibodies have been of the IgG type. The drug apparently acts as a hapten. In vivo, the interaction between the drug, antibody, and platelet leads to platelet injury and rapid sequestration with destruction. The in vitro demonstration of drug-induced platelet antibodies involves various serologic procedures.[233] One must have antibody, drug, and platelets in the system in order for the reactions to occur. Either the antibody or the drug alone are ineffective in terms of demonstrating platelet injury and destruction. Of the many drugs identified as causing immunologic thrombocytopenia, quinidine, quinine, and digitoxin, as well as thiazides have been most frequently implicated (Table 9).

Serologic verification of the presence of antibodies may be made by a variety of techniques. These include: complement fixation,[234] immune-injury,[233] platelet agglutination, and inhibition of clot retraction. Recently, the use of platelet aggregometry has been proposed as suitable for detection of platelet antibodies.[235]

Ordinarily, treatment is not needed since withdrawal of the offending drug is followed by rapid recovery. Platelet transfusion may be used during acute life threatening thrombocytopenia.

3. Posttransfusion Thrombocytopenia Due to Isoantibodies

Thrombocytopenia occurring approximately 1 week after blood transfusion is a unique entity in the immunologic group of thrombocytopenias. In the cases that have been studied to date, the antibody has been specific for a genetically determined platelet antigen: Pl^{A1}.[236] This antigen is present in approximately 98% of the normal population, but is lacking in the platelets of patients who develop posttransfusion purpura. The majority of cases have been women.[237] The anti-Pl^{A1} antibody, in most instances, can be detected by appropriate laboratory tests including agglutination, clot retraction inhibition, and complement fixation.

Transfused platelets are ineffective in the treatment of posttransfusion purpura. Plasmapheresis and exchange transfusion have been tried successfully.

4. Other Immunologic Thrombocytopenias

Many other disorders are associated with immunologic thrombocytopenia including systemic lupus erythematosus,[238] autoimmune hemolytic anemias (Evans syndrome),[239] chronic lymphocytic leukemia,[240] various lymphocytic lymphomas, rheumatoid arthritis, and hyperthyroidism.[241] In the case of systemic lupus erythematosus, the thrombocytopenia may precede by months or even years other manifestations of the disease. Platelet antibodies have been demonstrated in as many as 70% of these patients when more sensitive tests have been used.

5. Idiopathic Thrombocytopenic Purpura

When all known causes of thrombocytopenia are eliminated, one must consider the idiopathic variety of thrombocytopenia. The term idiopathic thrombocytopenic purpura (ITP) is usually employed to refer to instances with thrombocytopenia associated with no apparent exogenous etiologic factors or underlying disease states.[242] ITP is a diagnosis of exclusion and should be regarded as a syndrome that may arise in several different ways and one that undoubtedly encompasses a variety of fundamentally different disorders. ITP may occur in acute, chronic, or recurrent forms. By definition, the recurrent form is characterized by episodes of thrombocytopenia and periods in which the platelet count is normal. There are a number of differences between acute and chronic ITP (Table 10).

ITP is more common than all secondary forms of thrombocytopenia combined. The acute form occurs most frequently in children and young adults, while the chronic form occurs in patients of all ages, but is most common in adults of 20 to 40 years of age, with a marked female predominance.

There is now convincing evidence that the syndrome of ITP is due to platelet destruc-

TABLE 9
Drugs Causing Immunologic Thrombocytopenia[a]

Analgesics
    Salicylates*
    Acetaminophen
    Phenylbutazone*
    Antipyrine
Antibiotics
    Cephalothin
    Penicillin
    Streptomycin
    Para-aminosalicylic acid (PAS)
    Rifampin
    Novobiocin
    Various sulfa drugs*
Cinchona alkaloids
    Quinidine*
    Quinine*
Hypnotics
    Phenobarbital
    Meprobamate*
    Sedormid*
    Dilantin®
    Chlorpromazine
    Troxidone
    Methoin

Oral hypoglycemics
    Chlorpropamide*
    Tolbutamide
Heavy Metals
    Gold
    Mercury
    Bismuth
    Organic arsenicals*
Diuretics
    Acetazolamide
    Chlorothiazide*
    Mercurial diuretics
Others
    Digitoxin*
    Ergot
    Methyldopa
    Propylthiouracil
    Penicillamine
    Phenindione
    Disulfiram (Antabuse®)
    Chloroquine*
    Stibophen (Fuadin®)

[a] * = Drugs most frequently associated with immunologic thrombocytopenia.

TABLE 10
Clinical Picture of Acute and Chronic Idiopathic Thrombocytopenia

Clinical Characteristic	Acute	Chronic
Age	Less than 8 years old	20—40 years old
Sex predilection	None	Female over male 3:1
Prior infection	Common	Unusual
Onset of bleeding	Abrupt	Insidious
Platelet count	<20,000/mℓ mm³	30,000 to 80,000/mℓ mm³
Splenomegaly	Absent	Absent
Duration	2—6 weeks	Months to years
Spontaneous remissions	Occur in 90% of patients	Uncommon, fluctuating clinical course
Therapy		
Steroids	70% response	30% response
Splenectomy	70% response	90% response under age 45
		40% response over age 45

tion as a result of an immunologic process.[243] Platelet survival studies have yielded half-life results ranging from 2 to 3 days to minutes.[244] Isologous platelets survive no longer than autologous platelets, suggesting that the shortened half-life is due to a process extrinsic to the platelet. The infusion of plasma from patients with ITP will result in thrombocytopenia in a normal recipient.[245]

This "ITP Factor" is an IgG immunoglobulin that can be removed from the serum by absorption with normal human platelets and subsequently eluted.[246] This antibody

TABLE 11

Laboratory Tests for Platelet Antibodies

Platelet precipitation
Passive hemagglutination
Platelet lysis
Platelet complement fixation
Platelet agglutination
Antihuman globulin (AHG) techniques, direct and indirect
AHG agglutination
Mixed antiglobulin reaction
Antiglobulin consumption test
Fluorescent antibody techniques
Platelet electrophoresis
Platelet factor 3 availability test
Immunofluorescence microphotometry (IFMP)
^{14}C serotonin release
^{51}CR release from PNH platelets
^{131}I-FAB-Anti-F (ab)$_2$ test for quantitation of platelet-bound immunoglobulin
Inhibition of anti-IgG dependent lysis of sheep erythrocytes
Platelet indirect radioactive Coombs test
Platelet migration inhibition
Inhibition of platelet aggregation

has been produced by spleen cells in tissue cultures.[247] A number of laboratory tests for evaluating the presence of antiplatelet antibodies have been introduced in the past few years (Table 11).[248] There is, however, a relatively high incidence of negative results with these tests, despite the clinical picture of markedly accelerated platelet destruction.[246] Positive results are more frequently obtained in other clinical conditions associated with immunologic thrombocytopenias such as systemic lupus and lymphoreticular disorders.

In the acute idiopathic thrombocytopenic purpura syndrome, the disorder is usually self-limited, and spontaneous remissions occur in approximately 90 to 95% of the patients.[249] The duration of the illness may range from days to months. In contrast, chronic ITP is characterized by a fluctuating clinical course with episodes of bleeding lasting a few days or weeks and months of clinically asymptomatic periods.[250] Cessation of bleeding is often associated with a rapid increase in the number of platelets in these patients. Spontaneous remissions are uncommon and are usually incomplete.[251]

On examination of the peripheral blood, one typically finds platelets that are abnormally large, with some variation in shape.[252] The marrow is characterized by megakaryocytic hyperplasia.[176] Typically, the megakaryocytes are increased in size, and young forms with single nuclei and diminished cytoplasm are commonly present.[253]

Treatment of idiopathic thrombocytopenia purpura has included steroids, splenectomy, and, in occasional cases, immunosuppressive agents. In the acute form, often no treatment is indicated. As noted previously, as many as 90 to 95% of affected children will make a complete recovery without therapy. The mortality rate is extremely low. Consequently, in children with mild bleeding manifestations, particularly if the disorder has developed following an acute infection, only careful observation is indicated. Spontaneous recovery in older patients is less consistent, but in many circumstances these patients may also be managed expectantly.

Conservative management, however, is inadvisable if bleeding is severe or if a good follow-up cannot be assured. Serious bleeding is rare if the platelet count is greater than 50,000 per cubic milliliter in patients who have had the disease for more than 2 months. Expectant therapy should be limited to a period of not more than 6 months, since spontaneous remissions are exceedingly rare beyond this time.

Approximately 60 to 80% of patients with chronic ITP will respond to steroids with some increase in the platelet count.[254] The number of patients in whom these hormones will produce a complete remission or normalization of the platelet count is much smaller, ranging from 10 to 15%. The mechanism of action is not well understood, although steroids apparently reduce phagocytosis in the spleen and increase the platelet life span as a result.[255] Ordinarily, the dose of prednisone is approximately 60 mg/day in three to four divided doses. Steroid therapy may be maintained for a period of 2 weeks, and with the appearance of remission, dosage can be tapered over a period of several weeks. If relapse occurs, steroids should be increased or reinstituted at the initial dose and splenectomy considered.[254]

Splenectomy remains the treatment of choice for idiopathic thrombocytopenic purpura that does not remit following a trial of steroids. The response to splenectomy varies from 70 to 90%. The effectiveness of splenectomy in ITP presumably is the result of removal of the organ that is mainly responsible for sequestration of the antibody-sensitized platelets. Indications for splenectomy may be summarized as follows: (1) failure of spontaneous remission to occur after six or more months of observation in patients with moderate to severe clinical symptomatology, (2) failure to respond to steroid therapy and (3) when adequate follow-up cannot be assured.

Splenectomy is contraindicated in ITP in the following circumstances: (1) early in the first episode of bleeding, especially in children, (2) in patients with acute fulminating cases in which mortality following splenectomy has been high, (3) in patients with cardiac or other medical complications that contraindicate major surgery, (4) in children under 2 years of age in whom the hazard of fulminating infection following splenectomy is greater than at a later age and (5) in most cases of ITP in pregnant women.

In 5 to 20% of patients with ITP, splenectomy produces little or no lasting benefit. Unfortunately, there is no way of predicting this prior to the operation. The value of splenic sequestration studies is controversial, and currently they are not relied upon. Accessory spleens are mentioned frequently as the cause of failure of splenectomy. Most accessory spleens will be found in the area of the splenic pedicle and can be easily recognized and removed by the surgeon. However, occasionally, distant sites such as lower pelvis, lungs, and liver are encountered, and in these instances the spleen is not easily identified. Rupture of the spleen at surgery may produce splenosis — multiple small areas of splenic tissue in the peritoneum, representing implants of deposited cells. Surgical removal of the accessory spleen may in some instances result in a permanent remission, although not in all cases. Presumably, an exacerbation of the patient's immune process is responsible for recurrent thrombocytopenia in the majority of cases. In recent years, a number of immunosuppressive drugs have been used in cases of refractory ITP. These have included 6-mercaptopurine, azathioprine, alkylating agents such as Cytoxan® and chlorambucil, and vinka alkaloids such as vincristine.[256]

Ordinarily, in patients with ITP, platelet transfusions are not indicated. Even large numbers of platelets produce only a slight or transient increase in the platelet count, no doubt because of the rapidity with which they are sequestered and destroyed in vivo. Platelet transfusion should be reserved for life threatening emergencies such as subarachnoid hemorrhage.

PART 4: QUANTITATIVE DISORDERS OF PLATELETS — THROMBOCYTOSIS AND THROMBOCYTHEMIA

A platelet count greater than normal may be encountered in a variety of clinical circumstances. Thrombocytosis refers to a moderate, often short-lived and symptomless elevation of platelet count that occurs in association with several well-defined clinical states. The term "thrombocythemia", however, refers to a marked and persistent elevation in the platelet count occurring as a part of a myeloproliferative disorder.[257] By definition, thrombocythemia implies an unregulated proliferation of megakaryocytes, with an associated increased platelet production, in contrast to the reactive megakaryocytic proliferation and platelet production of thrombocytosis. Clinically, a clear cut distinction between thrombocytosis and thrombocythemia may sometimes prove difficult. However, because of the diagnostic, prognostic, and therapeutic implications, an attempt at differentiating these states is certainly worthwhile.

I. THROMBOCYTOSIS

Thrombocytosis is frequently a chance finding. The underlying cause is often readily detectable. Table 12 lists the most frequent causes of thrombocytosis and thrombocythemia. The postsplenectomy elevation in the platelet count typically reaches a peak after 2 weeks and tends to gradually subside in the following 2 to 3 months.[258] The mechanism of thrombocytosis is not entirely understood, although it is felt that removal of a humoral regulator normally produced by the spleen allows the bone marrow to temporarily undergo a megakaryocytic hyperplasia.[259] Subsequent return to normal levels is thought to be on the basis of a feedback inhibition of thrombopoiesis as a result of the high circulating platelet count. This has been experimentally demonstrated in animals following hypertransfusion of platelets.[260] Occasionally there is persistence of thrombocytosis following splenectomy.[258] Platelet function has not been well studied in postsplenectomy thrombocytosis, although increased platelet adhesiveness, i.e., retention, has been demonstrated in postoperative states in general.[261] This could possibly be related to the spleen's role in selectively sequestering more functionally active young platelets.[181]

Thrombocytosis is also seen postoperatively following major but not minor surgery.[262] Typically, the elevated platelet count is seen between the 3rd and 10th postoperative days and gradually will return to normal by the 10th to 16th postoperative day.[263] Counts may increase by 25 to 150% of the preoperative levels. Almost invariably, the thrombocytosis is preceded by a period of 2 to 6 days of thrombocytopenia, which will often begin within an hour after surgery. The mechanism for postoperative thrombocytosis has not been established, although hypoxia, in the course of general anesthesia, necrotic material from wound healing, and an elevation in circulating pulmonary megakaryocytes have all been postulated as possible etiological mechanisms. A recent study by Davis and Ross stress the frequent association of thrombocytosis with underlying malignancy.[264] This was first emphasized in the literature by Olef in 1936.[265] Levin and Conley recorded that in a series of 82 patients with thrombocytosis encountered in a survey of 14,000 patients in the Johns Hopkins Hospital, 31 (38%) had an underlying neoplastic disease.[266] The majority of the patients had carcinoma, but Hodgkin's disease and osteogenic sarcoma were also encountered. The finding of an unexplained thrombocytosis in a patient should suggest the possibility of an occult malignancy. The rather frequent association of thromboembolic disease and malignancy has not been related to the thrombocytosis. Platelet function studies in thrombocytosis associated with malignant disease have not been well evaluated.[267]

Acute blood loss is very frequently associated with the development of thrombocytosis. However, a consistent feature in this situation, as well as the postoperative thrombocytosis, is the prior occurrence of thrombocytopenia. Typically, the elevation in the platelet count occurs 36 hr following the acute hemorrhage.[268] This type of response can also be seen following phlebotomy in patients with polycythemia rubra vera, even though they will frequently have an elevated baseline platelet count.[269]

Iron deficiency anemia has also been associated with thrombocytosis.[270] However, this is a typical finding when the iron deficiency is of short duration. If there is pro-

TABLE 12

Causes of an Elevated Platelet Count

I. Thrombocytosis
    A. Secondary or reactive — transient
        1. Acute blood loss
        2. Postpartum
        3. Infection
        4. Posttraumatic
        5. Postsplenectomy
        6. Exercise
        7. Postoperative state
        8. Drugs — epinephrine
        9. Following thrombocytopenia
            a. Pernicious anemia (after treatment)
            b. Acute thrombocytopenic purpura
            c. Alcohol-induced thrombocytopenia
            d. Drug-induced thrombocytopenia
        10. Ovulation
        11. Sarcoidosis
        12. Adrenal hyperplasia
        13. Osteoporosis
        14. Vinblastine therapy
        15. Oral contraceptives
        16. 7-β-17-α-Dimethyl testosterone
        17. Citrovorum factor therapy
    B. Chronic
        1. Inflammatory bowel disease
            a. Ulcerative colitis
            b. Granulomatous colitis
        2. Rheumatoid arthritis
        3. Neoplasms
            a. Hodgkin's disease
            b. Carcinoma
            c. Osteogenic sarcoma
            d. Retinoblastoma
            e. Mesothelioma
        4. Iron deficiency (late in iron deficiency may see thrombocytopenia)
        5. Chronic hemolytc anemia with splenectomy
        6. Splenic atrophy
II. Thrombocythemia
    A. As a predominant feature — essential thrombocythemia
    B. As an accompanying feature of myeloproliferative disorder
        1. Polycythemia rubra vera
        2. Myeloid metaplasia
        3. Chronic myelocytic leukemia
        4. Myelomonocytic leukemia

found iron deficiency anemia, the patient will become thrombocytopenic. When oral iron therapy is begun, a reticulocytosis will develop that is accompanied by a fall in the platelet count; however, after 20 days a peak count higher than the initial count will be found. With parenteral iron, an increase in the platelet count will parallel the reticulocyte response.[271] The reason for thrombocytosis in early iron deficiency is not apparent, but a rather consistent finding in the bone marrow is megakaryocytic hyperplasia, irrespective of the peripheral platelet count.

Other causes of thrombocytosis are listed in Table 12. Of these, perhaps the most interesting are those that follow drug-induced thrombocytopenia. With the advent of intensive chemotherapeutic treatment of leukemias and lymphomas, one rather frequently encounters this phenomenon. Cytosine arabinoside has been the drug most frequently noted to be associated with the rebound thrombocytosis following marrow suppression. Also of interest is the recent use of the vinka alkaloids (vinblastine and vincristine) in the treatment of refractory patients with autoimmune thrombocytopenic purpura.

II. THROMBOCYTHEMIA

Thrombocythemia (i.e., autonomous production of platelets) is a feature of the myeloproliferative syndromes. To establish the diagnosis of thrombocythemia, one should rule out the clinical states associated with thrombocytosis. It should also be possible to define features of the myeloproliferative syndromes in a given patient. The typical bone marrow finding in the myeloproliferative thrombocythemias is the presence of an increased number of megakaryocytes with increased cytoplasmic size and nuclear lobe count.

In polycythemia rubra vera, one finds a peripheral thrombocytosis in about 50% of the patients at the time of diagnosis.[269] The degree of thrombocythemia is usually modest, being in the range of 450,000 to 1,000,000. However, patients with normal or only moderately elevated platelet counts may develop significant reactive thrombocytosis following phlebotomy or spontaneous bleeding. Thrombosis and/or hemorrhage together account for approximately 30 to 50% of the deaths in treated patients with polycythemia rubra vera.[272] The seemingly paradoxical occurrence of both hemorrhage and thrombosis in a patient with an elevated platelet count has been puzzling. However, in the recent literature a number of disorders of platelet function and morphology have been described in the myeloproliferative syndromes. In many cases, there can be either massive gastrointestinal bleeding requiring emergency surgery or occult gastrointestinal bleeding, which will result in an iron deficiency state with hypochromic microcytic red blood cells on the peripheral smear. The red blood cell count will remain in the vicinity of six to eight million, and often as a result of the iron deficiency, the hematocrit and hemoglobin will fall within the normal range.

Thrombocythemia can also be seen in myelofibrosis, although the finding is rather variable. Bouroncle and Doan found the platelet count to be high in 23 of 97 patients.[273] Although it is not unusual for a moderate to pronounced thrombocythemia to develop during the course of chronic myelogenous leukemia,[274] recent work indicates that perhaps this syndrome should not be classified as a member of the myeloproliferative family.[275]

Essential thrombocythemia or hemorrhagic thrombocytosis is also a member of the myeloproliferative family. This disease is most commonly seen in late middle age or old age, and there is a slight female sex predominance. These patients can present with either thrombotic or hemorrhagic symptoms, although bleeding problems predominate.[276] Typically, there is genitourinary bleeding, gastrointestinal bleeding, bleeding into the skin, or epistaxis. Prolonged bleeding following surgery, particularly dental extractions, is a rather frequent occurrence. Thrombosis of the carotid artery, femoral artery, coronary arteries, deep and superficial veins, pulmonary infarction, and hemorrhagic infarctions of the adrenal glands have all been reported. Ozer et al. outlined criteria for establishing the diagnosis of primary thrombocythemia in 1960.[277]

The bleeding that occurs in thrombocythemia is probably related to the high platelet count; for when the platelet levels are reduced to normal, bleeding will generally cease. The abnormal bleeding has been ascribed to a variety of qualitative platelet defects. Recently, Zucker and Mielke[278] and Ginsberg[279] have emphasized the importance of platelet function tests in the diagnosis and evaluation of an elevated platelet count. A finding of platelet functional abnormalities, particularly with respect to aggregation, is helpful in separating thrombocythemias from thrombocytosis. Also, the absence of epinephrine and collagen-induced aggregation, decreased platelet factor 3 activity, together with abnormalities of the bleeding time and platelet retention, are helpful in predicting which patients with an elevated platelet count are at a high risk for thrombotic or hemorrhagic complications. Defective platelet lipid peroxidation in myeloproliferative disorders has recently been described.[280] Low levels of lipid peroxidation have correlated well with clinical bleeding and bruising problems. In these studies, platelet lipid peroxidation was induced by the sulphydryl-blocking reagent n-ethylmaleimide (NEM). The low levels of lipid peroxidation could be due to: (1) an aged platelet population, (2) an abnormal cell line, (3) a reduction in the cyclo-oxygenase enzyme activity of the platelet prostaglandin synthetic pathway, (4) a reduction in the substrate for platelet prostaglandin synthesis, i.e., arachidonic acid and (5) an abnormality of the phospholipase A activation.

In addition, if one is contemplating using any of the antiplatelet drugs to control thrombotic complications (i.e., dipyridamole or aspirin), it is imperative that in such subjects with thrombocythemia, platelet function studies be undertaken early in order to detect the existence and the nature of platelet functional defects.[281]

Treatment of patients with active clinical bleeding associated with thrombocythemia may require the use of platelet concentrates. However, the other complication — that of thrombosis — is conventionally treated with anticoagulants (i.e., heparin and Coumadin®). The use of antiplatelet drugs in this situation has not been thoroughly evaluated.

REFERENCES

1. **Levin, J. and Bang, F. B.**, A description of cellular coagulation in the *Limulus, Bull. Johns Hopkins Hosp.,* 115, 337, 1964.
2. **Donne, A.**, De L'origine des globules du sang, de leur mode de formation et de leur fin, *C. R. Acad. Sci. Ser. D,* 14, 366, 1842.
3. **Bizzozero, G.**, Sur un nouvel element morphologique du sang chex les mamm: feres et sur son importance dans la trombose et dans la coagulation, *Arch. Ital. Biol.,* 1, 1, 1882.
4. **Eberth, J. D. and Schimmelbusch, C.**, Experimentelle Untersuchungen Uber Thrombose, *Virchows Arch. Pathol. Anat. Physiol.,* 103, 39, 1886.
5. **Wright, J. H.**, The origin and nature of blood plates, *Boston Med. Surg. J.,* 154, 643, 1906.
6. **Bowie, E. J. W. and Owen, C. A., Jr.**, Thrombocytopathy, *Semin. Hematol.,* 5, 73, 1968.
7. **Weiss, H. J.**, Platelet aggregation, adhesion and adenosine diphosphate release in thrombopathia (platelet factor 3 deficiency): in comparison with Glanzmann's thrombasthenia and von Willebrand's disease, *Am. J. Med.,* 43, 570, 1967.
8. **von Willebrand, E. A.**, Hereditar Pseudohamofili, *Fin. Laekaresaellsk. Handl.,* 68, 87, 1926.
9. **von Willebrand, E. A.**, Uber hereditare Pseudo-Hamophilie, *Acta Med. Scand.,* 76, 521, 1931.
10. **von Willebrand, E. A. and Jurgens, R.**, Uber ein neues verebbares Blutingubel: die konstitutionelle Thrombopathie, *Dtsch. Arch. Klin. Med.,* 175, 453, 1933.
11. **Alexander, B. and Goldstein, R.**, Dual hemostatic defects in pseudohemophilia, *J. Clin. Invest.,* 32, 551, 1953.
12. **Quick, A. J. and Hussey, C. V.**, Hemophilic condition in the female, *J. Lab. Clin. Med.,* 42, 929, 1953.
13. **Nilsson, I. M., Blomback, M., Jorpes, E., Blomback, B., and Johansson, S-A.**, von Willebrand's disease and its correction with human plasma fraction I-O, *Acta Med. Scand.,* 159, 179, 1957.
14. **Borchgrevink, C. F.**, Platelet adhesion in vivo in patients with bleeding disorders, *Acta Med. Scand.,* 179, 231, 1961.
15. **Salzman, E. W.**, Measurement of platelet adhesiveness: a simple in vitro technique demonstrating an abnormality in von Willebrand's disease, *J. Lab. Clin. Med.,* 62, 724, 1963.

16. Zimmerman, T. S., Ratnoff, O. D., and Powell, A. E., Immunologic differentiation of classic hemophilia (factor VIII deficiency) and von Willebrand's disease, with observations on combined deficiencies of antihemophiliac factor and proaccelerin (factor V) and an acquired circulating anticoagulant against antihemophiliac factor, *J. Clin. Invest.*, 50, 244, 1971.
17. Zimmerman, T. S. and Edgington, T. S., Molecular immunology of factor VIII, *Annu. Rev. Med.*, 25, 303, 1974.
18. Howard, M. A. and Firkin, B. G., Ristocetin: a new tool in the investigation of platelet aggregation, *Thromb. Diath. Haemorrh.*, 26, 362, 1971.
19. Gangarosa, E. J., Johnson, T. R., and Ramos, H. S., Ristocetin induced thrombocytopenia: site and mechanism of action, *Arch. Inter. Med.*, 105, 83, 1969.
20. Howard, M. A., Sawers, R. J., and Firkin, B. G., Ristocetin: a means of differentiating von Willebrand's disease into two groups, *Blood*, 41, 687, 1973.
21. Weiss, H. J., Hoyer, L. W., Rickles, F. R., Varma, A., and Rogers, J., Quantitative assay of a plasma factor, deficient in von Willebrand's disease, that is necessary for platelet aggregation. Relationship to factor VIII procoagulant activity and antigen content, *J. Clin. Invest.*, 52, 2708, 1973.
22. Baumgartner, H. R., The role of blood flow in platelet adhesion, fibrin deposition and formation of mural thrombi, *Microvasc. Res.*, 5, 167, 1973.
23. Tschopp, T. B., Weiss, H. J., and Baumgartner, H. R., Decreased adhesion of platelets to subendothelium in von Willebrand's disease, *J. Lab. Clin. Med.*, 83, 296, 1974.
24. Hoyer, L. W., de los Santos, R. P., and Hoyer, J. R., Antihemophiliac factor antigen: localization in endothelial cells by immunofluorescent microscopy, *J. Clin. Invest.*, 52, 2737, 1973.
25. Jaffe, E. A., Nachman, R. L., Becker, C. G., and Minick, R. C., Culture of human endothelial cells derived from umbilical veins: identification by morphologic and immunologic criteria, *J. Clin. Invest.*, 52, 2745, 1973.
26. Jaffe, E. A., Hoyer, L. W., and Nachman, R. L., Synthesis of von Willebrand factor by cultured human endothelial cells, *Proc. Natl. Acad. Sci. U.S.A.*, 71, 1906, 1974.
27. Holmberg, L., Mannucci, P. M., Turesson, I., Ruggeri, Z. M., and Nilsson, J. M., Factor VIII antigen in the vessel wall in von Willebrand's disease and haemophilia A, *Scand. J. Haematol.*, 13, 33, 1974.
28. Jaffe, E. A., Hoyer, L. W., and Nachman, R. L., Synthesis of antihemophiliac factor antigen by cultured human endothelial cells, *J. Clin. Invest.*, 52, 2757, 1973.
29. Jaffe, E. A., Endothelial cells and the biology of factor VIII, *N. Engl. J. Med.*, 296, 377, 1977.
30. Hoyer, L. W., von Willebrand's disease, *Prog. Hemostasis Thromb.*, 3, 231, 1976.
31. Gralnick, H. R., Coller, B. S., and Sultan, Y., Carbohydrate deficiency of the factor VIII/von Willebrand factor protein in von Willebrand's disease variants, *Science*, 192, 56, 1976.
32. Peake, I. R., Bloom, A. L., and Giddings, J. C., Inherited variants of factor VIII related protein in von Willebrand's disease, *N. Engl. J. Med.*, 291, 113, 1974.
33. Thomson, C., Forbes, C. D., and Prentice, C. R. M., Evidence for a qualitative defect in factor VIII related antigen in von Willebrand's disease, *Lancet*, 2, 594, 1974.
34. Sultan, Y., Simeon, J., and Caen, J. P., Detection of heterozygotes in both parents of homozygous patients with von Willebrand's disease, *J. Clin. Pathol.*, 28, 309, 1975.
35. Bowie, E. J. W., Fass, D. N., Olson, J. D., and Owen, C. A., Jr., The spectrum of von Willebrand's disease revisited, *Mayo Clin. Proc.*, 51, 35, 1976.
36. Veltkamp, J. J. and van Tilburg, N. H., Detection of heterozygotes for recessive von Willebrand's disease by the assay of antihemophiliac factor-like antigen, *N. Engl. J. Med.*, 289, 882, 1973.
37. Larrieu, M. J., Caen, J. P., Meyer, D. O., Vainer, H., Sultan, Y., and Bernard, J., Congenital bleeding disorders with long bleeding time and normal platelet count. II. von Willebrand's disease (report of 37 patients), *Am. J. Med.*, 45, 354, 1968.
38. Ahr, D. J., Rickles, F. R., Hoyer, L. W., O'Leary, D. S., and Conrad, M. E., von Willebrand's disease in hemorrhagic telangiectasia, *Am. J. Med.*, 62, 452, 1977.
39. Bennett, B. and Ratnoff, O. D., Changes in antihemophiliac factor (AHF, pregnancy and following exercise and pneumoencephalography, *J. Lab. Clin. Med.*, 80, 256, 1972.
40. van Royen, E. A. and ten Cate, J. W., Antigen/biologic activity ratio for factor VIII in late pregnancy, *Lancet*, 2, 449, 1973.
41. Egeberg, O. and Owren, P. A., Oral contraception and blood coagulability, *Br. Med. J.*, 1, 220, 1963.
42. Prentice, C. R. M., Forbes, C. D., and Smith, S. M., Rise of factor VIII after exercise and adrenalin infusion measured by immunologic and biologic techniques, *Thromb. Res.*, 1, 493, 1972.
43. Weiss, H. J., von Willebrand's disease — diagnostic criteria, *Blood*, 32, 668, 1968.
44. Mielke, C. H., Jr., Kaneshiro, M. M., Maher, I. A., Weiner, J. M., and Rapaport, S. I., The standardized normal Ivy bleeding time and its prolongation by aspirin, *Blood*, 34, 204, 1969.

45. **Sahud, M. A. and Cohen, R. J.**, Aspirin induced prolongation of the Ivy bleeding time. Its diagnostic usefulness, *Calif. Med.*, 115, 10, 1971.
46. **Quick, A. J.**, Minot-von Willebrand syndrome, *Am. J. Med. Sci.*, 253, 520, 1967.
47. **Bowie, E. J. W., Didisheim, P., and Thompson, J. H., Jr.**, von Willebrand's disease: a critical review, *Hematol. Rev.*, 1, 1, 1968.
48. **Zucker, M. B., Rifkin, P. L., Friedberg, N. M., and Coller, B. S.**, Mechanisms of platelet function as revealed by the retention of platelets in glass bead columns, *Ann. N. Y. Acad. Sci.*, 201, 138, 1972.
49. **Bowie, E. J. W., Owen, C. A., Jr., Thompson, J. H., Jr., and Didisheim, P.**, Platelet adhesiveness in von Willebrand's disease, *Am. J. Clin. Pathol.*, 52, 69, 1969.
50. **Meyer, D.**, In vitro platelet adhesiveness. Methods of study and clinical significance, *Adv. Exp. Biol. Med.*, 34, 123, 1972.
51. **Niessner, H.**, Measurement of platelet adhesiveness using a modified form of the Hellem II method with special reference to von Willebrand's-Jurgens syndrome, *Thromb. Diath. Haemorrh.*, 27, 434, 1972.
52. **Bowie, E. J. W. and Owen, C. A., Jr.**, The value of measuring platelet "adhesiveness" in the diagnosis of bleeding diseases, *Am. J. Clin. Pathol.*, 60, 302, 1973.
53. **Weiss, H. J., Rogers, J., and Brand, H.**, Defective ristocetin induced platelet aggregation in von Willebrand's disease and its correction by factor VIII, *J. Clin. Invest.*, 52, 2697, 1973.
54. **Olson, J. D., Brockway, W. J., Fass, D. N., Magnuson, M. A., and Bowie, E. J. W.**, Evaluation of ristocetin Willebrand factor assay and ristocetin induced platelet aggregation, *Am. J. Clin. Pathol.*, 63, 210, 1975.
55. **Brinkhous, K. M., Graham, J. E., Cooper, H. H., Allain, J. P., and Wagner, R. H.**, Assay of von Willebrand factor in von Willebrand's disease and hemophilia: use of a macroscopic platelet aggregation test, *Thromb. Res.*, 6, 267, 1975.
56. **Kattlove, H. E. and Gomez, M. H.**, Studies on the mechanism of ristocetin induced platelet aggregation, *Blood*, 45, 91, 1975.
57. **Holmberg, L. and Nilsson, I. M.**, Immunologic studies in haemophilia A, *Scand. J. Haematol.*, 10, 12, 1973.
58. **Stites, D. P., Hershgold, E. J., Perlman, J. D., and Fudenberg, H. H.**, Factor VIII detection by hemagglutination inhibition: hemophilia A and von Willebrand's disease, *Science*, 171, 196, 1971.
59. **Hoyer, L. W.**, Immunologic studies of antihemophiliac factor (AHF, factor VIII). IV. Radioimmunoassays of AHF antigen, *J. Lab. Clin. Med.*, 80, 822, 1972.
60. **Cornu, P., Larrieu, M. J., Caen, J., and Bernard, J.**, Transfusion studies in von Willebrand's disease. Effect on bleeding time and factor VIII, *Br. J. Haematol.*, 9, 189, 1963.
61. **Perkins, H. A.**, Correction of the hemostatic defects in von Willebrand's disease, *Blood*, 30, 375, 1967.
62. **Chediak, J. R., Telfer, M. C., and Green, D.**, Platelet function and immunologic parameters in von Willebrand's disease following cryoprecipitate and factor VIII concentrate infusion, *Am. J. Med.*, 62, 369, 1977.
63. **van Creveld, S. and Mochtar, I. A.**, von Willebrand's disease — a plasma deficiency cause of the prolonged bleeding time, *Ann. Pediatr. (Paris)*, 194, 387, 1960.
64. **Handin, R. I. and Moloney, W. C.**, Antibody induced von Willebrand's disease, *Blood*, 44, 933, 1974.
65. **Ingram, G. I. C., Kingston, P. J., Leslie, J., and Bowie, E. J. W.**, Four cases of acquired von Willebrand's syndrome, *Br. J. Haematol.*, 21, 189, 1971.
66. **Ingram, G. I. C., Prentice, C. R. M., Forbes, C. D., and Leslie, J.**, Low Factor VIII-like antigen in acquired von Willebrand's syndrome and response to treatment, *Br. J. Haematol.*, 25, 137, 1973.
67. **Mant, M. J., Hirsh, J., Gauldie, J., Bienenstock, J., Pineo, G. F., and Luke, K. H.**, von Willebrand's syndrome presenting as an acquired bleeding disorder in association with a monoclonal gammopathy, *Blood*, 42, 429, 1973.
68. **Poole-Wilson, T. A.**, Acquired von Willebrand's syndrome in systemic lupus erythematosus, *Proc. Royal Soc. Med.*, 65, 561, 1972.
69. **Simone, T. V., Cornet, J. A., and Abildgaard, C. F.**, Acquired von Willebrand's syndrome in systemic lupus erythematosus, *Blood*, 31, 806, 1968.
70. **Veltkamp, J. J., Stevens, P., Plas, M. V. D., and Loeliger, E. A.**, Production site of bleeding factor. (Acquired Morbus von Willebrand), *Thromb. Diath. Haemorrh.*, 23, 412, 1970.
71. **Sarji, K. E., Stratton, R. D., Wagner, R. H., and Brinkhous, K. M.**, Nature of von Willebrand factor: a new assay and a specific inhibitor, *Proc. Natl. Acad. Sci. U.S.A.*, 71, 2937, 1974.
72. **Bernard, J. and Soulier, J. P.**, Sur une nouvelle variete de dystrophie thrombocytaire hemorragipare congenitale, *Sem. Hop. Paris*, 24, 3217, 1948.

73. **Bithell T. C., Parokh, S. J., and Strong, R. R.**, Platelet function in the Bernard-Soulier syndrome, *Ann. N.Y. Acad. Sci.*, 201, 145, 1972.
74. **Cullum, C., Cooney, D. P., and Schrier, S. L.**, Familial thrombocytopenic thrombocytopathy, *Br. J. Haematol.*, 13, 147, 1967.
75. **Weiss, H. J., Tschopp, T. B., Baumgartner, H. R., Sussman, I. I., Johnson, M. M., and Egan, J. J.**, Decreased adhesion of giant (Bernard-Soulier) platelets to subendothelium: further implications of the role of the von Willebrand factor in hemostasis, *Am. J. Med.*, 57, 920, 1974.
76. **Caen, J., Levy-Toledano, S., and Sultan, Y.**, La dystrophic thrombocytaire hemorragipare (interaction des plaquettes et du facteur Willebrand), *Nouv. Rev. Fr. Hematol.*, 13, 595, 1973.
77. **Bosmann, H. B.**, Platelet adhesiveness and aggregation. II. Surface sialic acid, glycoprotein: N-acetylneuraminic acid transferase, neuraminidase of human blood platelets, *Biochim. Biophys. Acta*, 279, 456, 1972.
78. **Nurden, A. T. and Caen, J. P.**, Specific roles for platelet surface glycoproteins in platelet function, *Nature (London)*, 255, 720, 1975.
79. **Tobelem, G. M., Levy-Toledano, S., Bredoux, R., Michel, H., Nurden, A., and Caen, J. P.**, New approach for determination of the specific functions of platelet membrane sites, *Nature (London)*, 263, 427, 1976.
80. **Caen, J. P., Michel, H., Tobelem, G., Bodevin, E., and Levy-Toledano, S.**, Adhesion and aggregation of human platelets to rabbit subendothelium. A new approach for investigation: specific antibodies, *Experientia*, 33, 91, 1977.
81. **Walsh, P., Mills, D. C. B., Pareti, F. I., Stewart, G. J., Macfarlane, D. E., Johnson, M. M., and Egan, J. J.**, Hereditary giant platelet syndrome: absence of collagen induced coagulant activity and deficiency of factor XI binding to platelets, *Br. J. Haematol.*, 29, 639, 1975.
82. **Evensen, S. A., Solum, N. A., Grottum, K. A., and Hovig, T.**, Familial bleeding disorder with a moderate thrombocytopenia and giant platelets, *Scand. J. Haematol.*, 13, 203, 1974.
83. **Hirsh, J., Castelan, D. J., and Loder, P. B.**, Spontaneous bruising associated with a defect in the interaction of platelets and connective tissue, *Lancet*, 2, 18, 1967.
84. **Caen, J. and Legrand, Y.**, Abnormalities in the platelet collagen reaction, *Ann. N. Y. Acad. Sci.*, 201, 194, 1972.
85. **Glanzmann, E.**, Hereditare hamorrhagische thrombasthenie: ein beitrag zur pathologic der blutlattchen, *Jahrb. Kinderheilkd.*, 88, 113, 1918.
86. **Fonio, A. and Schwend, J.**, *Èner die Thrombocyten der Menschilchen Blutes*, Hans Huber, Bern, 1942.
87. **Braunsteiner, H. and Pakesch, F.**, Thrombocytoasthenia and thrombocytopathia: old names and new diseases, *Blood*, 11, 965, 1956.
88. **Zucker, M. B., Pert, J., and Hilgartner, M. W.**, Platelet function in a patient with thrombasthenia, *Blood*, 28, 524, 1966.
89. **Legrand, C. and Caen, J. P.**, Binding of ^{14}C-ADP by thrombasthenic platelet membranes, *Haemostasis*, 5, 231, 1976.
90. **Cronberg, S., Nilsson, I. M., and Zettergvist, E.**, Investigation of a family with members with both severe and mild degree of thrombasthenia, *Acta Paediatr. Scand.*, 56, 189, 1967.
91. **Weiss, H. J.**, Abnormalities of actor VIII and platelet aggregation: use of ristocetin in diagnosing the von Willebrand syndrome, *Blood*, 45, 403, 1975.
92. **Caen, J.**, Glanzmann thrombasthenia, *Clin. Haematol.*, 1, 383, 1972.
93. **Karpatkin, S. and Weiss, H. J.**, Deficiency of glutathione peroxidase associated with high levels of reduced glutathione in Glanzmann's thrombasthenia, *N. Engl. J. Med.*, 287, 1062, 1972.
94. **Moser, K., Lechner, K., and Vinazzer, H.**, A hitherto not described enzyme defect in thrombasthenia: glutathione reductase deficiency, *Thromb. Diath. Haemorrh.*, 19, 46, 1968.
95. **Rafelson, M. E. and Booyse, F. M.**, Molecular aspects of platelet aggregation, in *Platelet Aggregation*, Caen, J., Ed., Masson et Cie, Paris, 1971, 95.
96. **Nurden, A. T. and Caen, J. P.**, An abnormal platelet glycoprotein pattern in three cases of Glanzmann's thrombasthenia, *Br. J. Haematol.*, 28, 253, 1974.
97. **Caen, J. P., Vainer, H., and Gautier, A.**, Thrombasthenia, *Thromb. Diath. Haemorrh.*, 26 (Suppl.), 223, 1967.
98. **Borchgrevinck, C. F. and Waaler, B. A.**, The secondary bleeding time: a new method for the differentiation of hemorrhagic diseases, *Acta Med. Scand.*, 162, 361, 1958.
99. **Inceman, S., Asuman, U., and Aran, M.**, Essential athrombia, *Thromb. Diath. Haemorrh.*, 8, 502, 1962.
100. **Inceman, S. and Tangun, Y.**, Essential athrombia, *Thromb. Diath. Haemorrh.*, 33, 278, 1975.
101. **Weiss, H. J.**, Platelet aggregation, adhesion and adenosine diphosphate release in thrombopathia (platelet factor-3 deficiency): a comparison with Glanzmann's thrombasthenia and von Willebrand's disease, *Am. J. Med.*, 43, 570, 1967.

102. **Hardisty, R. M. and Hutton, R. A.**, Bleeding tendency associated with "new" abnormality of platelet behaviour, *Lancet,* 1, 983, 1967.
103. **O'Brien, J. R.**, Platelets: a Portsmouth syndrome? *Lancet,* 2, 258, 1967.
104. **Zucker, S., Mielke, C. H., Durocher, J. R., and Crosby, W. H.**, Oozing and bruising due to abnormal platelet function (thrombocytopathia), *Ann. Int. Med.,* 76, 725, 1972.
105. **Hardisty, R. M., Mills, D. C. B., and Kets-Ard, K.**, The platelet defect associated with albinism, *Br. J. Haematol.,* 23, 679, 1972.
106. **White, J. C., Edson, Desnick, S. J., and Witkop, C. J.**, Studies of platelets in a variant of the Hermansky-Pudlak syndrome, *Am. J. Pathol.,* 63, 319, 1971.
107. **Holmsen, H.**, The platelet: its membrane, physiology and biochemistry, *Clin. Haematol.,* 1, 235, 1972.
108. **Weiss, H. J., Chervenick, P. A., Zahiski, R., and Factor, A.**, A familial defect in platelet function associated with impaired release of adenosine diphosphate, *N. Engl. J. Med.,* 281, 1264, 1969.
109. **Pareti, F. I., Day, H. J., and Mills, D. C. B.**, Nucleotide and serotonin metabolism in patients with defective secondary aggregation, *Blood,* 44, 789, 1974.
110. **Holmsen, H. and Weiss, H. J.**, Further evidence for a deficient storage pool of adenine nucleotides in platelets from some patients with thrombocytopathia, "storage-pool disease", *Blood,* 39, 197, 1972.
111. **Lages, B., Scrutton, M. C., Holmsen, H., Day, J. H., and Weiss, H. J.**, Metal ion content of gel-filtered platelets from patients with storage pool disease, *Blood,* 46, 119, 1975.
112. **Safrit, H., Weiss, H. J., and Phillips, G. B.**, The phospholipid and fatty acid composition of platelets in patients with primary defects in platelet function, *Lipids,* 7, 60, 1972.
113. **Weiss, H. J., Tschopp, T. B., Rogers, J., and Brand, H.**, Studies of platelet 5-hydroxytryptamine (serotonin) in storage pool disease and albinism, *J. Clin. Invest.,* 54, 421, 1974.
114. **Holmsen, H., Setkowski, C. A., Lages, B., Day, J. H., Weiss, H. J., and Scrutton, M. C.**, Content and thrombin induced release of acid hydrolases in gel-filtered platelets from patients with storage pool disease, *Blood,* 46, 131, 1975.
115. **White, J. G. and Witkop, C. J.**, Effects of normal and aspirin platelets on defective secondary aggregation in the Hermansky-Pudlak syndrome: a test for storage pool deficient platelets, *Am. J. Pathol.,* 68, 57, 1972.
116. **Gerrard, J. M., White, J. G., Rao, G. H. R., Krivit, W., and Witkop, C. J.**, Labile aggregation stimulating substances (LASS): the factor from storage pool deficient platelets correcting defective aggregation and release of aspirin treated normal patients, *Br. J. Haematol.,* 29, 657, 1975.
117. **Weiss, H. J.**, Platelet physiology and abnormalities of platelet function, *N. Engl. J. Med.,* 293, 580, 1975.
118. **Baldini, M. G.**, Nature of the platelet defect in the Wiskott-Aldrich syndrome, *Ann. N. Y. Acad. Sci.,* 201, 437, 1972.
119. **Murphey, S., Oski, F. A., Naiman, J. L., Lusch, C. J., Goldberg, S., and Gardner, F. H.**, Platelet size and kinetics in hereditary and acquired thrombocytopenia, *N. Engl. J. Med.,* 286, 499, 1972.
120. **Kuramoto, A., Steiner, M., and Baldini, M. G.**, Lack of platelet response to stimulation in the Wiskott-Aldrich syndrome, *N. Engl. J. Med.,* 282, 475, 1970.
121. **Schaar, F. E.**, Familial idiopathic thrombocytopenic purpura, *J. Pediatr.,* 62, 546, 1963.
122. **Day, H. J. and Holmsen, H.**, Platelet adenine nucleotide "storage pool deficiency" in thrombocytopenia absent radii syndrome, *JAMA,* 221, 1053, 1972.
123. **Bell, T. G., Meyers, K. M., Prieur, D. J., Fauci, A. S., Wolff, S. M., and Padgett, G. A.**, Decreased nucleotide and serotonin storage associated with defective function in Chediak-Higashi syndrome cattle and human platelets, *Blood,* 48, 175, 1976.
124. **Corby, D. G. and Zuck, T. F.**, Newborn platelet dysfunction: a storage pool and release defect, *Thromb. Haemost.,* 36, 200, 1976.
125. **Weiss, H. J.**, Abnormalities in platelet function due to defects in the release reaction, *Ann. N. Y. Acad. Sci.,* 201, 161, 1972.
126. **Malmsten, C., Hamberg, M., Svenson, J., and Sammuelsson, B.**, Physiological role of an endoperoxide in human platelets: hemostatic defect due to platelet cyclo-oxygenase deficiency, *Proc. Natl. Acad. Sci. U.S.A.,* 72, 1446, 1975.
127. **Weiss, H. J. and Lages, B. A.**, Possible congenital defect in platelet thromboxane synthetase, *Lancet,* 1, 760, 1977.
128. **Weiss, H. J. and Ames, R. P.**, Ultrastructural findings in storage pool disease and aspirin-like defect of platelets, *Am. J. Pathol.,* 71, 447, 1973.
129. **Weiss, H. J.**, Abnormalities of factor VIII and platelet aggregation: use of ristocetin in diagnosing the von Willebrand's syndrome, *Blood,* 45, 403, 1975.
130. **Schwartz, J. P., Cooperberg, A. A., and Rosenberg, A.**, Platelet-function studies in patients with glucose-6-phosphate dehydrogenase deficiency, *Br. J. Haematol.,* 27, 273, 1974.

131. Sultan, Y., Brouet, J. C., and Devergie, A., Isolated platelet factor 3 deficiency, *N. Engl. J. Med.*, 294, 1121, 1976.
132. Alport, A. C., Hereditary familial congenital haemorrhagic nephritis, *Br. Med. J.*, 1, 504, 1927.
133. Epstein, C. J., Sahud, M. A., Piel, C. F., Goodman, J. R., Bernfield, M. R., Kushner, J. H., and Ablin, A. R., Hereditary macrothrombocytopathia, nephritis, and deafness, *Am. J. Med.*, 52, 299, 1972.
134. Eckstein, J. D., Filip, D. J., and Watts, J. C., Hereditary thrombocytopenia, deafness and renal disease, *Ann. Intern. Med.*, 82, 639, 1975.
135. Parsa, K. P., Lee, D. B. N., Zamboni, L., and Glassock, R. J., Hereditary nephritis, deafness and abnormal thrombopoiesis, *Am. J. Med.*, 60, 665, 1976.
136. Hegglin, V. R., Gleichzeitige konstitutionelle ver underungen an Neutrophilen und Thrombozyten, *Helv. Med. Acta*, 4, 439, 1945.
137. Lusher, J. M., Schneider, J., Mizukami, I., and Evans, R. K., The May-Hegglin anomaly: platelet function, ultrastructure and chromosome studies, *Blood*, 32, 950, 1968.
138. Godwin, H. A. and Ginsberg, A. D., May-Hegglin Anomaly: Defect in Megakaryocyte Fragmentation, 14th Annu. meeting Am. Soc. Hematology, San Francisco, 1971.
139. Estes, J. W., Carey, R. J., and Desai, R. G., Marfan syndrome: hematologic abnormalities in a family, *Arch. Intern. Med.*, 116, 889, 1965.
140. Estes, J. W., Platelet size and function in the inheritable disorders of connective tissue, *Ann. Intern. Med.*, 68, 1237, 1968.
141. Estes, J. W., Platelet abnormalities: inheritable disorders of connective tissue, *Ann. N. Y. Acad. Sci.*, 201, 445, 1972.
142. Czapek, E., Devkin, D., and Salzman, E. W., Platelet dysfunction in glycogen storage disease type I, *Blood*, 41, 235, 1973.
143. Weiss, H. J. and Rogers, J., Fibrinogen and platelets in the primary arrest of bleeding, *N. Engl. J. Med.*, 285, 369, 1971.
144. Inceman, S., Caen, J., and Bernard, J., Aggregation, adhesion and viscous metamorphosis of platelets in congenital fibrinogen deficiencies, *J. Lab. Clin. Med.*, 68, 21, 1966.
145. Lewis, J. H., Zucker, M. B., and Ferguson, J. H., Bleeding tendency in uremia, *Blood*, 11, 1073, 1956.
146. Larrain, C. and Langdell, R. D., The hemostatic defect of uremia. II. Investigation of dogs with experimentally produced acute urinary retention, *Blood*, 11, 1067, 1956.
147. Castaldi, P. A., Rozenberg, M. C., and Stewart, J. H., The bleeding disorder of uremia, *Lancet*, 2, 66, 1966.
148. Rabiner, S. F. and Hrodek, O., Platelet factor 3 in normal subjects and in patients with renal failure, *J. Clin. Invest.*, 47, 901, 1968.
149. Joist, H. H., Pechan, J., Schikowski, U., Hubner, G., and Gross, R., Studies on the nature and etiology of uremic thrombocytopathy, *Verh. Dtsch. Ges. Inn. Med.*, 75, 476, 1969.
150. Somer, J. B., Stewart, J. H., and Castaldi, P. A., The effect of urea on the aggregation of normal human platelets, *Thromb. Diath. Haemorrh.*, 19, 64, 1968.
151. Eknoyan, G., Wacksman, S. J., Glueck, H. I., and Will, J. J., Platelet function in renal failure, *N. Engl. J. Med.*, 280, 677, 1969.
152. Stewart, J. H. and Castaldi, P. A., Uraemic bleeding: a reversible platelet defect corrected by dialysis, *Q. J. Med.*, 36, 143, 1967.
153. Horowitz, H. I., Cohen, B. D., Martinez, P., and Papayoanou, M. F., Defective ADP-induced platelet factor 3 activation in uremia, *Blood*, 30, 331, 1967.
154. Horowitz, H. I., Stein, I. M., Cohen, B. D., and White, J. G., Further studies on the platelet-inhibiting effect of guanidinosuccinic acid and its role in uremic bleeding, *Am. J. Med.*, 49, 336, 1970.
155. Dunn, I., Weinstein, I. M., Maxwell, M. H., and Kleeman, C. R., Significance of circulating phenols in anemia of renal disease, *Proc. Soc. Exp. Biol. Med.*, 99, 86, 1958.
156. Michon, P., Larcan, A., Streiff, F., and Remigy, E., La diathse hemorragique ded la macroglobulinemia de Waldenstrom, *Sang*, 30, 447, 1959.
157. Perkins, H. A., MacKenzie, M. R., and Fudenberg, H. H., Hemostatic defects in dysproteinemias, *Blood*, 35, 695, 1970.
158. Vigliano, E. M. and Horowitz, H. I., Bleeding syndrome in a patient with IgA myeloma: interaction of protein and connective tissue, *Blood*, 29, 823, 1967.
159. Godal, H. C. and Borchgrevink, C. F., The effect of plasmapheresis on the hemostatic function in patients with macroglobulinemia of Waldenstrom and multiple myeloma, *Scand. J. Clin. Lab. Invest.*, 17, 133, 1965.
160. Bonnin, J. A., Platelet functional defects in thrombocytopenic purpura, *Blood*, 12, 726, 1967.

161. **Ulutin, O. J. and Ulutin, S. B.,** Yaygin damar ici pihtilasmasi, sarf olunma koagluopatisi ve fibrinolsis, *Turk. Tip Alemi*, 1, 16, 1971.
162. **Wilson, P. A. and Douglas, A. S.,** Platelet abnormality in human scurvy, *Lancet*, 1, 975, 1967.
163. **Maurer, H. M., McCue, C. M., Caul, J., and Still, W. J. S.,** Impairment in platelet aggregation in congenital heart disease, *Blood*, 40, 207, 1972.
164. **Larrieu, M. J.,** The effects of fibrinogen degradation products on platelets and coagulation, in *Trans. Conf. Int. Committee on Hemostasis and Thrombosis*, Brinkhouse, K. M., Ed., Schattauer, Stuttgart, 1966, 215.
165. **Stachurska, J.,** Inhibition of platelet aggregation by dialyzable fibrinogen degradation products (FDP), *Thromb. Diath. Haemorrh.*, 23, 91, 1970.
166. **Thomas, D. P.,** Abnormalities of platelet aggregation in cirrhosis, *Ann. N. Y. Acad. Sci.*, 201, 243, 1972.
167. **Weiss, H. J.,** The pharmacology of platelet inhibition, *Prog. Hemostasis Thromb.*, 1, 199, 1972.
168. **Mustard, J. F. and Parcham, M. A.,** Factors influencing platelet function: adhesion, release, and aggregation, *Pharmacol. Rev.*, 22, 97, 1970.
169. **Weiss, H. J.,** Antiplatelet drugs — a new pharmacologic approach to the prevention of thrombosis, *Am. Heart J.*, 92, 86, 1976.
170. **Salzman, E. W., Harris, W. H., and deSanctis, R. W.,** Reduction in venous thromboembolism by agents affecting platelet function, *N. Engl. J. Med.*, 284, 1287, 1971.
171. **Till, J. E. and McCulloch, E. A.,** A direct measurement of the radiation sensitivity of normal mouse bone marrow cells, *Radiat. Res.*, 14, 213, 1961.
172. **Ham, S. S. and Baker, B. L.,** The ultrastructure of megakaryocytes and blood platelets in the rat spleen, *Anat. Rec.*, 149, 251, 1964.
173. **Behnke, O.,** An electron microscopic study of megakaryocytes of rat bone marrow. I. Development of the demarcation membrane system and platelet surface coat, *J. Ultrastruct. Res.*, 24, 412, 1968.
174. **Nakao, K.,** Membrane surface specialization of blood platelet and megakaryocytes, *Nature (London)*, 217, 960, 1968.
175. **Harker, L. A.,** Kinetics of thrombopoiesis, *J. Clin. Invest.*, 48, 963, 1968.
176. **Harker, L. A. and Finch, C. A.,** Thrombokinetics in man, *J. Clin. Invest.*, 48, 963, 1969.
177. **Wright, J. H.,** The histogenesis of the blood platelet, *J. Morphol.*, 21, 263, 1910.
178. **Thiery, J. P. and Bessis, M.,** Mecanisme de la plaquettogenese: etude in vitro par la microtinematographie, *Rev. Hematol.*, 11, 162, 1956.
179. **Schulman, I., Pierce, M., Lukens, A., and Currimbhoy, Z.,** Studies on thrombopoiesis. I. A factor in normal human plasma required for platelet production, chronic thrombocytopenia due to its deficiency, *Blood*, 16, 943, 1960.
180. **Davey, N. G.,** *The Survival and Destruction of Human Platelets*, S. Karger, Basel, 1966, 99.
181. **Shulman, N. R., Watkins, S. P., Itscotz, S. B., and Students, A. B.,** Evidence that the spleen retains the youngest and hemostatically most effective platelets, *Trans. Assoc. Am. Physicians*, 81, 302, 1968.
182. **Steiner, M. and Baldini, N.,** Subcellular distribution of ^{51}Cr and characterization of its binding sites in human platelets, *Blood*, 35, 737, 1970.
183. **Bithell, T. C., Athens, J. W., Cartwright, G. E., and Wintrobe, M. M.,** Radioactive diisopropylfluorophosphate as a platelet label, an evaluation of the in vitro and in vivo techniques, *Blood*, 29, 354, 1967.
184. **Murphy, S. M. and Gardner, H.,** The labeling and preservation of human blood platelets, in *The Platelet*, Brinkhous, K. N., Mostofi, F. K., and Shermer, R. W., Eds., Williams & Wilkins, Baltimore, 1971.
185. **Aster, R. H.,** Pooling of platelets in the spleen: role in pathogenesis of "hypersplenic" thrombocytopenia, *J. Clin. Invest.*, 45, 645, 1966.
186. **Aster, R. H. and Jandl, J. H.,** Platelet sequestration in man. I. Method, *J. Clin. Invest.*, 43, 843, 1964.
187. **Leeksma, C. H. W. and Cohen, J. A.,** Determination of the life span of human blood platelet using labeled diisopropylfluorophosphate, *J. Clin. Invest.*, 35, 964, 1956.
188. **Adelson, E., Kaufman, R. M., Berdeguez, C., Lear, A. A., and Rheingold, J. J.,** Platelet tagging with tritium label diisopropylfluorophosphate, *Blood*, 26, 744, 1965.
189. **Aster, R. H.,** Studies of the fate of platelets in rats and man, *Blood*, 34, 117, 1969.
190. **Ebbe, S., Sapienza, P., Duffy, P., and Stohlman, F.,** DFP labeling of platelets during recovery from thrombocytopenia, *Blood*, 35, 613, 1970.
191. **Hirsh, J. and Dorey, J. C. G.,** Platelet function in health and disease, *Prog. Hematol.*, 7, 185, 1972.
192. **Linman, J. W.,** Factors controlling hemopoiesis: thrombopoietic and leukopoietic effects of "anemic" plasma, *J. Lab. Clin. Med.*, 59, 262, 1962.

193. **Brandt, P. W. T.**, Incidence of renal lesions in polycythemia: a study of 91 patients, *Br. Med. J.*, 1, 468, 1963.
194. **Siri, W. E., Van Dyke, D. C., Winchell, H. S., Pollycore, M., Parker, H. G., and Cleveland, A. S.**, Early erythropoietin, blood and physiologic responses to severe hypoxia in man, *J. Appl. Physiol.*, 21, 73, 1966.
195. **Gross, S., Keefer, B., and Newman, A. J.**, The platelets in iron deficiency anemia. I. The response to oral and parenteral iron, *J. Pediatr.*, 34, 315, 1964.
196. **Tyslowitz, R. and Dingemans, E.**, Effect of large doses of estrogen on the blood picture of dogs, *Endocrinology*, 29, 817, 1941.
197. **Shaper, A. G.**, Oestrogens, progesterone and platelets, *Lancet*, 2, 569, 1968.
198. **Fogel, B. J., Arias, D., and Kung, F.**, Platelet counts in healthy premature infants, *J. Pediatr.*, 73, 108, 1968.
199. **McBride, J. A. and Snodgrass, C. A.**, The effect of the normal menstrual cycle on the total platelet count, adhesive platelet count, and platelet adhesiveness, *J. Obstet. Gynaecol. Br. Commonw.*, 75, 367, 1968.
200. **Libre, L. P., Cowan, D. H., Watkins, S. P., and Shulman, N. R.**, Relationships between spleen, platelets and factor VIII levels, *Blood*, 31, 358, 1968.
201. **McClure, P. D., Ingram, G. I. C., and Jones, R. V.**, Platelet changes after adrenalin infusions with and without adrenalin blockers, *Thromb. Diath. Haemorrh.*, 13, 136, 1965.
202. **Bierman, H. R., Kelly, K. H., Cordes, F. L., Byron, R. L., Jr., Polhemus, J. A., and Rappaport, S.**, The release of leukocytes and platelets from the pulmonary circulation by epinephrine, *Blood*, 7, 653, 1952.
203. **Karpatkin, S.**, Heterogeneity of human platelets. I. Metabolic and kinetic evidence suggestive of young and old platelets, *J. Clin. Invest.*, 48, 1073, 1969.
204. **O'Neill, E. M. and Varadi, S.**, Neonatal aplastic anemia in Fanconi's anemia, *Arch. Dis. Child.*, 38, 92, 1963.
205. **Eisenstein, E. M.**, Congenital amegakaryocytic thrombocytopenic purpura, *Clin. Pediatr. (Philadelphia)*, 5, 143, 1966.
206. **Vossaugh, P., Leikin, S., Avery, G., Monit, G., and Sever, J.**, Neonatal thrombocytopenia in association with rubella, *Acta Haematol.*, 35, 158, 1966.
207. **Rodriquez, S. U., Leikin, S., and Hiller, N. P.**, Neonatal thrombocytopenia associated with antepartum administration of thiazide drugs, *N. Engl. J. Med.*, 270, 881, 1964.
208. **Nilsson, L. R.**, Chronic pancytopenia with multiple congenital abnormalities, *Acta Pediatr.*, 48, 518, 1960.
209. **Ackroyd, J. S.**, The pathogenesis of thrombocytopenic purpura due to hypersensitivity to sedormid, *Clin. Sci.*, 7, 249, 1949.
210. **Eisner, E. D. and Crowell, E. R.**, Hydrochlorothiazide dependent thrombocytopenia due to IgM antibody, *JAMA*, 215, 480, 1971.
211. **Kutti, J. and Linefield, A.**, The frequency of thrombocytopenia in patients with heart disease treated with oral diuretics, *Acta Med. Scand.*, 183, 245, 1968.
212. **Cooper, B. A. and Bigelow, F. S.**, Thrombocytopenia associated with the administration of diethylstilbestrol in man, *Ann. Intern. Med.*, 52, 907, 1960.
213. **Cowan, B. H.**, Thrombokinetics studies in alcohol related thrombocytopenia, *J. Lab. Clin. Med.*, 81, 64, 1972.
214. **Haut, M. J. and Cowan, D. H.**, The effect of ethanol on hemostatic properties of human blood platelets, *Am. J. Med.*, 56, 22, 1974.
215. **Japa, J.**, A study of the morphology and development of the megakaryocyte, *Br. J. Exp. Pathol.*, 24, 73, 1943.
216. **Kotilainen, M.**, Platelet kinetics in normal subjects and in haematological disorders, *Scand. J. Haematol. Suppl.*, 5, 1, 1969.
217. **Engstrom, K., Lindquist, A., and Soderstrom, N.**, Periodic thrombocytopenia or platelet dysgenesis occurring in man, *Scand. J. Haematol.*, 3, 290, 1966.
218. **Villalobos, T. J., Adelson, E., Riley, P. A., Crosby, W. H., and Glaucke, H.**, A cause of the thrombocytopenia and leukopenia that occurs in dogs during deep hypothermia, *J. Clin. Invest.*, 37, 1, 1958.
219. **McKay, D. G. and Margaretten, W.**, Disseminated intravascular coagulation in virus diseases, *Arch. Intern. Med.*, 120, 129, 1967.
220. **Corrigan, J. J., Ray, W. L., and May, N.**, Changes in the blood coagulation system associated with septicemia, *N. Engl. J. Med.*, 279, 851, 1968.
221. **Wilhelm, D. J. and Cherubin, C.**, Hypofibrinogenemia and thrombocytopenia with meningococcemia, *Am. J. Dis. Child.*, 113, 494, 1967.
222. **Carter, R. L.**, Platelet levels in infectious mononucleosis, *Blood*, 25, 817, 1965.

223. **Moschcowitz, E.,** An acute febrile pleiochromic anemia with hyaline thrombosis of terminal arterioles and capillaries: an undescribed disease, *Arch. Intern. Med.,* 36, 89, 1925.
224. **Baehr, G., Klemperer, T., and Schifrin, A.,** An acute febrile anemia and thrombocytopenic purpura with diffuse platelet thromboses of capillaries and arterioles, *Trans. Assoc. Am. Physicians,* 51, 43, 1936.
225. **Casale, A.,** Thrombocytic thrombocytopenic purpura: report of a case and review of 157 cases, *Hawaii Med. J.,* 25, 93, 1965.
226. **Brain, M. C.,** The hemolytic uraemic syndrome, *Semin. Hematol.,* 6, 162, 1969.
227. **Pearson, H. A., Shulman, N. R., Marder, V. J., and Cone, T. E.,** Isoimmune neonatal thrombocytopenia purpura: clinical and therapeutic considerations, *Blood,* 23, 154, 1964.
228. **Shulman, N. R., Marker, V. J., Hiller, M. C., and Collier, E. M.,** Platelet and leukocyte isoantigens and antibodies: serologic, physiologic, and clinical studies, *Prog. Hematol.,* 4, 222, 1964.
229. **Poley, J. R. and Stickler, G. B.,** Petechiae in the newborn infant, *Am. J. Dis. Child.,* 102, 365, 1961.
230. **Vipan, W. H.,** Quinine as a cause of purpura, *Lancet,* 2, 37, 1865.
231. **Rosenthal, N.,** The blood picture in purpura, *J. Lab. Clin. Med.,* 13, 303, 1928.
232. **Blajchman, J., Lowry, R. C., Pettit, J. E., and Stradling, P.,** Rifampicin-induced immune thrombocytopenia, *Br. Med. J.,* 3, 24, 1970.
233. **Shulman, N. R.,** Immunoreactions involving platelets, I, III, IV, *J. Exp. Med.,* 107, 665, 1958.
234. **Howell, E. and Perkins, H. A.,** Microtiter modification of the complement fixation test for platelet antibodies, *Transfusion,* 8, 33, 1968.
235. **Deykin, D. and Hellerstein, L. J.,** The assessment of drug dependence in isoimmune antiplatelet antibodies by the use of platelet aggregometry, *J. Clin. Invest.,* 51, 3142, 1972.
236. **Shulman, N. R., Aster, R. H., Leitner, A., and Hiller, M. C.,** Immunoreactions involving platelets. V. Post-transfusion purpura due to a complement fixing antibody against a genetically controlled platelet antigen. A proposed mechanism for thrombocytopenia and its relevance to "autoimmunity", *J. Clin. Invest.,* 40, 1597, 1961.
237. **Morrison, F. S. and Mollison, P. L.,** Post-transfusion purpura, *N. Engl. J. Med.,* 275, 243, 1966.
238. **Eversole, S. L.,** Cases of disseminated lupus erythematosus diagnosed as idiopathic thrombocytopenic purpura, *Johns Hopkins Med. J.,* 96, 210, 1955.
239. **Evans, R. S. and Duane, R. T.,** Acquired hemolytic anemia, *Blood,* 4, 1196, 1949.
240. **Ebbe, S., Wittels, B., and Dameshek, W.,** Autoimmune thrombocytopenic purpura (ITP type) with chronic lymphocytic leukemia, *Blood,* 19, 23, 1964.
241. **Marshall, J. S., Weisberger, A. S., Levy, R. P., and Breckenridge, R. T.,** Co-existent idiopathic thrombocytopenic purpura and hyperthyroidism, *Ann. Intern. Med.,* 67, 411, 1967.
242. **Baldini, M.,** Idiopathic thrombocytopenic purpura, *N. Engl. J. Med.,* 274, 1245, 1969.
243. **Shulman, N. R.,** Similarities between known antiplatelet antibodies, and factor responsible for thrombocytopenia in idiopathic thrombocytopenic purpura, *Ann. N.Y. Acad. Sci.,* 124, 499, 1965.
244. **Aster, R. H. and Keene, W. R.,** Sites of platelet destruction in idiopathic thrombocytopenic purpura, *Br. J. Haematol.,* 15, 61, 1969.
245. **Harrington, W. J., Mimick, V., Hollingsworth, J. W., and Moore, C. V.,** Demonstration of a thrombocytopenic factor in the blood of patients with thrombocytopenic purpura, *J. Lab. Clin. Med.,* 38, 1, 1951.
246. **Karpatkin, S., Strick, N., Karpatkin, M. B., and Siskind, G. W.,** Accumulative experience in the detection of anti-platelet antibody in 234 patients with idiopathic thrombocytopenic purpura, systemic lupus erythematosus and other clinical disorders, *Am. J. Med.,* 52, 776, 1972.
247. **Karpatkin, S., Strick, N., and Siskind, G. W.,** Detection of splenic antiplatelet antibody synthesis in idiopathic autoimmune thrombocytopenic purpura, *Br. J. Haematol.,* 23, 167, 1972.
248. **Shulman, N. R., Aster, R. H., Leitner, A., and Hiller, M. C.,** Immunoreactions involving platelets. V., *J. Clin. Invest.,* 40, 1597, 1961.
249. **Meyers, N. C.,** Results of treatment in 71 patients with idiopathic thrombocytopenic purpura, *Am. J. Med. Sci.,* 242, 295, 1961.
250. **Bernard, J., and Caen, J.,** Purpura thrombopenique et megacaryocytopenie cycliques nensuels, *Nouv. Rev. Fr. Hematol.,* 2, 378, 1962.
251. **Hirsch, E. O. and Dameshek, W.,** "Idiopathic" thrombocytopenia, *Arch. Intern. Med.,* 88, 701, 1951.
252. **Garg, S. K., Amorosi, E. L., and Karpatkin, S.,** Use of the megathrombocyte as an index of megakaryocyte number, *N. Engl. J. Med.,* 284, 11, 1971.
253. **Pisciotta, A. V., Stefanini, M., and Dameshek, W.,** Morphologic characteristics of megakaryocytes by phase-contrast microscopy in normals and in patients with idiopathic thrombocytopenic purpura, *Blood,* 8, 703, 1953.

254. Lacey, J. V. and Penner, J. A., Management of idiopathic thrombocytopenic purpura in the adult, *Semin. Thromb. Hemostasis,* 3, 160, 1977.
255. Shulman, N. R., Weinrach, R. S., and Libre, E. P., The role of the reticuloendothelial system in the pathogenesis of idiopathic thrombocytopenic purpura, *Trans. Assoc. Am. Physicians,* 78, 374, 1965.
256. Finch, S. C., Castro, O., Cooper, M., Covey, W., Erichson, R., and McPhedran, P., Immunosuppressive therapy of chronic idiopathic thrombocytopenic purpura, *Am. J. Med.,* 56, 4, 1974.
257. Epstein, E. and Goedel, A., Hamorrhagiche thrombocythanie bei vascularer schrumpfmitz, *Virchows Arch. A,* 293, 233, 1934.
258. Hirsh, J. and Dacie, J. V., Persistent post-splenectomy thrombocytosis and thromboembolism: a consequence of continuing anemia, *Br. J. Haematol.,* 12, 44, 1966.
259. Tarnuzi, A. and Smiley, R. K., Hematologic effect of splenic implants, *Blood,* 29, 373, 1967.
260. Evatt, B. L. and Levin, J., Measurement of thrombopoiesis in rabbits using ^{75}selenomethionine, *J. Clin. Invest.,* 48, 1615, 1969.
261. Wright, H. P., Changes in the adhesiveness of blood platelets following parturition and surgical operations, *J. Pathol. Bacteriol.,* 54, 461, 1942.
262. Petter, H. and Lindsay, S., Responses of platelets, eosinophils, and total leukocytes during and following surgical procedures, *Surg. Gynecol. Obstet.,* 110, 319, 1960.
263. Breslow, A., Kaufman, R. M., and Lawsky, A. R., The effect of surgery on the concentration of circulating megakaryocytes and platelets, *Blood,* 32, 393, 1968.
264. Davis, W. M. and Ross, A. O. M., Thrombocytosis and thrombocythemia, *Am. J. Clin. Pathol.,* 59, 243, 1973.
265. Olef, I., Differential platelet count, *Arch. Intern. Med.,* 57, 1163, 1936.
266. Levin, J. and Conley, D. L., Thrombocytosis associated with malignant disease, *Arch. Intern. Med.,* 114, 497, 1964.
267. Davis, R. B., Theologodes, A., and Kennedy, B. J., Comparative studies of blood coagulation and platelet aggregation in patients with cancer and non-malignant disease, *Ann. Intern. Med.,* 71, 67, 1969.
268. Desforges, J. F., Bigelow, F. S., and Chalmers, T. C., The effects of massive gastrointestinal hemorrhage on hemostasis, *J. Lab. Clin. Med.,* 43, 501, 1954.
269. Williams, J. W., Ed., *Hematology,* McGraw-Hill, New York, 1972, 530.
270. Schloesser, L. L., Kipp, M. A., and Wenzel, F. J., Thrombocytosis in iron deficiency anemia, *J. Lab. Clin. Med.,* 66, 107, 1965.
271. Gross, S., Keefer, V., and Newman, P. J., The platelets in iron deficiency anemia. I. The response to oral an parenteral iron, *Pediatrics,* 34, 315, 1964.
272. Wasserman, L. R., Polycythemia vera — its course and treatment: relation to myeloid metaplasia and leukemia, *Bull. N.Y. Acad. Med.,* 3, 343, 1954.
273. Bouroncle, B. A. and Doan, C. A., Myelofibrosis: clinical, hematologic and pathologic study of 110 patients, *Am. J. Med. Sci.,* 243, 697, 1962.
274. Minot, G. R. and Buckman, T. E., The blood platelets in the leukemias, *Am. J. Med. Sci.,* 169, 477, 1925.
275. Gilbert, H. S., A reappraisal of the "myeloproliferative disease" concept, *Mt. Sinai J. Med. N.Y.,* 37, 426, 1970.
276. Gunz, F. W., Hemorrhagic thrombocythemia: a critical review, *Blood,* 15, 706, 1960.
277. Ozer, F. L., Tranx, W. E., Miesch, D. C., and Levin, W. C., Primary hemorrhagic thrombocythemia, *Am. J. Med.,* 28, 807, 1960.
278. Zucker, S. and Mielke, C. H., Classification of thrombocytosis based on platelet function tests: correlation with hemorrhagic and thrombotic complications, *J. Lab. Clin. Med.,* 80, 385, 1972.
279. Ginsberg, A. D., Platelet function in patients with high platelet counts, *Ann. Intern. Med.,* 82, 506, 1975.
280. Keenan, J. P., Wharton, J., Shepherd, A. J. N., and Bellingham, A. J., Defective platelet lipid peroxidation in myeloproliferative disorders: a possible defect of prostaglandin synthesis, *Br. J. Haematol.,* 35, 275, 1977.
281. Ginsberg, A. D., Thrombocytosis and thrombocythemia, in *Physiologic Pharmacology,* Academic Press, New York, 1974, 199.
282. Triplett, D. A., Qualitative platelet disorders, in *Platelet Function: Laboratory Evaluation and Clinical Application,* Triplett, D. A., Ed., American Society of Clinical Pathology, Chicago, 1978.

Chapter 7

HEREDITARY PLASMA PROTEIN DISORDERS

Rodger L. Bick

TABLE OF CONTENTS

I. Introduction to the Three Hemophilias 150

II. Hemophilia A 150
    A. Pathophysiology of Factor VIII 150
    B. Clinical Aspects of Hemophilia A 152
    C. Clinical and Laboratory Diagnosis of Hemophilia A 152
    D. Management of Hemophilia A 152

III. Hemophilia B (Christmas Disease, PTC Deficiency, Factor IX Deficiency) 154
    A. Clinical and Laboratory Aspects of Hemophilia B 154
    B. Pathophysiology of Hemophilia B 154
    C. Management of Hemophilia B 155

IV. Hemophilia C (PTA Deficiency, Rosenthal's Disease) 155
    A. Clinical Aspects of Hemophilia C 155
    B. Pathophysiology of Hemophilia C 155
    C. Management of Hemophilia C 155

V. Rare Congenital Coagulation Protein Defects 156
    A. Congenital Fibrinogen (Factor I) Deficiency 156
        1. Afibrinogenemia and Hypofibrinogenemia 156
        2. Dysfibrinogenemia 156
            a. Clinical Manifestations 156
            b. Pathophysiology 156
            c. Laboratory Diagnosis 157
            d. Treatment 157
    B. Congenital Prothrombin (Factor II) Deficiency 157
    C. Congenital Factor V Deficiency (Parahemophilia) 157
    D. Congenital Factor VII or X Deficiency 157
    E. Congenital Factor XIII (Fibrin Stabilizing Factor, Laki Lorand Factor, Transglutaminase) Deficiency 159
    F. Contact Activation Defects 159
        1. Factor XII (Hageman) Deficiency 159
        2. Fletcher Factor Deficiency 159
        3. Fitzgerald Factor Deficiency 160

References 161

I. INTRODUCTION TO THE THREE HEMOPHILIAS

The hemophilias are characterized as hereditary coagulation factor defects with a clinical bleeding tendency, a prolonged activated partial thromboplastin time and a normal prothrombin time. Hemophilia was first recognized in Talmud writings of the second century. It was forbidden to circumcise the sibling male of a male who had bled at circumcision. These ancient Jewish writings not only recognized hemophilia, but also recognized its mode of transmission from mother to son, as this law applied only to the same mother; the father could differ.[1] Hemophilia has experienced an extremely interesting history. All are familiar with the hemophilia gene in Queen Victoria and its subsequent spread into Spanish and Russian royalties. The disease was first noted in the medical literature in 1803 after being recognized by Otto, a Philadelphia physician. The name hemophilia, however, was not attached to these disorders until 1828, and it is credited to a German physician named Hopff. In the 1800s the diagnosis of hemophilia was established by demonstrating a positive family history and abnormal whole blood clotting time, which became the standard diagnostic criteria for hemophilia. In 1947, antihemophiliac factor (Factor VIII, AHF, or AHG) was recognized.[2] This began an era of active investigation into the nature of classical hemophilia and led to the development of efficacious therapeutic products.

In 1952, a form of hemophilia differing from classical hemophilia was described.[3] The new missing clotting factor was named plasma thromboplastin component (Factor IX or PTC). In the same year, a similar case was found in England. The surname of the family was Christmas and the disorder became known as Christmas disease or hemophilia B.[4]

In 1953 a third form of hemophilia was reported. The thromboplastic factor missing in this disorder was called plasma thromboplastic antecedent (Factor XI or PTA).[5] The disorder is now known as hemophilia C. There are thus three recognized forms of hemophilia. Hemophilia A (classical hemophilia or AHF deficiency) is inherited as a sex-linked recessive trait, i.e., transmitted by the female and manifested in the male. This disorder accounts for approximately 85% of all forms of hemophilia. It can theoretically occur in females through nondisjunction of the X chromosome or from a marriage between a male hemophiliac and female carrier. Hemophilia B (Christmas disease or Factor IX deficiency) accounts for approximately 10% of hemophiliacs. It also has a sex-linked recessive pattern of inheritance. Hemophilia C, (PTA deficiency or Factor XI deficiency) accounts for only about 5% of all hemophilias, is inherited as an autosomal dominant trait, and is manifest in both males and females. This disease is most commonly seen in Jewish people of Russian descent. All three forms of hemophilia occur in approximately 1 out of every 10,000 male births. Regional variations have been noted. In the U.S., the incidence is 1 in 12,000 male births and in Scandinavian countries it is 1 in every 8000 male births.

II. HEMOPHILIA A (CLASSICAL HEMOPHILIA, FACTOR VIII DEFICIENCY)

A. Pathophysiology of Factor VIII

In order to thoroughly understand and appreciate the differences between classical hemophilia and von Willebrand's disease, a familiarity with current concepts of the Factor VIII molecule is necessary. It is now recognized and generally accepted that there are at least three discrete functions that can be attributed to the Factor VIII macromolecular complex (Chapter 6). Procoagulant activity is measured in the routine partial thromboplastin time (PTT) assay system or the specific Factor VIII assay. This function is depicted as VIII_{COAG}. It is this protein that is abnormal in classical hemo-

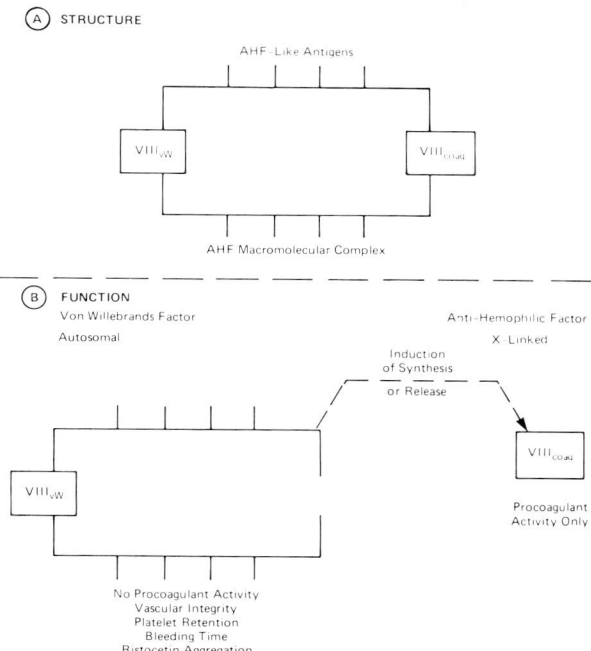

FIGURE 1. Structure-function relationship of the Factor VIII macromolecular complex. A = structure and B = function.

philia. This small procoagulant portion is attached to a larger portion of the Factor VIII complex, which has immunological activity and is commonly referred to as cross-reacting material. This function is depicted as VIII_{AGN}. Attached to or a part of the larger immunological part of the protein is the so-called von Willebrand factor, which is depicted as VIII_{vWF}[6] (Chapter 6). It can be found attached to platelet surfaces in the normal patient, but not in the von Willebrand's patient and, in addition, it normally circulates associated with the procoagulant portion. Factor VIII_{vWF} is responsible for vascular integrity and normal platelet function, and may play a major role in allowing platelets to attach to endothelium. Current concepts of the Factor VIII macromolecular complex are illustrated in Figure 1. Appreciating the nature of the Factor VIII macromolecular complex provides an explanation for the numerous clinical and laboratory differences between patients with classical hemophilia and von Willebrand's disease.

Techniques for the immunological detection of Factor VIII have allowed for the detection of carriers for classical hemophilia. Discriminant analysis and comparison of functional Factor VIII activity vs. immunological activity in a particular female, allows for the detection of a carrier state in greater than 80% of carriers of hemophilia A.[7] Determination of procoagulant activity alone cannot be used for this purpose, as the normal range is too wide (50 to 150% of normal). From the theoretical standpoint, and consistent with the Lyon hypothesis, the female carrier will have 100% of the X chromosomes coding for the synthesis of immunological Factor VIII. However, only one half of the X chromosomes will be coding for the synthesis of procoagulant activity. Another use of immunological assays is to define the rare patient with von Willebrand's disease who has extremely low Factor VIII procoagulant activity as well. This allows for the differential diagnosis between von Willebrand's disease or hemophilia A. In hemophilia A there will be normal VIII_{AGN} and VIII_{COAG} will be decreased.

B. Clinical Aspects of Hemophilia A

The clinical picture of hemophilia A is characterized by intra-articular, intramuscular, and intracerebral bleeding. The disease is usually diagnosed in early childhood when the youngster begins to crawl and subsequently suffers intra-articular bleeding, which later develops into crippling hemarthroses. Some cases are diagnosed at circumcision or tonsillectomy, where profuse bleeding is suddenly noted. In general, classical hemophilia exists in three forms (severe, moderate, and mild), with the clinical course correlating quite well with levels of functional Factor VIII.

Severe hemophiliacs have between 0 and 5% of functional Factor VIII. These individuals suffer numerous spontaneous intramuscular, intra-articular, and, at times, intracerebral bleeds. Usually they require no trauma to initiate hemorrhage. They suffer profuse bleeding with minor trauma or surgery. Moderate hemophiliacs have about 5 to 10% functional Factor VIII circulating. These individuals also suffer spontaneous intra-articular, intramuscular, and, at times, intracerebral bleeding, but less frequently than the severe patients. They also have major bleeding with trauma or surgery. Mild hemophiliacs have 10 to 25% functional Factor VIII levels. These individuals rarely have spontaneous bleeding, but may bleed profusely when subjected to trauma or surgery.

C. Clinical and Laboratory Diagnosis of Hemophilia A

The diagnosis of hemophilia A is suggested by a positive family history. However, only 60% of hemophilia A patients have a positive family history. In approximately 40% of patients the gene appears spontaneously. As noted above, the bleeding manifestations are characteristic. The finding of an abnormal activated partial thromboplastin time in the face of a normal prothrombin time in a patient with a *positive* bleeding history is highly suggestive of Factor VIII (85%), Factor IX (10%), or Factor XI (5%) deficiency. It should be mentioned that an abnormal activated partial thromboplastin time in the face of a normal prothrombin time and a *negative* bleeding history is suggestive of Factor XI deficiency, Factor XII deficiency, or Fletcher factor deficiency. These diseases will be covered in detail in subsequent sections in this chapter. The use of a differential PTT will allow one to differentiate between Factor VIII, IX, and XI deficiency.[8]

In the differential PTT system, one corrects the abnormal PTT with reagents that are either rich in Factor VIII or rich in Factor IX. The latter reagent consists of aged normal human serum (rich in Factor IX and depleted of Factor VIII). If the Factor VIII-rich reagent corrects the PTT, the disorder may be assumed to be hemophilia A. If the Factor IX reagent corrects the abnormal PTT, hemophilia B may be assumed to be present. If both reagents partially correct the abnormal PTT, Factor XI deficiency is present. If both reagents totally correct the activated PTT, Hageman (Factor XII) deficiency is present. Differential PTT findings in the hemophilias are summarized in Table 1. Once a diagnosis of hemophilia A is established by the differential PTT method, the actual level of Factor VIII should be determined. If the patient is a severe hemophiliac with Factor VIII levels approximately 1% of normal, an inhibitor screen should be performed and, if present, its concentration quantitated by appropriate assay procedures.

D. Management of Hemophilia A

In general, mild hemophilic bleeds are best managed by cold compresses and topical thrombin, if needed. Minor bleeds usually do not require infusion of fresh plasma, cryoprecipitate, or Factor VIII concentrate. The management of life-threatening bleeding has changed in the past several years. Initially, only fresh whole blood or fresh plasma was available. This is seldom used for management of hemophilic bleeding

TABLE 1

Differentiation of the Hemophilias (Differential PTT)

Defect	PTT	PT	AHF reagent	PTC reagent
Hemophilia A	Long	Normal	Total correction	No correction
Hemophilia B	Long	Normal	No correction	Total correction
Hemophilia C	Long	Normal	Partial correction	Partial correction
Factor XII Deficiency	Long	Normal	Total correction	Total correction

TABLE 2

Formula for the Calculation of the Amount of Concentrate Needed (Factor VIII or Factor IX)

$$U_t = (L_D - L_i) \times 0.6 \times W$$

and

$$C = \frac{U_t}{U_c}$$

where U_t = total units needed, L_D = desired level, L_i = initial level, W = weight in kilograms, C = milliliters of concentrate needed, and U_c = units per milliliter in concentrate.

today. The discovery of cryoprecipitate and its subsequent use in hemophilia was a major milestone in the management of these patients.[9] The disadvantage of using cryoprecipitate is the high protein content and the variable Factor VIII content in each preparation. Most centers now utilize commercially available and potent Factor VIII concentrates for the management of significant hemorrhage. Concentrates offer the advantage of low volume, low protein content, and a predictable Factor VIII titer.[10] By knowing the initial level of Factor VIII, one can calculate the amount of Factor VIII concentrate needed for infusion. Serious hemophilic bleeding will cease when the patient's Factor VIII level reaches approximately 30% of normal. As a general rule, the infusion of 25 units of Factor VIII concentrate per kilogram will increase the Factor VIII level to approximately 50% of normal.[11] The exact amount of Factor VIII needed to raise the patient's level to a predetermined "desired level" can be calculated by a rationale similar to that used for calculating electrolyte replacement. For example, the desired level of Factor VIII, minus the initial level, represents the percent of Factor VIII required. Thus the desired level minus the initial level multiplied by 0.6 times body weight in kilograms will give the exact number of units required to take the patient to the desired level of Factor VIII activity. This formula is given in Table 2.

Approximately 10% of hemophilia A patients develop antibodies to Factor VIII.[12] In most instances, these are IgG type 4 with a kappa light chain.[13] They usually develop spontaneously, and a classical anamnestic response may be seen if these individuals are treated with Factor VIII concentrates, cryoprecipitate, or any other source of Factor VIII. Immunosuppressive therapy with cyclophosphamide, Imuran®, or prednisone appears to have little effect in controlling patients with high inhibitor titers.[14] A newer approach in the therapy of these patients has been to use activated prothrombin complex concentrates containing an active principle which will bypass the necessity of Factor VIII and allow for hemostasis to occur.[15,16] The clinical trials that have been completed using several of the commercially available prothrombin complex concentrates in patients with high inhibitor titers have proven successful. Screening tests for the detection of anti-VIII antibodies are now available and quite simple to perform.[17] It is imperative to define inhibitor titers, as only in this way can one decide whether to try to "overdrive" the Factor VIII deficiency and control hemorrhage with massive amounts of Factor VIII concentrate in patients with low titers or, alternatively, in high-titer patients, to resort to the use of activated prothrombin complex concentrates.

III. HEMOPHILIA B (CHRISTMAS DISEASE, PTC DEFICIENCY, FACTOR IX DEFICIENCY)

A. Clinical and Laboratory Aspects of Hemophilia B

The clinical manifestations of Factor IX deficiency are similar to classical hemophilia. The patient often experiences intra-articular and intramuscular bleeding when he begins to crawl in infancy. The disease, like classical hemophilia, can be present in severe or mild forms, with mild patients experiencing few if any spontaneous bleeds, but suffering profuse bleeding with trauma or surgery. Unlike classical hemophilia, however, there is poor correlation between the level of circulating Factor IX and clinical bleeding. Like classical hemophilia, Factor IX deficiency should be suspected in the face of a positive bleeding history, an abnormal activated partial thromboplastin time, and a normal prothrombin time. The disease is inherited as a sex-linked recessive trait and is therefore manifest in males and carried by females. This disorder is much less common than Factor VIII deficiency and accounts for approximately 10% of hemophilia. A diagnosis of Factor IX deficiency is made by utilizing the differential partial thromboplastin time as described previously (Factor VIII-rich reagent will not correct the prolonged PTT, but Factor IX-rich reagent — aged normal serum — does corect the PTT. Once a diagnosis of Factor IX deficiency has been made, a specific Factor IX assay should be performed to quantitate the level of circulating Factor IX. This is done in a manner similar to a Factor VIII assay. Patients with very low levels of Factor IX should be screened for the presence of an inhibitor. The incidence of inhibitors to Factor IX is less frequent than that for inhibitors to Factor VIII. In hemophilia B, only 5 to 6% of patients have inhibitors to Factor IX.

B. Pathophysiology of Hemophilia B

Much less is known about the pathophysiology of this disorder in comparison to hemophilia A. It is known, however, that variants of hemophilia B do exist. The first variants were discovered using Ox brain thromboplastin times. Previous work revealed that some patients with Factor IX deficiency had a prolonged Ox brain thromboplastin time, while others had normal times. These patients with a prolonged Ox brain thromboplastin time have been designated hemophilia B_m, the "m" being derived from the surname of the first family found with this disorder.[18]

It has been established that some patients with Factor IX deficiency resemble classical hemophilia in that Factor IX-like antigen or nonfunctioning Factor IX protein is present. Thus these patients are cross-reacting material (CRM) positive. The majority of patients with hemophilia B, however, have no detectable Factor IX levels by currently available immunologic techniques. Thus there are hemophilia B patients who are CRM⁺ and CRM⁻. Therefore, at least four genetic variants of hemophilia B exist. These are delineated in Table 3. The clinical significance of these variances is not known. Evidence suggests that patients who are CRM⁺ have a milder form of the disease.[19]

TABLE 3

Variants of Hemophilia B

Immunological (CRM)[a]	Ox-brain thromboplastin time	Designation
CRM⁺	Normal	B⁺
CRM⁺	Long	B⁺$_m$
CRM⁻	Normal	B⁻
CRM⁻	Long	B⁻$_m$

[a] Immunological "cross-reacting material".

C. Management of Hemophilia B

As with hemophilia A, minor bleeding is best managed by supportive therapy, cold compresses, and topical thrombin, when necessary. For life-threatening bleeding, several Factor IX-containing concentrates are commercially available (prothrombin complex concentrates).[20-22] These preparations are not without hazard of hepatitis, and clinical use should be weighed against this danger.[23,24] In addition, numerous reports have indicated that these materials can be thrombogenic and may lead to the development of a disseminated intravascular coagulation-type syndrome.[25,26] As with hemophilia A, the exact amount of concentrate needed can be calculated according to the formula given in Table 2. Also as in hemophilia A, these patients need only be increased to 30 or 40% of normal assayable Factor IX activity before bleeding usually ceases. Elective surgery procedures should be managed in a similar way.

IV. HEMOPHILIA C (PTA DEFICIENCY, ROSENTHAL'S DISEASE FACTOR XI DEFICIENCY)

A. Clinical Aspects of Hemophilia C

Hemophilia C differs significantly from hemophilia A or B. It is inherited as an autosomal dominant trait and can be expressed in both males and females. In addition, the clinical course can be highly variable, with some patients experiencing no bleeding tendency and other patients suffering profuse bleeding.[27] Interestingly, there appears to be no correlation between the levels of assayable circulating Factor XI and the bleeding tendency of the patient. Indeed, many patients are noted to change their clinical course, with bleeders becoming nonbleeders and vice versa. This may or may not be correlated with any change in the Factor XI levels. Hemophilia C need not necessarily become manifest in early childhood. Commonly, it becomes manifest as a bleeding disorder in adult life.

B. Pathophysiology of Hemophilia C

Very little is known about the pathophysiology of hemophilia C. There are no data to indicate whether individuals suffering from this disease have an absolute lack of Factor XI or a circulating, dysfunctional Factor XI. Variants of the disease have not yet been described.

C. Management of Hemophilia C

The mainstay of therapy for clinically significant bleeding is the infusion of plasma, usually fresh frozen material. A dose of 10 ml/kg usually suffices to control significant bleeding.[28] It has recently been noted that certain lots of commercial prothrombin complex concentrate contain high levels (10 to 30 units per ml) of Factor XI. This has been used to control life-threatening bleeding in patients who fail to respond to infusions of plasma.[29] Prothrombin complex concentrates are potentially thrombogenic, and a stability check should always be performed on every bottle before this material is infused. The stability check consists of adding 0.1 ml of concentrate to 1 ml of citrated patient's plasma and observing for clot formation for a period of 5 min. If no clot forms during that period of time, it can be assumed that no thrombin is generated. A more predictive assay of thrombogenicity of these concentrates has been advocated by Blatt and coworkers.[30] They have further noted that prothrombin complex concentrates are far less thrombogenic if antithrombin III is added to them.[25]

V. RARE CONGENITAL COAGULATION PROTEIN DEFECTS

A. Congenital Fibrinogen (Factor I) Deficiency

1. Afibrinogenemia and Hypofibrinogenemia

Congenital afibrinogenemia is extremely rare, with only 60 cases having been reported. This disorder is inherited as an autosomal recessive trait. It is thought that afibrinogenemia represents the homozygous state and hypofibrinogenemia represents the heterozygote.[31] Afibrinogenemic patients may suffer severe hemophilia-like bleeding, including intra-articular bleeding with crippling hemarthroses. In addition, umbilical stump bleeding at childbirth is characteristic. These patients also suffer cutaneous bruising and have life-threatening bleeding following trauma or surgery. Hypofibrinogenemic patients may suffer only mild bleeding, usually never spontaneous, but may bleed significantly with surgery or trauma. The diagnostic laboratory findings of afibrinogenemia are an infinite thrombin time, reptilase time, prothrombin time, and partial thromboplastin time.

2. Dysfibrinogenemia

Congenital dysfibrinogenemia is a disorder characterized by normal fibrinogen levels (immunologically), but the molecule is abnormal. There have been several types of dysfibrinogenemias described.[32] By international agreement, these are named by the city where first discovered. All appear to be inherited by autosomal dominance, and all are characterized by a long or infinite thrombin time, with the exception of fibrinogen Oslow, which demonstrates a short thrombin time, and fibrinogen Oklahoma, which has a normal thrombin time.

a. Clinical Manifestations

Greater than 50% of patients with congenital dysfibrinogenemias demonstrate no clinical bleeding diathesis. Of the remainder, however, many do demonstrate bleeding similar to that seen with hypofibrinogenemic states. Several of the dysfibrinogenemias are characterized by thrombosis only.[33,34]

b. Pathophysiology

In most of these disorders the pathophysiology is poorly understood. There are a variety of different types of dysfibrogenemias, and varying characteristics are noted for each. Immunologic methods always reveal fibrinogen levels to be normal or increased. Various defects have been described for each particular type of dysfibrinogenemia and have included such findings as abnormal immunoelectrophoretic mobility, abnormal carbohydrate content, and slow release of fibrinopeptide A or B with thrombin. The most completely characterized dysfibrinogenemia is fibrinogen Detroit.[35] In this instance, the amino acid serine is substituted for arginine in position 19 of the A α chain (Figure 4 in Chapter 3). This unique and laborious discovery represents the second disease state to be defined by a single amino acid substitution — the first, of course, being sickle cell anemia. Table 4 lists the congenital dysfibrinogenemias thus far described.

c. Laboratory Diagnosis

Except for fibrinogen Oslow and fibrinogen Oklahoma, all of the congenital dysfibrinogenemias have a prolonged or infinite thrombin and reptilase time. In these disorders a normal amount of immunological fibrinogen is noted.

d. Treatment

Fibrinogen concentrates were previously used; now cryoprecipitate or fresh plasma is usually used to treat bleeding episodes in patients with afibrinogenemia. Whole blood may also be used, but in the case of whole blood it must be relatively fresh — not older than 5 days. To achieve hemostasis, it is only necessary to raise and maintain the fibrinogen level to 50 to 100 mg/dl. Since the half-life of fibrinogen is about 4 days, infusions need not be frequent. It is of interest to note that, usually, bleeding episodes do not recur as soon as all of the infused fibrinogen disappears from the patient's plasma.

B. Congenital Prothrombin (Factor II) Deficiency

This disorder[37] is extremely rare, with only 15 to 16 cases having been reported. Congenital prothrombin deficiency appears to be inherited as an autosomal recessive trait. Clinically, these patients have numerous hematomata and ecchymoses. In addition, they experience mucosal membrane bleeding and may manifest severe bleeding with surgery and trauma. Intra-articular bleeding and hemarthroses have not been reported. In those instances where appropriate studies have been performed, a true prothrombin deficiency (CRM⁻) has been found, but at least two cases of dysfunctional Factor II (CRM⁺) have been reported.

C. Congenital Factor V Deficiency (Parahemophilia)

This extremely rare disorder was first found in Oslow in 1947.[38] Subsequently, 30 more cases have been noted. Some have been associated with classical hemophilia and von Willebrand's syndrome.[39] Like congenital prothrombin deficiency, many of these individuals have mucosal membrane bleeding as well as hematomata and ecchymoses. Intra-articular bleeding and hemarthroses have not been reported. Thus far, evidence suggests this to be a true deficiency (CRM⁻), rather than a dysfunctional Factor V. This deficiency must be treated with fresh plasma when significant bleeding occurs.

D. Congenital Factor VII or X Deficiency

These two disorders[40] are extremely rare, with only 60 to 70 cases of congenital Factor VII deficiency having been reported. One in 100,000 has Factor X deficiency. Both are inherited as autosomal recessive traits and both manifest a similar clinical bleeding diathesis. The patients suffer intra-articular bleeding and hemarthroses, but, more commonly, demonstrate only mild mucosal bleeding, manifest by epistaxis, genitourinary and gastrointestinal bleeding. Significant bleeding can occur with surgery or trauma. In several instances, no bleeding manifestations whatsoever have been present. In both congenital Factor VII and congenital Factor X deficiency two variants exist. Some patients with congenital Factor VII deficiency have been reported to have a true deficiency (CRM⁻), while others have a dysfunctional Factor VII molecule (CRM⁺). The same situation appears to exist for congenital Factor X deficiency. In both of these disorders the prothrombin time is prolonged. The differential diagnosis is made by the utilization of the Stypven® time (prothrombin time performed with Russell's viper venom). The Stypven® time will be normal in congenital Factor VII

TABLE 4

Dysfibrinogenemias

		Defect, if known						
Name	Date	F.P.A.	F.P.B.	Polymerization	Hexose	Hexosamine	Sialic acid	Total carbohydrate
Parma	1958			?				
Vancouver	1963			?				
Paris I	1963			+				
Baltimore	1964	+						
Zurich I	1965			+	?	?	↓	?
Cleveland I	1967	+		+				
Detroit	1968			+	↓	→	N	↓
Paris II	1968			+	↓	N	→	↓
St. Louis	1968			+	→	N	↓	↓
Zurich II	1970			+	N	N	N	N
Louvain	1970			+				
Oklahoma	1970							
Los Angeles	1970	+		+	?	?	N	?
Bethesda I	1970		+					↓
Amsterdam	1971			+	N	→	↓	
Nancy	1971			+				
Wiesbaden	1971			+				
Troyes	1972							
Metz	1972	+						
Giessen	1972	+						
Bethesda II	1972			+	N	?	N	?
Montreal	1972			+				
Vienna	1973			+				
Iowa City	1973							
Cleveland II	1973	+						
Philadelphia	1974			+				

deficiency and will be prolonged in Factor X deficiency. Bleeding in both of these disorders, if it reaches significant or life-threatening proportions, can be controlled with prothrombin complex concentrates.

E. Congenital Factor XIII (Fibrin Stabilizing Factor, Laki Lorand Factor, Transglutaminase) Deficiency

Factor XIII deficiency[44] is extremely rare, with only 50 cases having been reported. This disorder is inherited as an autosomal recessive trait. The clinical hallmark of this disorder is poor wound healing after trauma or surgery, which is found in at least 50% of patients. Similar to the congenital afibrinogenemias, umbilical cord bleeding at birth is also extremely common. Other bleeding manifestations that occur are hematomata, ecchymoses, and, more rarely, intra-articular bleeding. Mucosal membrane bleeding has not been described in this disorder. In the vast majority of these patients, a true deficiency does not exist, but a dysfunctional Factor XIII is present. Thus the patients are CRM⁺. A few cases have been reported that are truly deficient in Factor XIII (CRM⁻). In congenital Factor XIII deficiency, platelets, as well as plasma, are void of functional Factor XIII. This is in distinction to acquired Factor XIII deficiency, where plasma is void of functional Factor XIII, but Factor XIII is found in platelets.

Factor XIII levels of between 3 and 5% are adequate for normal hemostasis. Since the half-life of Factor XIII is 4 to 6 days, clinically significant hemorrhage due to Factor XIII deficiency can usually be managed with infusion of plasma given at 10 ml/kg every 7 to 10 days.[45] The laboratory diagnosis of Factor XIII deficiency is noted by the finding of fibrin solubility in 1% monochloroacetic acid or in 5 M urea.[46]

F. Contact Activation Defects

1. Factor XII (Hageman) Deficiency

Factor XII deficiency was first described by Ratnoff and Colopy in 1955.[41] This disorder is relatively rare; since the original description, only 160 to 180 cases have been described. Hageman deficiency is inherited as an autosomal recessive trait and usually is not associated with any bleeding diathesis. However, several patients with a mild bleeding tendency have been reported. Of particular significance, however, is the noting that an inordinately high number of patients with Hageman trait have died as a consequence of thrombosis (usually acute coronary artery thrombosis or acute pulmonary embolization).[42] This may be related to the known role of Factor XII in activation of the fibrinolytic system (Chapter 3).

Hageman factor is also involved in activation of the complement system, generation of kinins, and appears to be involved in neutrophil chemotaxis. This may assume paramount importance in acute disseminated intravascular coagulation.[43]

The pathophysiology of Hageman deficiency is poorly understood; however, in all patients studied thus far, this disorder appears to be a true deficiency of Hageman factor, as all have been CRM⁻ when subjected to immunochemical studies. Hageman deficiency assumes major importance, since it causes marked prolongation of the activated partial thromboplastin time. The disorder is also characterized by an abnormal whole blood clotting time and a prolonged clotting time in glass or siliconized tubes. The prothrombin time is normal. Numerous patients with Hageman trait have undergone major surgical procedures and not only have required no preoperative treatment, but have not demonstrated any significant bleeding during or after surgery.

2. Fletcher Factor Deficiency

A new coagulation factor was described in 1965. In this interesting disorder, a family from eastern Kentucky was involved in a fire, necessitating hospitalization of several children. During hospitalization adenoidectomy was contemplated for one child. A preoperative hemostasis screen revealed a markedly prolonged PTT. In all, four of fourteen siblings had markedly prolonged activated partial thromboplastin times. Careful investigation of the family failed to reveal evidence of any hemorrhagic tendency. The family surname is Fletcher and the defect is now known as Fletcher factor deficiency.[46] Subsequently, six to eight es of Fletcher factor deficiency have been found. Investigations into Fletcher factor deficiency have revealed this defect to be characterized by a normal prothrombin time, a long activated partial thromboplastin time, and plasma recalcification time. Both of these latter tests are completely corrected by longer incubation with kaolin, celite, or glass. A screening test for Fletcher factor deficiency is simple and consists of correcting a markedly prolonged PTT by incubating the mixture with kaolin for 10 min, rather than 2 to 3 min.

Decreased Fletcher factor has been found in newborns, patients with severe liver disease, uremia, and in patients with Fitzgerald factor trait, which is discussed below. Fletcher factor is the same as plasma prekallikrein (see Chapter 3).

3. Fitzgerald Factor Deficiency

It has been noted that a mixture of Factor XII, Factor XI, Fletcher factor, and kaolin fail to give activation of Factor XI. Because of this, it has been proposed that other "factors" must also be necessary. Fitzgerald factor appears to be one such factor. This factor was first reported in 1964.[47] This deficiency was found after noting a normal prothrombin time and a markedly prolonged activated partial thromboplastin time in an asymptomatic 71 year old male. Approximately five cases of Fitzgerald factor deficiency have now been reported, and preliminary evidence suggest it to be an autosomal recessive trait. This disorder is characterized by a prolonged activated partial thromboplastin time, which is not corrected by longer incubation of kaolin. The defect is, however, corrected with the addition of plasmas that are deficient in Factor XII, Fletcher factor, and Factor XI. In addition, kallikrein ("activated" Fletcher factor) also does not correct the defect. However, activated XI or XII will give correction. Similar to Fletcher factor and Factor XII deficiency, these patients have defects in surface-activated fibrinolysis, in kaolin-induced kinin generation, and in vascular permeability (PF/Dil).[48] The exact relationship of Fitzgerald factor to Factors XII, Fletcher factor, and Factor XI is described in Chapter 3. Fitzgerald factor has now been shown to be identical to high molecular weight kininogen.

An additional "activation phase" factor was reported in 1974 by Bick, and coworkers.[49] In this instance, a patient with the Hughes-Stoven syndrome (pulmonary arterial aneurysms, deep-vein thrombophlebitis, and dural sinus thromboses) was found to have a markedly prolonged kaolin-activated partial thromboplastin time. This individual had a normal bleeding time and normal levels of other known clotting factors, including Fletcher factor. The abnormal kaolin-activated PTT was partially corrected and the celite-activated PTT was completely corrected by longer incubation times. The addition of normal plasma, aged serum, or barium sulfate-absorbed plasma all shortened the activated PTT by 15 to 20 sec, but never corrected it to normal. Circulating anticoagulants could not be found in this patient, suggesting an additional factor in the contact activation phase.

REFERENCES

1. **Rosher, F.**, Hemophilia in the Talmud and Rabbinic writings, *Ann. Intern. Med.*, 70, 833, 1969.
2. **Brinkhous, K. M.**, Clotting defect in hemophilia: deficiency in plasma factor required for platelet utilization, *Proc. Soc. Exp. Biol. Med.*, 66, 117, 1947.
3. **Aggeler, P. M., White, S. G., Glendening, M. B., Page, E. W., Leake, T. B., and Bates, G.**, Plasma thromboplastin component (PTC) deficiency: a new disease resembling hemophilia, *Proc. Soc. Exp. Biol. Med.*, 79, 692, 1952.
4. **Biggs, R., Douglas, A. M., Macfarlane, R. A., Dacie, J. V., Pitney, W. R., Merskey, C., and O'Brien, J. R.**, Christmas disease: a condition previously mistaken for haemophilia, *Br. Med. J.*, 2, 1378, 1952.
5. **Rosenthal, R. L., Dreskin, O. H., and Rosenthal, N.**, New hemophilia-like disease caused by deficiency of a third plasma thromboplastin factor, *Proc. Soc. Exp. Biol. Med.*, 82, 171, 1953.
6. **Gralnick, H. R., Sultan, Y., and Coller, B. S.**, von Willebrand's disease: combined qualitative and quantitative defects, *N. Engl. J. Med.*, 296, 1024, 1977.
7. **Klein, H. G., Aledort, L. M., Bouma, B. H., Hoyer, L. W., Zimmerman, T. S., and de Mets, D. L.**, A cooperative study for the detection of the carrier state of classic hemophilia, *N. Engl. J. Med.*, 296, 959, 1977.
8. **Fekete, L. F.**, The partial thromboplastin time and related assays, in *Modern Concepts and Evaluation of Hemostasis and Thrombosis*, Bick, R. L., Ed., Publ. No. 548, American Society of Clinical Pathologists, Chicago, 1978, chap. 6.
9. **Pool, J. G. and Shannon, A. E.**, Production of high-potency concentrates of antihemophilic globulin in a closed-bag system, *N. Engl. J.Med.*, 273, 1443, 1965.
10. **Brinkhous, K. M., Shanbrom, E., and Roberts, H. R.**, A new high-potency glycine-precipitated antihemophilic factor (AHF) concentrate, *JAMA*, 205, 613, 1968.
11. **Abildgaard, C. F., Simone, J. V., Corrigan, J. J., Seeler, R. A., Edelstein, G., Vanderheiden, J., and Schulman, I.**, Treatment of hemophilia with glycine-precipitated Factor VIII, *N. Engl. J. Med.*, 275, 471, 1966.
12. **Nilsson, I. M., Blomback, M., and Wichel, B.**, Inhibitors in Hemophilia, in Proc. 7th Congr. World Fed. Hemophilia, Tehran, 1971.
13. **Anderson, B. R. and Terry, W. D.**, Gamma G4-globulin antibody causing inhibitor of clotting factor VIII, *Nature (London)*, 217, 174, 1968.
14. **Penner, J. A. and Kelly, P. E.**, Management of patients with factor VIII or IX inhibitors, *Semin. Thromb. Hemostas.*, 1, 386, 1975.
15. **Fekete, L. F., Holst, S. L., Peetoom, F., and de Veber, L. L.**, "Auto" Factor IX Concentrate: A New Therapeutic Approach to Treatment of Hemophilia A Patients with Inhibitors, 14th Int. Cong. Hematol., San Paolo, Brazil, July 16 to 21, 1972, Abstr. 295.
16. **Kruczynski, E. M. and Penner, J. A.**, Activated prothrombin concentrate for patients with factor VIII inhibitors, *N. Engl. J. Med.*, 291, 164, 1974.
17. **Tse, D., Fekete, L. F., and Shanbrom, E.**, A simple procedure for accurate quantitation of factor VIII inhibitors, *Thromb. Diath. Haemorrh.*, 23, 19, 1970.
18. **Elodi, S. and Puskas, E.**, Variants of hemophilia B, *Thromb. Diath. Haemorrh.*, 28, 489, 1972.
19. **Bloom, A. L.**, Coagulation factor variants, *Br. J. Haematol.*, 23, 643, 1972.
20. **Breen, F. A. and Tullis, J. L.**, Prothrombin concentrate in treatment of Christmas disease and allied disorders, *JAMA*, 208, 1848, 1969.
21. **Tullis, J. L., Melin, M., and Jurigian, P.**, Clinical use of human prothrombin complexes, *N. Engl. J. Med.*, 273, 667, 1965.
22. **Soulier, J. P., Josso, F., Steinbuch, M., and Cosson, A.**, The therapeutical use of fraction P.P.S.B., *Bibl. Haematol. (Basel)*, 29, 1127, 1968.
23. **Biggs, R.**, Jaundice and antibodies directed against factors VIII and IX in patients treated for hemophilia or Christmas disease in the United Kingdom, *Br. J. Haematol.*, 26, 313, 1974.
24. **Kingdon, H. S.**, Hepatitis after konyne, *Ann. Intern. Med.*, 73, 656, 1970.
25. **White, G. C., Roberts, H. R., Kingdon, H. S., and Lundblad, R. L.**, Prothrombin complex concentrates: potentially thrombogenic materials and clues to the mechanism of thrombosis in vivo, *Blood*, 49, 159, 1977.
26. **Triantaphyllopoulos, D. C.**, Intravascular coagulation following injection of prothrombin complex, *Am. J. Clin. Pathol.*, 57, 603, 1972.
27. **Rosenthal, R. L.**, Factor XI: general review, *Bibl. Haematol. (Basel)*, 23, 1350, 1965.
28. **Shulman, N. R.**, Surgical care of patients with hereditary disorders of blood coagulation, *Mod. Treat.*, 5, 61, 1968.
29. **Bick, R. L., Adams, T., and Radack, K.**, Surgical hemostasis with a Factor XI-containing concentrate, *JAMA*, 229, 163, 1974.

30. **Blatt, P. M., Lundbald, R. L., Kingdon, H. S., McLean, G., and Roberts, H. R.**, Thrombogenic materials in prothrombin complex concentrates, *Ann. Intern. Med.*, 81, 766, 1974.
31. **Jackson, D. P., Beck, E. A., and Charache, P.**, Congenital disorders of fibrinogen, *Fed. Proc.*, 24, 816, 1965.
32. **Mammen, E. F.**, Congenital abnormalities of the fibrinogen molecule, *Semin. Thromb. Hemostas.*, 1, 184, 1974.
33. **Beck, E. A.**, Abnormal fibrinogen (fibrinogen Baltimore) as a cause of a familial hemorrhagic disorder, *Blood*, 24, 853, 1964.
34. **Samama, M., Soria, J., Soria, C., and Bousser, J.**, Congenital and Familial Dysfibrinogenemia without Bleeding Tendency, Abst. 13th Cong. Int. Soc. Hematol., International Society of Hematology, Caracas, 1968, 179.
35. **Mammen, E. F., Prasad, A. S., Barnhart, M. I., and Au, C. C.**, Congenital dysfibrinogenemia: fibrinogen Detroit, *J. Clin. Invest.*, 48, 235, 1969.
36. **Blomback, M., Blomback, B., Mammen, E. F., and Prasad, A. S.**, Fibrinogen Detroit: a molecular defect in the N-terminal disulfide knot of human fibrinogen, *Nature (London)*, 218, 134, 1968.
37. **Hougie, C.**, Hemophilia and hemophilioid diseases, in *Fundamentals of Blood Coagulation in Clinical Medicine*, McGraw-Hill, New York, 1963, chap. 4.
38. **Owren, P. A.**, Parahemophilia: hemorrhagic diathesis due to absence of a previously unknown clotting factor, *Lancet*, 2, 446, 1947.
39. **Quick, A. J.**, Hypoprothrombinemic states, in *Hemorrhagic diseases and thrombosis*, Lea & Febiger, Philadelphia, 1966, chap. 3.
40. **van Crevald, S. and Veder, H. A.**, Congenital hypoproconvertinemia, *Ann. Paediatr.*, 190, 316, 1958.
41. **Ratnoff, O. D. and Colopy, J. E.**, A familial hemorrhagic trait associated with a deficiency of clot-promoting fraction of plasma, *J. Clin. Invest.*, 34, 602, 1955.
42. **McPherson, R. A.**, Thromboembolism in Hageman trait, *Am. J. Clin. Pathol.*, 68, 420, 1977.
43. **Kaplan, A. P., Meier, H. L., and Mandle, R.**, The Hageman factor dependent pathways of coagulation, fibrinolysis, and kinin-generation, *Semin. Thromb. Hemostas.*, 3, 1, 1976.
44. **Duckert, F.**, Documentation of the plasma Factor XIII deficiency in man, *Ann. N.Y. Acad. Sci.*, 202, 190, 1972.
45. **Ikkala, E.**, Transfusion therapy in congenital deficiencies of plasma Factor XIII, *Ann. N.Y. Acad. Sci.*, 202, 200, 1972.
46. **Hathaway, W. E., Belhasen, L. P., and Hathaway, H. S.**, Evidence for a new plasma thromboplastin factor. I. Coagulation studies and physiocochemical studies (case report), *Blood*, 26, 521, 1965.
47. **Saito, H., Ratnoff, O. D., Waldmann, R., and Abraham, J. P.**, Fitzgerald trait: deficiency of a hitherto unrecognized agent, Fitzgerald factor, participating in surface — mediated reactions of clotting, fibrinolysis, generation of kinins, and the property of diluted plasma enhancing vascular permeability (PF/DIL), *J. Clin. Invest.*, 55, 1082, 1975.
48. **Schreiber, A. D.**, Plasma inhibitors of the Hageman factor dependent pathways, *Semin. Thromb. Hemostas.*, 3, 43, 1976.
49. **Bick, R. L., Adams, T., and Goldberg, L. S.**, Evidence for a new activation phase clotting abnormality in a patient with the Hughes-Stoven syndrome, *Beitr. Pathol.*, 153, 310, 1974.

Chapter 8

DISSEMINATED INTRAVASCULAR COAGULATION (DIC) AND RELATED SYNDROMES

Rodger L. Bick

TABLE OF CONTENTS

I. Introduction 164

II. Pathophysiology 165

III. Diagnosis 168
    A. Clinical Diagnosis 168
    B. Laboratory Diagnosis 168

IV. Therapy 172

V. Related Syndromes 174
    A. Microangiopathic Hemolytic Anemia 175
    B. Hemolytic-Uremic Syndrome (HUS) 175
    C. Respiratory Distress Syndrome (RDS) 176
    D. Thrombotic Thrombocytopenic Purpura (TTP) 176

VI. Summary 177

References 177

I. INTRODUCTION

Disseminated intravascular coagulation (DIC), also known as consumption coagulopathy or defibrination syndrome, is not a single disease entity, but rather an intermediary mechanism of disease.[1] It is usually, but not always, associated with well-defined clinical entities.[2] In addition, it can be manifest as a wide clinical spectrum. For example, if the intravascular clotting process is dominant and secondary fibrino(geno)lysis minimal, DIC may be expressed primarily as diffuse thromboses, as in malignancy. Alternatively, if the secondary fibrinolysis that occurs with DIC is dominant and the drive toward procoagulant activity minimal, the clinical manifestitations will be hemorrhage, the more common expression of DIC.[3,4] Patients often demonstrate combinations of these two clinical manifestations. Thus DIC represents a wide spectrum of clinical findings, with patients presenting anywhere in the continuum between diffuse thromboses and/or hemorrhage. The clinical conditions most commonly associated with DIC are depicted in Table 1.

A common trigger for DIC is an obstetrical accident, primarily: amniotic fluid embolism, retained fetus syndrome, placental abruption, and, less commonly, placenta previa. Amniotic fluid has procoagulant (clot-promoting) activity and can initiate the clotting sequence, thus leading to DIC. When a dead fetus remains in utero for greater than 5 weeks, the incidence of DIC approaches 50%.[5] The trigger is thought to be necrotic fetal tissue released into the uterine and, subsequently, into the systemic maternal circulation. Necrotic fetal tissue has procoagulant or thromboplastin-like activity and is able to initiate the clotting sequence. In cases of placental abruption, placental tissue and/or placental enzymes with procoagulant activity may be released into the uterine and then systemic maternal circulation to provide a trigger for initiating the clotting sequence.[6,7]

Another common triggering event for DIC is intravascular hemolysis, whether it be minor hemolysis due to multiple transfusions with banked whole blood, frank hemolytic transfusion reactions, or intravascular hemolysis of any etiology. Two mechanisms have been proposed. The release of red cell ADP may initiate a platelet release reaction with generation of platelet factor 3 activity and subsequent activation of the coagulation system. Additionally, the release of red cell membrane phospholipoprotein during hemolysis may independently initiate the clotting sequence and perhaps also a platelet release reaction. Sepsis is not uncommonly associated with acute DIC, although the exact mechanism(s) remain unclear. The first organism to be associated with DIC was the meningococcus.[8,9] Later, other Gram-negative organisms were described in association with DIC. Thus it was thought that bacteremias triggered DIC by release of endotoxin that induced both coagulation and the platelet release reaction. However, DIC has now been described with Gram-positive organisms as well, so other mechanisms, in addition to endotoxin, must also be involved. Other potential mechanisms for initiation of DIC in septicemia involve initiation of platelet release or "contact phase" activation of coagulation by materials from bacterial coats (lipopolysaccharides).[10-12] Viremias may also be associated with DIC, most commonly varicella. During viremia, DIC may be initiated by antigen-antibody complex activation of platelet release and/or the coagulation system. In addition, antigen-antibody complexes may damage the endothelium, which in turn may initiate platelet release and subsequent coagulation or direct activation of coagulation through endothelium/collagen-induced Factor XII_a generation.[13]

Burns and crush injuries are not uncommonly associated with acute DIC. It seems reasonable that, in significant burns, the microhemolysis with subsequent release of red cell phospholipid and/or ADP may provide the trigger for DIC. In patients suffer-

TABLE 1

Conditions Associated with DIC

Obstetrical accidents
    Amniotic fluid embolism
    Placental abruption
    Retained fetus syndrome
Intravascular hemolysis
    Hemolytic transfusion reaction
    Multiple transfusions (banked whole blood)
Septicemia
    Gram-negative (endotoxin)
    Gram-positive (mucopolysaccharides ?)
Viremia (varicella)
Solid malignancy
Leukemias
    Promyelocytic
    Other
Acidosis/alkalosis
Burns
Crush injury and tissue necrosis
Vascular disorders

ing massive tissue necrosis from crush injuries, the release of necrotic tissue with procoagulant (thromboplastin-like) activity may trigger the clotting sequence, as well as initiate the platelet release reaction.

Most patients with disseminated malignancy have some laboratory evidence of DIC, however many never develop clinical manifestations. Malignancy represents a special situation in that DIC may be *acute, subacute,* or *chronic,* and may be manifest as local thromboses, diffuse thromboses, minor hemorrhage, diffuse hemorrhage, or any combination.[14] The acute leukemias are also associated with DIC. This was first noted in acute promyelocytic leukemia. The release of procoagulant enzymes from promyelocytes appears responsible for triggering the clotting sequence.[15,16] In many instances, the initiation of cytotoxic chemotherapy may initiate or significantly enhance the disseminated intravascular clotting process. For this reason, some have advocated the use of prophylactic heparin or mini-heparin before initiating cytotoxic chemotherapy.[17]

The malignancies most commonly associated with *acute* DIC are depicted in Table 2. As noted, the most common malignancy in which DIC occurs is acute promyelocytic leukemia.[15,16] However, acute DIC may also be seen in almost any type of solid tumor. There are numerous potential mechanisms by which malignancy may provide triggers for DIC. The patient with malignancy and associated DIC presents a major problem in management, and thus a clear understanding and definition of possible triggering events is desirable and often necessary for efficacious control of the intravascular clotting process.

II. PATHOPHYSIOLOGY

Figure 1 summarizes the manner in which various disease states can provide a wide variety of triggering events to initiate disseminated intravascular coagulation. The net result of any of these triggering mechanisms is the ultimate generation of systemic thrombin and systemic plasmin. Figure 2 depicts the pathophysiology of DIC once the trigger has been provided and generation of systemic thrombin and plasmin has occurred. As thrombin circulates, it enzymatically attacks fibrinogen, systemically rather than locally, creating fibrin monomer. Under physiological conditions, fibrin mon-

TABLE 2

Malignancies Most Commonly Associated with Acute DIC

Acute promyelocytic leukemia
Lung
Gall bladder
Stomach
Colon
Breast
Ovary
Melanoma
Prostate

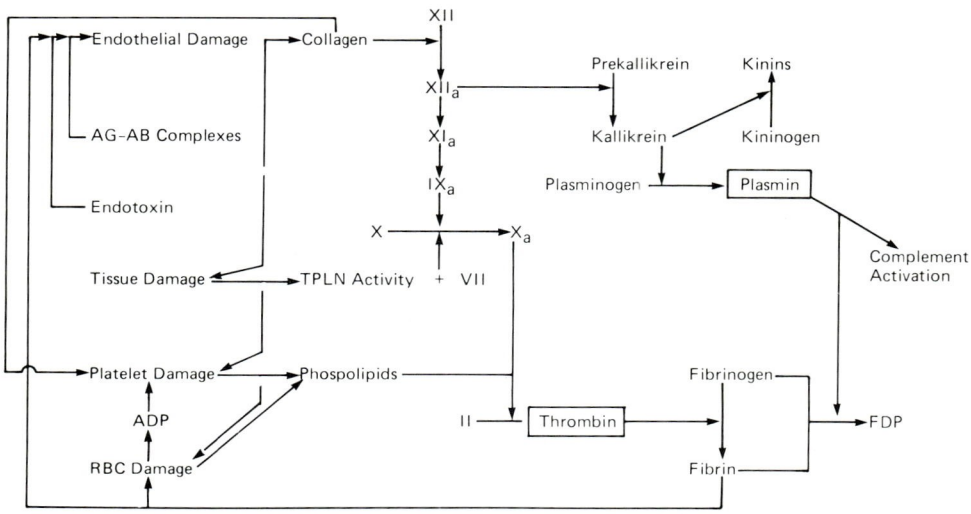

FIGURE 1. Triggering pathophysiology in disseminated intravascular coagulation (DIC).

omer subsequently polymerizes into fibrin (Chapter 3). However, in the face of plasmin generation, fibrinogen is simultaneously being degraded, creating fibrinogen/fibrin degradation products, the X, Y, D, and E fragments[18] (Figures 25 and 26 in Chapter 3). Some of these fragments have a high affinity for fibrin monomer and the two complex before much of the fibrin monomer can polymerize into fibrin. This combination of degradation products and fibrin monomer form the so-called *soluble fibrin monomer,* the presence of which provides the basis of paracoagulation reactions (the protamine sulfate test and the ethanol gelation test), which are aids in diagnosing disseminated intravascular coagulation.[19,20] When protamine sulfate is added to citrated plasma that contains soluble fibrin monomer, it acts to dissociate degradation products, allowing fibrin monomer to polymerize, and resultant fibrin strands are observed in the test tube. While some fibrin monomer is complexing with degradation products to form soluble fibrin monomer, other fibrin monomers polymerize primarily in the microvasculature, leading to impedence of blood flow, tissue hypoxia, and resultant ischemia and necrosis in multiple end organs. In addition, polymerized fibrin deposited in the microvasculature leads to entrapment of platelets, attendant thrombocytopenia, and may cause microangiopathic hemolytic anemia from fibrin-red cell contact.[21] The microhemolysis can provide more triggering material for continued intravascular co-

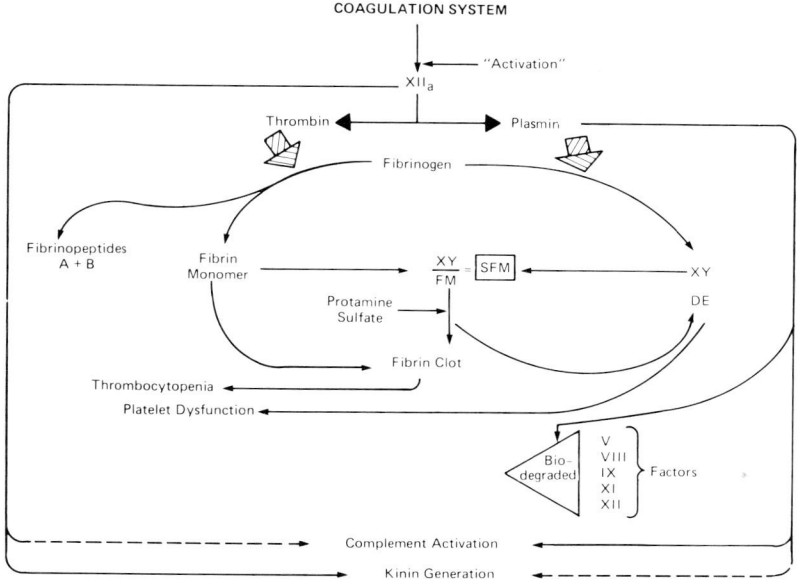

FIGURE 2. Pathophysiology of disseminated intravascular coagulation (DIC).

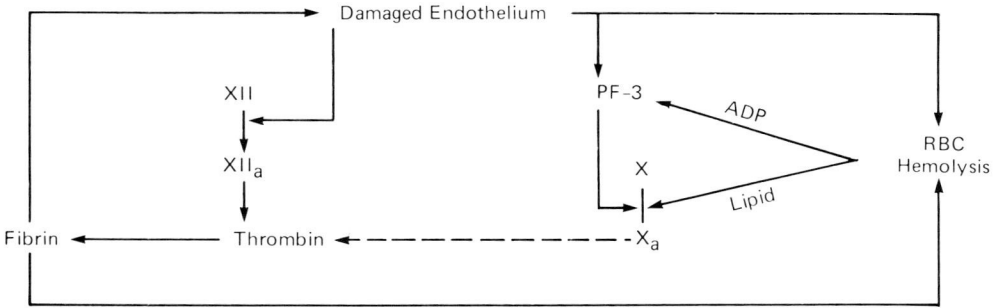

FIGURE 3. Selected "pathocybernetics" in disseminated intravascular coagulation (DIC).

agulation (ADP and red cell membrane phospholipid), thus creating a pathologic cycle (Figure 3).

Plasmin is also capable of degradation and/or inactivation of Factors V, VIII, IX, XI, ACTH, growth hormone, complement, insulin, and other plasma proteins. This may occur systemically in DIC. The syndrome of acute disseminated intravascular coagulation with hemorrhage might be more aptly referred to as "acute disseminated intravascular proteolysis", as it is the systemic plasmin generation that appears to account for the majority of hemorrhage. This occurs through the creation of fibrinogen/fibrin degradation products that interfere with fibrin monomer polymerization, the presence of platelet dysfunction by coating of platelet membranes with degradation products,[22] and plasmin biodegradation of Factor V, VIII, IX, and other plasma proteins. By understanding the circular pathophysiology of DIC (thrombin + plasmin generation), one can appreciate that if thrombin generation is moderate to maximum and the secondary fibrinolytic response (plasmin generation) minimal, the same pathophysiology will be more commonly associated with polymerization of fibrin, minimal lysis, and diffuse thromboses, (commonly seen in the patient with malignancy). Alternatively, if plasmin activity is dominant over thrombin activity, then hemorrhage, the more common expression of DIC, will result.

Another important consideration in appreciating the pathophysiology of DIC is the interrelationship between the intravascular clotting process and other plasma protein enzyme systems (Figure 28 in Chapter 3). During an intravascular clotting episode initiated by a variety of triggers (abnormal endothelium, exposed collagen, foreign surfaces, phospholipids, etc.), the activation of Factor XII often occurs (Figure 1). Factor XII$_a$, via the kallikrein system, indirectly activates the fibrinolytic system, which may be an alternate or major route of secondary fibrinolysis in DIC.[23] Plasmin activates the first and third component of complement, thus initiating the complement sequence with subsequent cell lysis, immunoadherence, and other immune phenomena.[24] Kallikrein generates kinins from kininogens, leading to hypotension, increased vascular permeability, pain, and other manifestations.[25] This complex pathophysiology must be considered when dealing with, and trying to explain, many of the clinical and laboratory findings in patients with acute, subacute, and chronic DIC.

III. DIAGNOSIS

A. Clinical Diagnosis

The clinical diagnosis of disseminated intravascular coagulation need not be difficult. The key to a high index of suspicion is to simply note the appropriate *type of bleeding* in the appropriate *clinical setting*. The usual clinical settings associated with DIC are depicted in Table 1. If the patient has one of these clinical conditions with hemorrhage or thromboses, DIC should be suspected. The type of bleeding manifest by most patients with acute or subacute DIC is suggestive of multiple hemostatic compartment defects.[26] For example, most patients with acute DIC will bleed from at least three points at once.[27] This may be manifest in a wide variety of ways and commonly is seen as melena and hematemesis, or epistaxis, or hemoptysis, in association with oozing from intravascular sites, hematuria, and associated findings of petechiae and purpura. This type of bleeding suggests that multiple hemostatic compartments (i.e., plasma coagulation protein and/or platelets and/or the vasculature) are involved. Most patients also display shock and associated end organ hypoxia and/or ischemic changes. This may be manifest in a wide variety of ways, depending upon end organ involvement and degree of occlusive changes. Renal failure, due to fibrin thrombi deposited in the renal microvasculature, is not an unusual manifestation. Additionally, one must recall the interplay between coagulation, fibrino(geno)lysis, kinin generation, and complement activation in these patients, thus accounting for many attendant signs and symptoms. Many patients with malignancy and subacute or chronic DIC will not display fulminant and multiple site type bleeding, such as is seen in those with acute DIC. In malignancy, they more commonly complain of minor mucosal membrane bleeding, often manifest as excessive gingival bleeding with toothbrushing, minor hemoptysis, bothersome epistaxis, and, at times, hematuria. In addition, they will usually complain of easy and, more significantly, spontaneous bruisability. Petechiae and purpura are usually present, but may be minimal findings. When the patient with malignancy presents with diffuse thrombosis, this may be a manifestation of the opposite clinical spectrum of DIC, and the patient should be appropriately studied for confirmatory evidence.

B. Laboratory Diagnosis

Although noting the appropriate type of bleeding in the appropriate clinical setting can virtually assure a diagnosis of DIC, laboratory confirmation is desirable, if not

TABLE 3

Laboratory Findings in Acute DIC

Abnormal prothrombin time
Abnormal partial thromboplastin time
Abnormal thrombin time
Abnormal platelet count
Abnormal tourniquet test
Abnormal clot retraction
Abnormal Factors V and VIII
Positive fibrin(ogen) split products
Positive protamine sulfate test
Antithrombin III consumption
Leukocytosis
Schistocytosis

mandatory, before committing a patient to heparin or other anticoagulant type of therapy. In view of the pathophysiology of DIC, it is clear that these patients will have numerous abnormal laboratory tests of hemostasis, particularly in acute DIC. In subacute or chronic DIC, especially when associated with malignancy, many laboratory parameters may be difficult to interpret or may be within normal limits. Table 3 depicts the laboratory tests that are typically abnormal in acute DIC.

The prothrombin time is prolonged for several reasons: (1) hypofibrinogenemia is usually present, (2) Factor V is often digested by plasmin, and (3) products of fibrino(geno)lysis (FDP) interfere with fibrin polymerization. Occasionally, the prothrombin time is normal or "super normal", however, this does not rule out a diagnosis of acute DIC. The reason(s) for a normal or shortened prothrombin time in DIC remain unclear.

Similarly, the partial thromboplastin time (PTT) is usually prolonged in greater than 50% of patients with acute DIC, for the same reasons as the prothrombin time and, in addition, is prolonged by plasmin digestion of Factors VIII, IX, and XI. As with the prothrombin time, the PTT may also be normal or "super normal".

The thrombin time likewise is usually prolonged in acute DIC due to hypofibrinogenemia and inhibition of the test system by FDP.

Like the prothrombin time and partial thromboplastin time, the thrombin time can also be normal or "super normal". Performance of a thrombin time and, alternatively/additionally, a reptilase time can add additional information if the resultant thrombin time clot (or reptilase time clot) is observed for evidence of lysis for 5 to 10 min. To observe the clot is of no additional expense, requires a minimum of laboratory time, is faster than plasminogen/plasmin assays or a euglobulin lysis time and provides evidence for significant fibrino(geno)lysis, thus aiding the diagnosis. A reptilase time is often helpful as a baseline when diagnosing DIC, since it is one of the few laboratory modalities that can be used to follow the patient with acute DIC once heparin has been given.

In most instances of acute DIC there is significant thrombocytopenia, which may be noted by careful observation of a peripheral smear or performance of a platelet count. Additional findings on a peripheral smear will often be a mild leukocytosis, usually between 12,000 to 15,000 per cubic millimeter and a slight shift to the left. Furthermore, one will see red cell fragments (schistocytes) in approximately 50% of patients with acute DIC. The mechanism(s) for these microangiopathic changes have been well described.[28] Tests of platelet function will usually be abnormal in acute DIC, because of thrombocytopenia and the coating of platelet membranes by fibrino(geno)lytic degradation products. Thus clot retraction, a tourniquet test, or template bleeding time will be abnormal. These last two tests should not be performed when suspecting acute DIC, as they will add little, if anything, to the diagnosis and may cause unnecessary bleeding. Tests of platelet adhesion and aggregation will usually be abnormal. Any combination of aggregation defects may be seen.

If factor assays are performed, low levels of Factors V, VIII, and IX will usually be noted due to plasmin digestion. Factor assays are rarely, if ever, indicated or necessary for diagnosing acute DIC. The vast majority of patients will have significantly elevated fibrinogen/fibrin degradation products (FDP). The actual titer may bear little relationship to the clinical course of the intravascular clotting process, since the titer of FDP will depend upon an interplay between degree of procoagulant activity, degree of fibrino(geno)lytic response, and other factors such as poor renal clearance (degree of renal failure) and activity of the reticuloendothelial system. Some patients with acute DIC (approximately 15% in our experience) will have minimal or no elevation of FDP. This is thought to be due to overwhelming fibrino(geno)lysis (perhaps by nonspecific proteases) that has simply biodegraded FDPs past the point where they are detectable by commercially available kits, which measure only fragments D and E. In addition, if there is minimal fibrino(geno)lytic response and fibrinogen/fibrin degradation products are early species (intermediates between fibrinogen and X fragment) (Figure 25 in Chapter 3), they also will not be detected due to limitations of commercial kits. Thus the finding of minimal or absent FDP in the face of a strongly suspected diagnosis of DIC cannot be used to rule out the diagnosis.

The paracoagulation reactions for detecting the presence of soluble fibrin monomer (protamine sulfate or ethanol gelation test) are simple to perform and are usually positive in the presence of acute DIC. Both tests are reported to have attendant advantages and disadvantages. These variables have recently been described, but the best test or methodology remains unclear.[29] The protamine sulfate test, as described by Kidder et al.,[30] detects soluble fibrin monomer, even after heparinization. As with all other laboratory modalities, paracoagulation reactions, especially the protamine sulfate test, must be interpreted in the appropriate clinical setting. Soluble fibrin monomer may also be seen in some instances of acute myocardial infarction, pulmonary embolism, extensive deep vein thrombophlebitis, and in contraceptive pill users. Some 5 to 10% of patients with acute DIC have a negative paracoagulation reaction. The reasons for this remain unclear.

A newer laboratory modality that is helpful in confirming a diagnosis of DIC is an Antithrombin III (AT-III) determination.[31] Consumption of this inhibitor due to generation of thrombin and other serine proteases occurs early on and, to a significant degree, in most instances of DIC.[32] AT-III consumption may not be seen in some patients with malignancy, since this alpha-2-globulin may behave as an acute phase reactant and may only be consumed down to normal or near normal levels. The AT-III assay is of additional benefit in monitoring the patient with DIC, as the system is uneffected by FDP or heparin. When one sees cessation of AT-III consumption, it can usually be assumed that therapy has been reasonably efficacious at either blunting or stopping the intravascular clotting process.[32] Table 4 depicts AT-III levels before and after therapy in a series of patients with acute DIC.

Another laboratory modality that is becoming available and may be quite useful for a diagnosis of DIC is the radioimmunoassay of fibrinopeptide A.[33] From the clinical standpoint, the difficulty with this modality is the length of time required to perform the assay. An additional modality that may prove quite useful for both diagnosing and monitoring DIC is that of fibrinogen chromatography as described by Fletcher and Alkjaersig[34,35] (or fibrinogen electrophoresis on a polyacrylamide gel system). Both of these modalities will allow for the detection of *fibrin monomer* (fibrinogen minus fi-

TABLE 4

Antithrombin III Profiles in DIC — Before and After Treatment (Normal Range: 89—120%)

Patient	Pretreatment AT-III (%)	Posttreatment AT-III (%)	Type of therapy	Diagnosis (trigger)
1	90	130	ASA/dipyridamole[a]	Malignancy
2	105	176		
3	80	97		
4	65	99		
5	60	98		PRV/hepatitis
6	77	100		CVD
7	66	104		Malignancy
8	80	160		
9	145	163		
10	47	104	Heparin[b]	Sepsis
11	68	93		Shock/cardiac arrest
12	36	103		Shock
13	73	124		Shock/hemolysis
14	50	90	Mini-heparin[c]	Shock
15	75	107		Shock/cardiac arrest
16	50	98		Hemolysis
17	75	93		Kasabach-Merritt
18	137	167		Malignancy
19	31	86		Sepsis/malignancy
20	76	105		
21	68	98		
22	47	68		
23	80	114		
24	58	100		Transfusion reaction
25	12	110		CVD/sepsis
26	80	148		HHT
27	72	115		HHT
28	65	95		Hip fract./retroperit. bleed
29	65	128		HHT
30	55	76		Malignancy/sepsis
31	73	100	D and C	Missed abortion

[a] ASA: 600 mg b.i.d., dipyridamole: 50 mg q.i.d.
[b] Heparin: 20,000—30,000 U./24, constant infusion.
[c] Mini-heparin: 2500—5000 U. q 8—12 hr, subcutaneously.

brinopeptides A and B), *fibrinogen dimer,* and *fibrinogen polymer* (high molecular weight subspecies consisting of fibrinogen complexed with various fibrinogen/fibrin fragments). In addition, these systems may allow for the detection of fibrinogen "first derivative", the high solubility species (I-8, I-9) described by Mosesson and Sherry.[36] These consist of high solubility (low thrombin clottability) fibrinogen derivatives that have undergone minimal plasmin cleavage at the carboxyterminal end of the A-alpha chain. During an episode of excessive procoagulant activity with generation of systemic thrombin, an early increase in fibrinogen/fibrin complexes may be expected. When a secondary fibrinolytic response begins to occur, a decrease in fibrinogen/fibrin complexes, an increase in FDP, and an increase in the fibrinogen first derivatives may be seen. At the present time, these research tools remain laborious and time consuming procedures and are formidable for the clinical laboratory, but may prove highly useful for both diagnosing and monitoring acute, subacute, or chronic DIC in the near future.

IV. THERAPY

In the past, acute DIC has been associated with a high mortality. Reasons for this are several fold. Efficacious therapy has been slow in developing, and many disease states associated with DIC are in themselves often fatal. However, many patients are now surviving as more rational and effective therapy is being developed. The therapy of acute DIC should be approached in a logical and sequential fashion. Clearly, the most important therapeutic modality that can be delivered to the patient is to remove or treat the triggering process.[37,38] In many instances this may not be possible, as in malignancy. However, in many diseases associated with DIC, some reasonable attempts can be made to effectively treat the procoagulant triggering process. This may in itself stop the intravascular clotting process. If it does not, it will usually blunt the process and afford the patient a reasonable chance of responding to heparin or other therapy aimed at stopping intravascular clotting. On the other hand, if reasonable attempts are not directed to the triggering event or disease state, the patient often is unable to respond to heparin or other therapy. For example, obstetrical accidents seldom, if ever, require heparinization. Evacuation of the uterus will almost always stop the intravascular clotting process within 3 to 4 hr. It is often difficult to convince an obstetrician-genecologist to take a bleeding patient to the operating room, but prompt cessation of hemorrhage after evacuation of the uterus is usually quite striking.

In sepsis and DIC, specific antimicrobial and usual supportive therapy should be instituted before considering therapy aimed specifically at DIC. As in obstetrical accidents, many patients with sepsis will also partially or completely correct their intravascular clotting process with specific antimicrobial therapy. If antibiotic and supportive therapy alone does not stop the intravascular clotting process, it will usually blunt the process enough for the patient to have a chance of responding to heparin therapy. In patients with shock and DIC, the infusion of fluids, stabilization of cardiac status, pH, electrolytes, and other measures to expand vascular volume and improve cardiac output may stop DIC, but more often will significantly blunt the clotting process to allow the patient an opportunity to respond to heparin therapy.

In malignancy, removal of the triggering process(es) is often not possible. However, surgical, chemotherapeutic, or radiotherapeutic modalities to shrink the tumor mass may be of significant benefit in blunting or stopping the intravascular clotting process. In rarer instances, the initiation of chemotherapy or radiation therapy will cause further tissue necrosis and worsening of, or triggering of, a DIC process. Table 5 outlines the sequential therapy of DIC.

If, after reasonable attempts have been made to treat the underlying disease (and thus the triggering process), the patient continues to bleed, consideration must be given to therapy that will stop the intravascular clotting process. In our experience, the patient is afforded about a 4 hr trial (after attempting to treat the triggering event) before initiating heparin or other therapy. The time element is empirical and depends upon the degree and type of hemorrhage. Traditional methods for stopping the intravascular clotting process have consisted of heparinizing the patient. This has usually been delivered at 20,000 to 30,000 units over 24 hr. Our past approach was to give 7000 to 10,000 units intravenous push, followed by 20,000 units by constant infusion over the ensuing 24 hr. Once this is initiated, there is usually partial or complete correction of the laboratory modalities in 2 to 3 hr, followed shortly thereafter by significant slowing or cessation of clinical hemorrhage. Again, it must be emphasized that heparinizing the patient is often without avail if the underlying disease state has not first been treated in as effective a manner as possible. More recently it has been noted that "mini-heparin" therapy may be as efficacious as larger medical doses of heparin.[32] Our approach

TABLE 5

Sequential Therapy of Acute DIC

Reasonable attempts to treat or remove triggering event
  Evacuate uterus
  Antibiotics
  Electrolytes
  Volume replacement
  Maintain blood pressure
  Antineoplastic therapy
Stop clotting process
  Mini-heparin
  Heparin
  Antiplatelet drugs
  Antithrombin III concentrates (investigational)
Component therapy
  Packed red cells
  Platelets
  Prothrombin complex
  Factor VIII, Factor V
  Volume expanders (albumin)
Inhibit residual fibrino(geno)lysis
Amino caproic acid[a]

[a] Caution: ventricular arrhythmias, hypotension, hypokalemia.

now is to initiate anticoagulant therapy for acute DIC with the administration of 2500 to 5000 units subcutaneously every 8 to 12 hr, depending upon the nature and severity of bleeding. With this regimen, one usually sees cessation of AT-III consumption, lowering of FDP, increase in fibrinogen, and correction of the other usual laboratory modalities of acute DIC, in 2 to 3 hr, followed shortly thereafter by blunting or cessation of clinical bleeding. The initiation of mini-heparin therapy, rather than the usual medical doses of heparin, appears rational for several reasons: (1) if the patient fails to respond, larger doses of heparin can always be administered, (2) unlike the medical doses of heparin, mini-heparin is associated with no or minimal chance of increasing the patient's hemorrhage, and (3) most importantly, in our experience, mini-heparin has been as efficacious as large dose heparin therapy. In light of current understanding of the heparin/AT-III/thrombin-serine protease/fibrinogen axis (COAX)* mini-heparin, from a theoretical standpoint, should be equally effective as large dose heparin.

Another recent, and still investigational approach, is the administration of AT-III concentrates. A few patients have been treated with plasma fractions containing AT-III, and this appears to be as effective as mini-heparin or medical doses of heparin in stopping the intravascular clotting process.[39] Similar findings have been noted in dogs treated with AT-III for endotoxin-induced DIC.[40] Hopefully, in the near future, AT-III concentrates will become available for more widespread investigation to establish efficacy. Often, when patients fail to respond to heparin therapy, it is because AT-III has been depleted, thereby minimizing anticoagulant efficacy. It is particularly in these patients that AT-III therapy would be expected to offer maximum efficacy in stopping the intravascular clotting process. Like mini-heparin therapy, the use of AT-III concentrates should be associated with little or no danger of increasing clinical hemorrhage.

* Coagulant-anticoagulant axis (COAX), see Chapter 14.

Going through the first two sequential steps as outlined above for the therapy of DIC, i.e., therapy aimed at the triggering disease state and the initiation of heparin or other therapeutic modalities to stop the intravascular clotting process, will cause cessation of DIC in the majority of patients. Occasionally, however, patients will continue to bleed after these two steps. The most common reasons are failure to control the triggering disease or coagulation factor depletion due to plasmin digestion and, to a lesser extent, consumption of factors. In this situation, the third sequential step to be considered is blood component replacement. All reasonable attempts should be made to define which components are lacking and most likely contributing to continued hemorrhage. *Only* those thought necessary to control hemorrhage should be delivered. The patient may be treated with fresh frozen plasma, cryoprecipitate, prothrombin complex concentrates, and/or platelets as indicated, but replacement should be as specific as possible. It should be emphasized at this point that component therapy should never be used (with the exception of packed red cells, AT-III, and platelets) until the patient has been heparinized or treated with other modalities, and it is reasonably certain that the intravascular clotting process has been controlled.[42] The addition of components in the face of continued DIC may "add fuel to the fire". If the patient is given fresh frozen plasma or clotting factor concentrates this may provide more fibrinogen/fibrin degradation products, further inhibition of fibrin monomer polymerization, further interference with platelet function, and further plasmin-induced biodegradation of clotting Factors V, VIII, and IX. This may exaggerate DIC, and clinical hemorrhage will often become much more pronounced.

Rarely, patients will continue to bleed after going through the three steps outlined above. When this occurs, it is most often due to continued residual fibrino(geno)lysis. In this *rare* instance, antifibrinolytic therapy (usually aminocaproic acid) may be considered. This is used in DIC in the usual doses: 5 g initial slow intravenous push, followed by 2 g every 1 to 2 hr for 24 hr or until clinical bleeding stops. This agent should always be given slowly, as it may be associated with hypokalemia, hypotension, ventricular arrhythmias, and diffuse intravascular thromboses, especially if the intravascular clotting process has not been arrested first. Monitoring of cardiac status, electrolytes, and renal output is essential. It must be reemphasized that only in rare instances do patients with DIC require antifibrinolytic therapy (less than 5% of patients, in our experience). As in the case of component therapy, antifibrinolytic therapy should *never* be used in acute DIC unless one is first assured that the intravascular clotting process has been successfully controlled with heparin or other therapy. If the intravascular clotting process is ongoing, the patient requires fibrinolysis for clearing of fibrin microthrombi. Thus if antifibrinolytic therapy is used in the face of continuing clotting, the consequences are obviously catastrophic. The problem of managing chronic DIC in the patient with malignancy is discussed in Chapter 11.

V. RELATED SYNDROMES

Appreciating the cybernetic nature of normal hemostasis, i.e., the numerous complex and delicate interplays between coagulation proteins, other plasma protein systems, the platelets, the vasculature, and all of the attendant inhibitors to these various components, one cannot help but be impressed by similar, although exaggerated, interplays that must be occurring in a "pathocybernetic" manner in DIC. It is evident that numerous circular events are occurring in DIC. Thus in many instances the point at which the process starts may not be necessarily relevant with respect to the end clinical results. For example, endothelial damage may occur via numerous mechanisms. Damaged endothelium may, in turn, activate coagulation and/or lead to red cell microangiopathic hemolysis, which may then lead to release of red cell ADP and membrane phospholipid, which may cause further triggering of coagulation and/or platelet release, with subsequent activation of coagulation. These singular isolated circular systems in DIC are depicted in Figure 3. Understanding these as well as numerous other potential circular events in DIC explains how many different starting points, via similar or related pathophysiology, oan lead to similar clinical manifestations. The process may be local (organ specific) or systemic. It may start with platelets, endothelium, or coagulation proteins, and may represent dominant procoagulant activity with minimal or inadequate secondary fibrinolytic response (i.e., thrombosis) or minimal procoagulant activity and overwhelming secondary fibrino(geno)lysis (i.e., hemorrhage). Appreciating this wide spectrum of clinical manifestations allows for considering other syndromes to be probably related to what we label classical DIC. These potentially similar syndromes include thrombotic thrombocytopenia purpura, microangiopathic hemolytic anemia, respiratory distress syndrome (hyaline membrane disease), hemolytic uremic syndrome, and shock lung.

A. Microangiopathic Hemolytic Anemia

Microangiopathic red cell changes (RBC fragments, schistocytes, Heilmeyer-Helmet cells) may be seen in a variety of disorders, including DIC, TTP, hypertension, eclampsia, and hemolytic uremic syndrome. These changes may arise from RBC contact with fibrin or damaged endothelium (Figure 3). When fibrin and/or endothelium induces RBC fragmentation, a resultant release of RBC membrane phospholipids and RBC adenosine diphosphate (ADP) may initiate subsequent activation of the procoagulant system and/or platelets. This can result in further fibrin deposition and endothelial damage, thus recycling the pathophysiology. Alternatively, when RBC fragmentation occurs before endothelial damage (cardiac valves, intravascular hemolysis, fibrin deposition), resultant RBC membrane phospholipids and ADP release may lead to platelet release, procoagulant drive, fibrin deposition, and subsequent resultant endothelial damage, with further RBC fragmentation and, again, a recycling of pathophysiology. Thus the starting points may differ, but the cycling pathophysiology is similar, namely: endothelial damage, RBC fragmentation, procoagulant drive, fibrin deposition, resultant secondary fibrinolytic response, and back to endothelial damage.

It is obvious that any of the above may be the starting point. However, the interplays and the balance between the endothelial damage, procoagulant drive, and secondary fibrinolytic response will determine whether the clinical manifestations will be hemorrhage or thrombosis, or both. In addition, the DIC process may be systemic or localized to an individual organ system, as the following disorders illustrate.

B. Hemolytic-Uremic Syndrome (HUS)

Renal vascular damage of any etiology may initiate microangiopathic hemolysis, with subsequent red cell ADP and/or membrane phospholipid-induced platelet release and/or procoagulant activity. This leads to fibrin deposition, further endothelial damage, and a perpetuation of the cycle. The salient clinical manifestations are (1) uremia from renal vascular damage and (2) RBC fragments from damaged endothelium and/or fibrin. More rarely, the cycle may start with procoagulant activity, fibrin deposition, and subsequent vascular endothelial damage to the kidney with resultant uremia. HUS, therefore, shares similar if not identical pathophysiology with DIC, but in most instances the process begins with and is localized to the kidney. In some instances, the same pathophysiology may exist in the usual *disseminated* or systemic intravascular coagulation, with uremia (resulting from renal microvascular damage) being only one of the many systemic clinical manifestations of more classical DIC.

C. Respiratory Distress Syndrome (RDS)

It has now become clear that the hyaline membrane of RDS represents excessive fibrin deposition. Triggers for the procoagulant drive in these infants at high risk for RDS (prematures and infants of diabetic mothers) remain unclear. However, it appears that the usual secondary fibrinolytic response that usually accompanies excessive fibrin deposition (such as in DIC) is lacking in these infants. Current evidence suggests that infants from diabetic mothers have markedly elevated fibrinolytic inhibitors (alpha-2-macroglobulin) and premature infants have decreased plasminogen levels, thus explaining the lack of a fibrinolytic response to the procoagulant drive in RDS.[43] Therefore, like HUS, RDS maybe a DIC-like syndrome that is localized (lungs) rather than systemic and characterized by excessive procoagulant activity (fibrin deposition), without the usual fibrinolytic response (lysis and hemorrhage).

D. Thrombotic Thrombocytopenic Purpura (TTP)

TTP, like DIC, appears to be an intermediary mechanism of disease rather than a strict disease entity. It is often associated with several well-recognized clinical settings, especially a strong allergic history, antibiotic therapy (sulfas, penicillin, and tetracyclines), collagen vascular disorders, and, less commonly, viremia, pregnancy, and excessive sun exposure. The salient clinical features of TTP represent a classical pentad and consist of thrombocytopenic purpura, hemolytic anemia, neurological defects that may or may not be waxing and waning, fever, and hematuria. The most common chief complaints in TTP are either neurologic, hemorrhagic episodes, malaise, fatigue, or fever. The types of bleeding and thrombosing in TTP represent a wide spectrum of manifestations, as in DIC. Petechiae and purpura are by far the most common signs of hemorrhage. Retinal hemorrhage occurs in approximately 20% of patients, gross hematuria occurs in 18%, and epistaxis, gingival bleeding, and melena occur less frequently.

The classical laboratory findings of TTP are schistocytosis, reticulocytosis, anemia, thrombocytopenia, a leukocytosis with a shift to the left, microscopic hematuria, proteinuria, and indirect hyperbilirubinemia. Marrow examination usually reveals erythroid and myeloid hyperplasia, with normal to increased young megakaryocytic forms. Coagulation changes reported in association with TTP have been inconsistent. Commonly, most tests are within normal limits, except tests of platelet and vascular function and platelet counts. Some investigations have reported increased coagulation factors as may be appreciated in chronic compensated DIC.[45] Others have reported decreased coagulation factors, and the most uniform coagulation abnormality, other than thrombocytopenia, appears to be elevated FDP.[46]

The organs most commonly involved with characteristic thrombi are the myocardium, adrenals, posterior pituitary, pancreas, kidneys, and gray matter of the central nervous system.[47] Diagnostic biopsies are most rewarding if they are done in gingival tissue adjacent to the upper incisors where the area is very accessible, highly vascular, and control of hemostasis can be easily achieved. The rewards will also be high if a blind cervical node biopsy is performed. The bone marrow is positive for classical thrombi in about 50% of patients. The classical pathological findings in TTP are PAS positive hyaline deposits in the subendothelium (commonly seen in preterminal arterioles), capillary dilations and intraluminal thrombi.[48] There is classically an absence of platelet material in the subendothelial hyaline deposits, and there is typically endothelial proliferation with a notable absence of inflammatory areas. In most cases there is an absence of immunoglobulins in the hyaline deposits.

The sequential pathogenesis of these lesions has been well studied and appear to consist of subendothelial deposits consisting of fibrinogen, fibrin monomer, fibrin, fibrinogen/fibrin intermediates, and an absence of platelet material. This is followed by development of deposits consisting of the above, plus platelet aggregates and inconsistent amounts of IgG. These deposits are usually noted between the muscularis and subendothelium, with some interconnections. Following this, there is endothelial proliferation and then intraluminal thrombi, which are often noted to interconnect with subendothelial and intramural deposits. Kwaan and co-workers[49] have provided additional insight into possible pathophysiological events in TTP. These investigators have studied plasminogen activator activity in patients with TTP and have found that endothelial plasminogen activator activity is totally absent in all involved vessels in patients with classical TTP. However, endothelial plasminogen activator activity appears to be normal in uninvolved vessels in the same group of patients. It appears that TTP, like DIC, is an intermediary mechanism of disease and may share similar pathophysiology with DIC, i.e., a primary procoagulant drive being provided by a variety of potential triggers with decreased or absent secondary fibrino(geno)lysis, thus being manifest primarily as a thrombotic rather than a primary hemorrhagic disorder. This could explain the clinical manifestations of thromboses and thrombocytopenic-type bleeding only. Since minimal or no fibrinolysis is occurring, the absence of uniformly abnormal coagulation tests (due to plasmin digestion of coagulation factors as in classical DIC) is also explained. It remains unclear whether procoagulant drive begins in the vessel wall and a secondary fibrinolytic response is impossible, or whether a procoagulant drive leads to changes in the vessel wall, resulting in an impeded fibrinolytic response.

In summary, it appears that TTP, like many other disorders, may share a common pathophysiology with DIC, the clinical manifestations differing because (1) the procoagulant drive supersedes the secondary fibrino(geno)lytic response and (2) the process is localized. Current concepts of TTP have been recently reviewed and summarized.[50,51]

VI. SUMMARY

Current concepts of the etiology, pathophysiology, diagnosis, and management of DIC have been presented. Considerable attention has been devoted to interrelationships that have remained confusing for some time. Only by clearly understanding these interrelationships can one appreciate the divergent and wide spectrum of often confusing clinical and laboratory findings in these patients. This review has also pointed out that other syndromes, not clinically considered in the spectrum of DIC, may really represent similar or identical pathophysiology and, although organ specific (as in HUS or RDS) may, in fact, be variants of DIC.

REFERENCES

1. **Muller-Berghaus, G.,** Pathophysiology of disseminated intravascular coagulation, *Thromb. Diath. Haemorrh.,* Suppl. 36, 45, 1969.
2. **Bick, R. L. and Adams, T.,** Disseminated intravascular coagulation: etiology pathophysiology, diagnosis and management, *Med. Counterpoint,* 6, 38, 1974.
3. **Mersky, C.,** Defibrination syndrome, in *Human Blood Coagulation, Hemostasis and Thrombosis,* Biggs, R., Ed., Blackwell Scientific, London, 1976, 492.
4. **Damus, P. S. and Salzman, E. W.,** Disseminated intravascular coagulation, *Arch. Surg. (Chicago),* 104, 262, 1972.

5. **Waxman, B. and Gamrin, R.**, Use of heparin in disseminated intravascular coagulation, *Am. J. Obstet. Gynecol.*, 112, 434, 1972.
6. **Steichele, D. F.**, Consumption coagulopathy in obstetrics and gynecology, *Thromb. Diath. Haemorrh. Suppl.*, 36, 177, 1969.
7. **Hafter, R. and Graeff, H.**, Molecular aspects of defibrination in a reptilase-treated case of "dead fetus syndrome", *Thromb. Res.*, 7, 391, 1975.
8. **McGehee, W. H., Rapaport, S. I., and Hjort, P. F.**, Intravascular coagulation in fulminant meningiococcaemia, *Ann. Intern. Med.*, 67, 250, 1967.
9. **Abildgaard, C. F., Corrigan, J. J., Seeler, R. A., Simone, J. V., and Schulman, I.**, Meningiococcemia associated with intravascular coagulation, *Pediatrics*, 40, 78, 1967.
10. **Corrigan, J. J.**, Changes in the blood coagulation system associated with septicemia, *N. Engl. J. Med.*, 279, 851, 1968.
11. **Yoshikawa, T., Tanaka, R., and Guze, L. B.**, Infection and disseminated intravascular coagulation, *Medicine (Baltimore)*, 50, 237, 1971.
12. **Cronberg, S., Skansberg, P., and Nivenios-Larsson, K.**, Disseminated intravascular coagulation in septicemia caused by beta hemolytic streptococci, *Thromb. Res.*, 3, 405, 1973.
13. **Mason, J. W., Kleeberg, U., Dolan, P., and Colman, R. W.**, Human plasma killikrein and Hageman factor in endotoxin shock, *Ann. Intern. Med.*, 73, 545, 1970.
14. **Bick, R. L.**, Treatment of bleeding and thrombosis in the patient with cancer, in *Management of the Patient with Cancer*, Nealon, T., Ed., W.B. Saunders, Philadelphia, 1976, 48.
15. **Gralnick, H. R. and Tan, H. K.**, Acute promyelocytic leukemia: a model for understanding the role of the malignant cell in hemostasis, *Human Pathol.*, 5, 661, 1974.
16. **Matsuoka, M. and Onishi, Y.**, Pathologic cells as procoagulant substance of disseminated intravascular coagulation syndrome in acute promyelocytic leukemia, *Thromb. Res.*, 8, 263, 1976.
17. **Gralnick, H. R., Bagley, J., and Abrell, E.**, Heparin treatment for the hemorrhagic diathesis of acute promyelocytic leukemia, *Am. J. Med.*, 52, 167, 1972.
18. **Mosesson, M. W.**, Fibrinogen catabolic pathways, *Semin. Thromb. Hemostas.*, 1, 63, 1974.
19. **Breen, F. A. and Tullis, J. Z.**, Ethanol gelation, a rapid screening test for intravascular coagulation, *Ann. Intern. Med.*, 69, 1197, 1968.
20. **Gurewich, V. and Hutchinson, E.**, Detection of intravascular coagulation by a serine dilution protamine sulfate test, *Ann. Intern. Med.*, 75, 895, 1971.
21. **Surgenor, D. M.**, Erythrocytes and blood coagulation, *Thromb. Diath. Haemorrh.*, 32, 247, 1974.
22. **Kopec, M., Wegrzynowiczy, Z., Budzynski, A., Latallo, Z., Lipinski, B., and Kowalski, E.**, Interaction of fibrinogen degradation products with platelets, *Exp. Biol. Med.*, 3, 73, 1968.
23. **Laake, K. and Vennerod, A.**, Factor XII-induced fibrinolysis: studies on the separation of prekallikrein, plasminogen proactivator, and Factor XI in human plasma, *Thromb. Res.*, 4, 285, 1974.
24. **Ratnoff, O. D. and Naff, G. B.**, The conversion of Cls to Cl' esterase by plasmin and trypsin, *J. Exp. Med.*, 125, 337, 1961.
25. **Kaplan, A., Meier, H., and Mandle, R.**, The Hageman factor dependent pathways of coagulation, fibrinolysis, and kinin generation, *Semin. Thromb. Hemostas.*, 3, 6, 1976.
26. **Bick, R. L. and Shanbrom, E.**, A systemic approach to the diagnosis of bleeding disorders, *Med. Counterpoint*, 4, 27, 1972.
27. **Bowie, E. J. W., Cooper, H., Fuster, V., Kazmier, F., and Owen, C. A.**, The diagnosis of intravascular coagulation, *Thromb. Diath. Haemorrh., Suppl.*, 36, 137, 1973.
28. **Bull, B., Rubenberg, M., Dacie, J., and Brain, M. C.**, Microangiopathic hemolytic anemia: mechanisms of red-cell fragmentation, *Br. J. Haematol.*, 14, 643, 1968.
29. **Marder, V. J., Matchett, M. O., and Sherry, S.**, Detection of serum fibrinogen and fibrin degradation products: comparison of six techniques using purified products and application in clinical studies, *Am. J. Med.*, 51, 71, 1971.
30. **Kidder, W. R., Logan, L. J., Rapaport, S. I., and Patch, M. J.**, The plasma protamine paracoagulation test: clinical and laboratory evaluation, *Am. J. Clin. Pathol.*, 58, 675, 1972.
31. **Bick, R. L., Kovacs, I., and Fekete, L. F.**, A new two stage functional assay for Antithrombin III: clinical and laboratory evaluation, *Thromb. Res.*, 8, 745, 1976.
32. **Bick, R. L., Dukes, M., Wilson, W. L., and Fekete, L. F.**, Antithrombin III (AT-III) as a diagnostic aid in disseminated intravascular coagulation, *Thromb. Res.*, 10, 721, 1977.
33. **Nossel, H. L., Ti, M., Kaplan, K. L., Spandonis, K., Soland, T., and Butler, V. D.**, The generation of fibrinopeptide-A in clinical blood samples: evidence for thrombin activity, *J. Clin. Invest.*, 58, 1136, 1976.
34. **Alkjaersig, N., Roy, L., and Fletcher, A. P.**, Analysis of gel exclusion chromatographic data by chromatographic plate theory analysis: application to plasma fibrinogen chromatography, *Thromb. Res.*, 3, 525, 1973.

35. **Fletcher, A. P. and Alkjaersig, N.**, Blood hypercoagulability, intravascular coagulation, and thrombosis: new diagnostic concepts, *Thromb. Diath. Haemorrh. Suppl.*, 45, 389, 1971.
36. **Mosesson, M. W. and Sherry, S.**, The preparation of properties of human fibrinogen of relatively high solubility, *Biochemistry*, 5, 2829, 1966.
37. **Bick, R. L.**, Disseminated intravascular coagulation, in *Difficult Diagnostic Problems in Hemostasis and Thrombosis*, Bick, R. L., Ed., American Society of Clinical Pathologists, Chicago, 1976.
38. **Mersky, C.**, Diagnosis and treatment of intravascular coagulation, *Br. J. Haematol.*, 15, 523, 1968.
39. **Bick, R. L., Fekete, L. R., and Wilson, W. L.**, Treatment of disseminated intravascular coagulation (DIC) with Antithrombin III, *Trans. Am. Soc. Hematol.*, 167, 1976.
40. **Penner, J. A., Leach, K., and Rohwedder, J.**, Thrombogenic characteristics of prothrombin complex and the effect of Antithrombin III, *Trans. Am. Soc. Hematol.*, 177, 1976.
41. **Yin, E. T.**, Effect of heparin on neutralization of factor X_a and thrombin by the plasma alpha-2-globulin inhibitor, *Thromb. Diath. Haemorrh.*, 33, 43, 1974.
42. **Bick, R. L., Schmalhorst, W. R., and Fekete, L. F.**, Disseminated intravascular coagulation and blood component therapy, *Transfusion (Philadelphia)*, 16, 361, 1976.
43. **Ambrus, C. M., Weintraub, D. H., Durphy, D., Dowd, J. E., Pickren, J. W., Niswander, K. R., and Ambrus, J. L.**, Studies on hyaline membrane disease. I. The fibrinolytic system in pathogenesis and therapy, *Pediatrics*, 32, 10, 1963.
44. **Goldenfarb, P. B. and Finch, S. C.**, Thrombotic thrombocytopenic purpura: a ten year study, *JAMA*, 226, 644, 1973.
45. **Barnhart, M. I., McCutcheon, S. A., Riddle, J. M., and Ohorodnik, J. M.**, Thrombotic thrombocytopenic purpura as a model of accelerated protein synthesis, *Thromb. Diath. Haemorrh.*, 12, 211, 1964.
46. **Lerna, R. G., Rapaport, S. I., and Metzer, J.**, Thrombotic thrombocytopenic purpura: several clotting studies, relation to the generalized Schwartzman reaction, and remission after adrenal steroid and dextran therapy, *Ann. Intern. Med.*, 66, 1180, 1967.
47. **Amorosi, E. L. and Ultmann, J. E.**, Thrombotic thrombocytopenic purpura: report of 16 cases and review of the literature, *Medicine (Baltimore)*, 45, 139, 1966.
48. **Gore, I.**, Disseminated arteriolar and capillary platelet thrombosis: a morphological study of its histogenesis, *Am. J. Pathol.*, 26, 155, 1950.
49. **Kwaan, H. C., Gallo, G., Potter, E., Cutting, H., and Stanzler, R.**, The nature of the vascular lesion in thrombotic thrombocytopenic purpura, *Ann. Intern. Med.*, 68 (Abstr.), 1169, 1968.
50. **Nalbandian, R. M., Henry, R. L., and Bick, R. L.**, Thrombotic cytopenic purpura: an extended editorial, *Semin. Thromb. Hemostas.*, 5, 216, 1979.
51. **Kwaan, H. C.**, The pathogenesis of thrombotic thrombocytopenic purpura, *Semin. Thromb. Hemostas.*, 5, 184, 1979.

Chapter 9

PRIMARY HYPERFIBRINO(GENO)LYTIC SYNDROMES

Rodger L. Bick and Genesio Murano

TABLE OF CONTENTS

I. Introduction 182

II. Pathophysiology of Primary Hyperfibrino(geno)lysis 182

III. Alterations of Hemostasis in Chronic Liver Disease 183
    A. Introduction 183
    B. Etiology and Pathophysiology 184
        1. Coagulation Protein Changes 184
        2. Hyperfibrino(geno)lysis 184
        3. Platelet Changes 185
        4. Other Defects 185
    C. Clinical Diagnosis 185
    D. Laboratory Diagnosis 186
    E. Management 187
    F. Summary 187

IV. Alterations of Hemostasis Associated with Cardiopulmonary Bypass 188
    A. Introduction 188
    B. Pathophysiology 188
        1. Thrombocytopenia 188
        2. Functional Platelet Defects 189
        3. Vascular Defects 190
        4. Isolated Coagulation Factor Defects 191
        5. Disseminated Intravascular Coagulation 192
        6. Primary Hyperfibrino(geno)lysis 192
        7. Other Defects 193
        8. Summary of Pathophysiology 194
    C. Prevention 194
        1. Historical Information 194
        2. Physical Findings 195
        3. Pre-CPB Laboratory Screen 197
    D. Clinical and Laboratory Diagnosis 197
    E. Management 198
    F. Summary 200

V. Hyperfibrino(geno)lysis in Malignancy 201

VI. Summary 201

References 202

I. INTRODUCTION

Until recently, primary activation of the fibrinolytic system was considered uncommon, and the only situations in which clinical fibrinolysis existed were assumed to be those secondary to disseminated intravascular coagulation (DIC). However, these considerations were formulated in an era when there were insufficient clinical laboratory tools to assess fibrinolytic activity in patients. Early work in clinical fibrinolysis was limited to the use of the euglobulin lysis time (EGLT), which is of questionable clinical significance in assessing fibrinolytic activity.[1,2] With the advent of newer and more sophisticated techniques, such as the fibrin plate technique,[3,4] the caseinolytic assay technique,[5] and chromogenic substrates,[6] it is now recognized that primary activation of the fibrinolytic system is not an uncommon clinical event. The conditions in which primary activation of the fibrinolytic system may occur are generally well defined and include cardiopulmonary bypass, chronic liver disease, and malignancy. Each of these clinical situations will be discussed separately in this chapter.

II. PATHOPHYSIOLOGY OF PRIMARY HYPERFIBRINO(GENO)LYSIS

Primary hyperfibrino(geno)lysis usually occurs in well-defined clinical entities in which there is direct or indirect activation of plasminogen into systemically circulating plasmin. In most disorders, the precise mechanism by which this occurs is not known. In several types of malignancies, tumor extracts are capable of activating the fibrinolytic system either directly or indirectly. In other disorders, mechanisms that may be involved include poor hepatic clearance of plasminogen activators or a decrease or dysfunction of inhibitors such as the alpha-2-macroglobulin fraction.[7] In chronic liver disease, alpha-2-macroglobulin is often increased, but appears to lose significant biologic function in inhibiting the fibrinolytic system. Table 1 lists various mechanisms through which the fibrinolytic system could be activated. Figure 1 depicts the pathophysiology of primary hyperfibrino(geno)lysis.

As the fibrinolytic system becomes activated, there is systemic circulating plasmin (systemic proteolytic activity). Plasmin degrades fibrin(ogen) into the fibrinogen degradation products (FDP): X,Y,D, and E fragments. As in DIC (Chapter 8), the presence of circulating plasmin and FDP results in compromised hemostatic function. Figure 2 compares and contrasts the salient features of DIC and primary hyperfibrino(geno)lysis, which can present in exactly the same manner as DIC and are often manifested as catastrophic hemorrhage. Since in primary hyperfibrino(geno)lysis there has been no thrombin generated, as occurs in DIC, there is no fibrin monomer for FDP to attach to, thus there is *no* soluble fibrin monomer.

Since there has been little or no activation of the major serine proteases, there is little or no consumption of Antithrombin III (AT-III), as is commonly seen in DIC. In addition, no fibrin is deposited in the microcirculation, and, consequently, there is no thrombocytopenia. However, the presence or absence of thrombocytopenia should *not* be used to establish a differential diagnosis, because many disorders that are usually associated with a primary activation of the fibrinolytic system are often associated with thrombocytopenia via unrelated mechanisms. At present, an AT-III determination as well as a paracoagulation reaction test, such as the protamine sulfate test, appear to be good differential diagnostic tools for distinguishing between primary hyperfibrino(geno)lytic syndromes and DIC with secondary fibrino(geno)lysis. As discussed in Chapter 8, the protamine sulfate test or ethanol gelation test may, on occasion, be negative in DIC. Thus the careful interpretation of laboratory data in the appropriate clinical setting provides the hallmark of making a differential diagnosis.

TABLE 1

Mechanisms of Fibrino(geno)lytic System Activation

Increased activators
    Plasma activators
    Endothelial activators
    Other (pathological) activators
Decreased inhibitors
    Alpha-2-macroglobulin
    Alpha-2-antiplasmin
    Alpha-1-antitrypsin
Decreased activator inhibitors
Increased plasminogen?

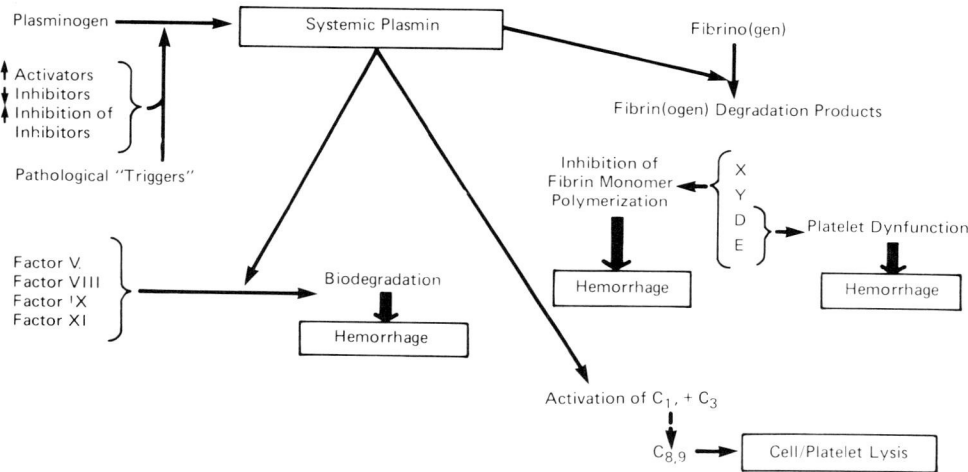

FIGURE 1. Pathophysiology of primary hyperfibrino(geno)lysis.

III. ALTERATIONS OF HEMOSTASIS IN CHRONIC LIVER DISEASE

A. Introduction

Patients with chronic liver disease commonly experience significant hemorrhage, which presents a major challenge in clinical care, taxes the laboratory and local blood banking facilities, and is often the terminal event in the patient.[8,9] The alterations of hemostasis that occur in these patients are complex and multifaceted.

Classically, it has been thought that hemorrhage in chronic liver disease is due to decreased synthesis of the vitamin K-dependent prothrombin complex factors, Factors II, VII, IX, and X.[10] However, numerous additional hemostatic alterations must be appreciated in order to render efficacious therapy. The most common sequence of events in these patients is that a localized bleed often develops, usually from a ruptured esophageal varix, peptic ulcers, or hemorrhagic gastritis.[11] These bleeds tend to cascade into massive hemorrhage, which is usually poorly responsive to the usual therapeutic modalities of Sengstaken-Blakemore tamponade, massive transfusions with whole blood/fresh frozen plasma, and vasopressin infusion. Unsuccessful management is usually attributed to the fact that, while some defects are treated and partially or completely corrected, other defects are left essentially unattended.

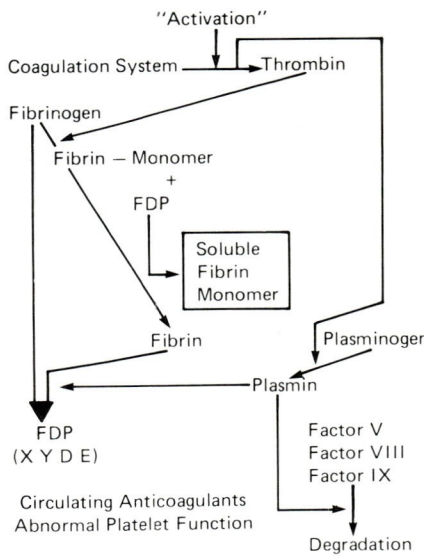

FIGURE 2. A comparison of mechanism of activation and products formed in primary fibrino(geno)lysis and disseminated intravascular coagulation.

B. Etiology and Pathophysiology

1. Coagulation Protein Changes

The patient with chronic liver disease often demonstrates an early and significant decreased synthesis of the prothrombin complex Factors (II, VII, IX, and X). From the laboratory standpoint, these patients behave similarly to those on warfarins. The decrease in Factor VII best correlates with the prothrombin time determination. However, the decreases in Factors IX and X best correlate with predisposition to clinical hemorrhage.[12] The patient with chronic liver disease may also synthesize dysfunctional prothrombin complex factors (Chapter 3), the so-called "PIVKA" derivatives (proteins induced by vitamin K absence/antagonism).[13,14]

Hypofibrinogenemia may occur. However, it rarely reaches a level of clinical significance. Normal or increased fibrinogen levels may also be seen in these patients, as fibrinogen may behave as an acute-phase reactant. In addition, many patients have an acquired dysfibrinogenemia, reflected by abnormal fibrin monomer polymerization[15,16] and/or abnormal carbohydrate content.[17]

As the disease becomes terminal, there may also be decreased synthesis of Factors V and VIII. Early in the clinical course, these two factors may actually be elevated. The synthesis of prekallikrein is also decreased; however, the clinical significance of this defect remains unclear. Patients with chronic liver disease of any etiology usually demonstrate significantly decreased levels of AT-III. The pathophysiology of this remains unclear, as this may represent either a true decreased synthesis or synthesis of a dysfunctional AT-III molecule.[18,19] Some patients may have normal or high AT-III levels, since this alpha-2-globulin, like fibrinogen, may behave as an acute-phase reactant. The clinical significance of this finding remains unclear with respect to developing hypercoagulability or thrombosis.

2. Hyperfibrino(geno)lysis

The majority of patients with chronic liver disease experience a hyperfibrino(geno)lytic syndrome[20,21] due to increased quantities of circulating plasmin. Primary hyperfibrino(geno)lysis (circulating plasmin) causes numerous hemostatic defects. Hypofibrinogenemia and "pseudodysfibrinogenemia" occurs in the presence of fibrino(geno)lysis. Pseudodysfibrinogenemia is manifest in several forms; one is the creation of high solubility (I-8, I-9) fractions,[22] low thrombin clottability fibrinogen subspecies. This represents fibrinogen that has undergone minimal cleavage by plasmin (Chapter 3). Because of fibrino(geno)lysis, patients with chronic liver disease usually demonstrate elevated FDP. The early degradation products also create a pseudodysfibrinogenemia by complexing with native fibrinogen and thus interfering with fibrin monomer polymerization. In addition, the latter degradation products coat the surfaces of platelets, rendering them dysfunctional.[23] Circulating plasmin can also cause the proteolysis of Factor V, Factor VIII, Factor IX, and Factor XI. Thus these factors may be decreased. These additional fibrino(geno)lytic insults to hemostasis must always be borne in mind when clinical care is being rendered to the patient with chronic liver disease.

3. Platelet Changes

About 35% of patients with chronic liver disease develop thrombocytopenia via several mechanisms[24] (Chapter 6). The most pronounced of these is splenic sequestration secondary to congestive splenomegaly associated with portal hypertension. However, if the patient has disease due to alcoholism, ethanol itself is toxic to megakaryocytes. It suppresses the bone marrow and bone marrow reserves, including megakaryopoiesis. Of equal importance, but commonly neglected clinically, is the recognition of a platelet dysfunction in these patients. The precise reason(s) for abnormal platelet function remains unclear. The decreased uptake of palmate and stearate in the platelet membrane in these individuals may account for significant dysfunction.[25] Abnormal platelet factor 3 release in many patients has also been noted. This may be a reflection of abnormal platelet membrane lipids or may be due to coating of platelet membranes by FDP, as previously discussed. Thus the patient with chronic liver disease may demonstrate thrombocytopenia, as well as dysfunctional platelets. Both processes contribute to clinical hemorrhage.

4. Other Defects

The patient with chronic liver disease often demonstrates poorly defined vascular defects.[26] This has been ascribed to an estrogen effect on the vasculature, as these individuals do have abnormal metabolism and increased levels of estrogen. The vascular defect may reach clinical significance, especially if the patient is subjected to surgery or trauma. DIC rarely, if ever, occurs *de novo* as a hemostatic defect in chronic liver disease. However, these patients are candidates for DIC if provided with one of the usual appropriate triggering events for this syndrome (Chapter 8). Table 2 outlines the alterations of hemostasis associated with chronic liver disease.

C. Clinical Diagnosis

The clinical diagnosis of hemorrhage associated with chronic liver disease is usually obvious. Most often, the patient presents with or develops fulminant hemorrhage in the form of massive hemoptysis, hematochezia, and melena, often in association with epistaxis, all in the face of the usual attendant clinical manifestations such as ascites and other signs of portal hypertension. In addition, most patients presenting in this manner demonstrate petechiae, purpura, spider telangiectasia, and ecchymoses. The clinical bleeding often progresses into a more generalized disorder, with associated hematuria, oozing from intravenous sites, and similar bleeding. More rarely, a patient who is clinically free of obvious hemorrhage, when questioned will admit to sponta-

TABLE 2

Alterations of Hemostasis in Chronic Liver Disease

Coagulation protein defects
    Decreased synthesis of Factors II, VII, IX, and X
    PIVKA synthesis of Factors II, VII, IX, and X
    Hypofibrinogenemia (rarely of clinical significance)
    Decreased synthesis of Factors V and VIII (at terminal stage)
    Decreased synthesis of Fletcher factor
    Decreased/dysfunctional synthesis of AT-III
Hyperfibrino(geno)lysis
    Abnormal fibrinolytic inhibitors (α-2-macroglobulin)
    Abnormal hepatic clearance of plasminogen activators
    Hypofibrinogenemia (lysis)
    "Pseudodysfibrinogenemia"
    Elevated FDP
        Defective fibrin monomer polymerization
        Platelet dysfunction
    Proteolysis of Factors V, VIII, IX, and XI
Platelet defects
    Thrombocytopenia
    Platelet dysfunction (FDP, PF-3)
Other defects
    Vascular defects (poorly defined)
    DIC? — usually not present without another trigger

neous and/or easy bruising in association with periodic hematuria, periodic epistaxis, and gingival bleeding with toothbrushing.

D. Laboratory Diagnosis

Most tests of hemostasis, including the screening tests outlined in Chapter 4, will be abnormal in the face of the significant changes associated with chronic liver disease. The mainstay laboratory test for assessing the function of the prothrombin complex factors is the prothrombin time.

In significantly decreased or dysfunctional synthesis of Factors II, VII, IX, and X, the prothrombin time will be abnormal. The decrease in Factor VII most closely correlates with prothrombin time prolongation, while the decreased synthesis of Factor IX and Factor X most closely correlate with clinical bleeding. The prothrombin time may be also abnormal for additional reasons. In the presence of elevated FDP or plasmin-induced degradation of Factor V, the prothrombin time will be prolonged.

The activated partial thromboplastin time is likewise often abnormal in the patient with chronic liver disease. This occurs for reasons similar to those described for the prothrombin time. Specific factor assays will usually reveal low values. However, values that are high, or normal, depending upon the particular defect, have been noted. High levels of Factor VIII may be found unless significant plasmin is present, in which case, very low levels of Factors VIII, V, and/or XI may be seen.

Tests of fibrinolysis will be abnormal in about 75% of patients. Plasmin and FDP will be found circulating at increased levels and plasminogen decreased due to depletion. Tests of platelet function will likewise be abnormal for reasons outlined in Part III.B.3 of this chapter. The aggregation patterns are similar to those seen in DIC (Chapter 8).

The template bleeding time will often be prolonged due to a functional platelet defect, thrombocytopenia, and/or the vascular defect that is present in many of these patients. In fact, a template bleeding time should *not* be performed in the face of thrombocytopenia (less than 100,000 platelets per cubic millimeter) as it may cause bleeding and will render results that are meaningless.[27] The use of a thrombin time and reptilase time will offer some indication as to degree of pseudodysfibrinogenemia that may be present. However, both of these laboratory modalities will also be prolonged in the face of elevated FDP, rendering the results difficult to interpret.

It is clear that most tests of hemostasis can be abnormal in the patient with chronic liver disease. It is only with the use of a well-chosen hemostatic profile that each component of hemostasis can be assessed, the precise defect, or combination thereof, delineated, and a logical approach to treatment of hemorrhage planned.

E. Management

All clinicians are well aware of the catastrophic hemorrhage that can occur in chronic liver disease and the major challenge this presents for the laboratory, blood bank, pathologist, and surgeon. The mainstay of therapy in most of these patients is still limited to infusions of fresh frozen plasma, Sengstaken-Blakemore tamponade, gastric lavage, and vasopressin infusion. However, as pointed out earlier, many patients fail to respond to these modalities of therapy. If the patient has significant fibrino(geno)lysis, the concomitant or subsequent use of antifibrinolytic agents, usually aminocaproic acid, may be indicated. This is used in the usual manner of 5 to 10 g slow intravenous push, followed by 1 to 2 g/hr for 24 hr or until cessation of clinical hemorrhage. If the patient is significantly thrombocytopenic, the use of platelet concentrates may also be considered. This will correct the thrombocytopenia and will alleviate bleeding from the functional platelet defect, which may also be present. With patients who fail to respond to the aforementioned modalities, the use of prothrombin complex concentrates[28,29] in conjunction with other components, such as platelet concentrates, may have to be resorted to. An additional, although somewhat heroic, approach is to treat patients with exchange transfusions. The use of exchange transfusion or the infusion of prothrombin complex concentrates is probably not indicated in the patient with chronic liver disease and fulminant hemorrhage, unless a surgically correctable bleeding point is demonstrable.

In reality, many patients with fulminant hemorrhage survive if they are approached in a logical manner, i.e., if the precise hemostatic defects present are diagnosed in the laboratory and treated individually. This approach usually allows for successful blunting or arrest of hemorrhage to the point where the patient may become a reasonable candidate for surgical correction of the initiating event, which is usually peptic ulcer disease, a ruptured esophageal varix, or hemorrhagic gastritis.

F. Summary

One must no longer attribute hemorrhage in the patient with chronic liver disease only to a decrease in the synthesis of Factors II, VII, IX, and X. Numerous defects may occur and when significant or life-threatening hemorrhage develops, this may be due to any one or a combination of the defects that have been defined in the preceeding sections. When approaching the patient with hemorrhage in chronic liver disease, it is a major clinical and clinical laboratory challenge to precisely define those defects that are most likely at fault and to then deliver specific and efficacious therapy. If primary hyperfibrino(geno)lysis is the major contributor to hemorrhage, as it often is, the appropriate therapy would be antifibrinolytic (aminocaproic acid). Fresh frozen plasma will usually correct bleeding associated with decreased and/or defective synthesis of Factors II, VII, IX, and X. If significant thrombocytopenia or platelet dysfunction is present, infusions of platelet concentrates are indicated. When the patient fails to respond to specific therapy directed at clearly defined defects, the use of prothrombin complex concentrates in combination with other components may have to be resorted to. However, this remains investigational and those choosing to use this therapeutic modality should be aware of the potential for disseminated thromboses as well as hepatitis.

IV. ALTERATIONS OF HEMOSTASIS ASSOCIATED WITH CARDIOPULMONARY BYPASS

A. Introduction

Cardiac surgery using cardiopulmonary bypass (CPB) is now performed in most community hospitals. Catastrophic intraoperative or postoperative hemorrhage may be associated with this procedure and may place undue demands on local blood bank facilities[30] and lead to prolonged hospitalization and significantly altered morbidity and mortality. The actual incidence of life-threatening hemorrhage associated with CPB varies between 5 and 25%.[31]

Many instances of CPB hemorrhage are clearly due to inadequate surgical technique. However, a significant number are also secondary to alterations in hemostasis created by CPB. When managing a hemorrhaging CPB patient, it is important to quickly distinguish between surgical and nonsurgical bleeding. This key question must be answered before deciding upon surgical vs. medical control of hemorrhage.

B. Pathophysiology

Until recently, the pathophysiology of altered hemostasis created by CPB remained poorly defined. Failure to do this has precluded the development of uniform concepts of successful prevention, adequate and rapid diagnosis, and efficacious control of hemorrhage. The most frequently cited abnormalities to account for CPB hemorrhage have included: (1) inadequate heparin neutralization, (2) protamine excess, (3) heparin rebound, (4) thrombocytopenia, (5) hypofibrinogenemia, (6) primary hyperfibrinolysis, (7) disseminated intravascular coagulation (DIC), (8) isolated coagulation factor deficiencies, (9) transfusion reactions, and (10) hypocalcemia.[32]

The suggestion that all these defects may contribute to CPB hemorrhage clearly demonstrates that the basic pathophysiology of hemostasis during CPB remains confusing to many.

1. Thrombocytopenia

Some early studies of hemostasis during CPB noted significant thrombocytopenia, in the range of 50,000 platelets per cubic millimeter. This was thought to be responsible for CPB hemorrhage. The degree of thrombocytopenia was related to time on bypass, becoming much more pronounced with perfusions lasting longer than 60 min. Later studies noted similar findings. Porter and Silver[33] found the majority of patients undergoing CPB to have platelet counts decreasing to 33% of preoperative counts. In addition, the thrombocytopenia did not abate until several days after CPB. Some investigators, finding thrombocytopenia during CPB, concluded that this represents thrombocytopenia of DIC.[34]

Other investigators have failed to find significant thrombocytopenia during CPB.[35-37] This wide variety in experience most likely represents different surgical and pumping techniques, such as flow rate, normothermic vs. hypothermic perfusion, particular oxygenation mechanism used, time on bypass, and priming solution used. In our experience, a flow rate of 40 ml/kg/min and a pump prime of 20 ml/kg of 5% dextrose in Ringer's lacate plus 5% dextrose in water in a ratio of 2:1 mix[35] produces only minimal thrombocytopenia. Figure 3 demonstrates changes in platelet number with this pumping technique. The particular type of oxygenation mechanism used appears to play little role, if any, in causing thrombocytopenia. The most commonly cited mechanisms for the development of CPB thrombocytopenia are (1) hemodilu-

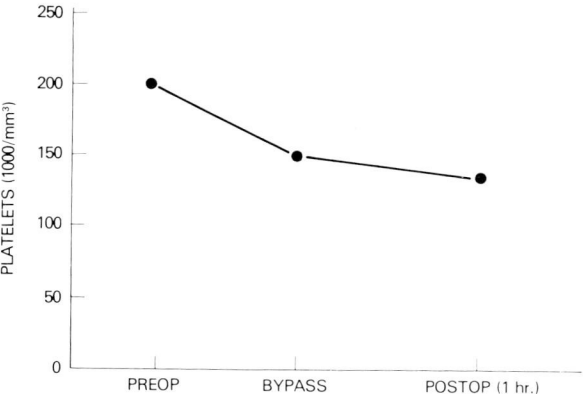

FIGURE 3. Platelet numbers during cardiopulmonary bypass. (From Bick, R. L., *Semin. Thromb. Hemostas.*, 3, 59, 1976. With permission).

tion, (2) formation of intravascular platelet thrombi, (3) platelet utilization in the pump and/or oxygenation system, and (4) peripheral utilization due to DIC. One study[35] has failed to find a correlation between CPB hematocrit and platelet count, suggesting that hemodilution is not a major factor. Indeed, the role, if any, of these mechanisms in producing CPB thrombocytopenia remains unclear.

2. Functional Platelet Defects

In spite of numerous investigations regarding platelet number during CPB, there has been a surprising lack of interest in assessing platelet function. Early investigators[38] suspected development of abnormal platelet function by noting faulty clot retraction. These results were of unclear significance, however, since other abnormal parameters known to effect clot retraction, such as hypofibrinogenemia and thrombocytopenia, were also present. Another early study[39] assessed platelet adhesion before placing patients on CPB, but failed to evaluate platelet function during or after bypass. In this study, abnormal preoperative platelet adhesion was associated with increased postoperative bleeding. Salzman[40] studied platelet adhesion before, during, and after CPB and noted abnormal adhesion in all patients during bypass. However, the significance of this defect was difficult to evaluate since all patients were markedly thrombocytopenic, and this is known to alter adhesion studies.[41] Further information obtained from this study was that heparin, in doses used during CPB, does not alter platelet adhesion. It was concluded that a circulating anticoagulant might be responsible for this functional platelet defect, since the plasma from CPB patients altered adhesion when added to normal platelets. This anticoagulant probably represented FDP.

More recently, platelet adhesion studies have been performed in patients without thrombocytopenia[35] undergoing CPB. Platelet function, assessed by adhesion, becomes profoundly abnormal (decrease to 50% of preoperative levels) in most patients at the initiation of bypass. Little correlation is noted between hematocrit, fibrinogen level, or FDP titer and abnormal platelet adhesion. In addition, there is poor correlation between chest tube blood loss and abnormal platelet adhesion. Figure 4 depicts platelet adhesion changes during CPB. This degree of abnormal platelet function would be expected to significantly compromise hemostasis.

Many factors, some possibly altered by CPB, may affect platelet function as assessed by adhesion. These include: (1) pH, (2) absolute platelet count, (3) hematocrit, (4) drugs, and (5) the presence of FDP. Although recent studies[35] do not clearly define

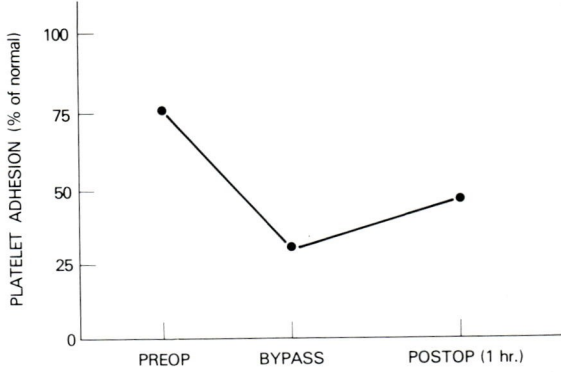

FIGURE 4. Platelet function during cardiopulmonary bypass. (From Bick, R. L., Semin. Thromb. Hemostas., 3, 59, 1976. With permission).

reasons for abnormal platelet function during CPB, they do suggest that several of the above-mentioned mechanisms are most likely not involved. The finding of platelet counts greater than 100,000 per cubic millimeter and hematocrits greater than 30% in most patients with markedly abnormal platelet function at 1 hr post-CPB, sugest that these two parameters do not account for altered platelet function. In addition, patients have normal or near normal pH at 1 hr post-CPB. Heparin, in levels higher than that attained in patients undergoing CPB, has been shown not to alter platelet adhesion. Circulating FDP are known to interfere with platelet function, and these are often present during CPB. However, there has been poor correlation noted between levels of circulating FDP and degree of abnormal platelet function during CPB.[35]

Other possible mechanisms for abnormal platelet function during CPB include platelet membrane damage by shearing forces or contact with foreign material resulting in partial release of platelet contents, platelet membrane coating with nonspecific proteins, incomplete platelet release, or nonspecific platelet damage induced by fast flow rates. No studies done thus far allow conclusions to be drawn regarding the contribution of any of these mechanisms. Only one preliminary report[42] has noted platelet aggregation anomalies during CPB. In this series of 29 patients, only 20% developed aggregation abnormalities. However, following heparin reversal with protamine sulfate, 90% of patients developed aggregation abnormalities. It was concluded that this was due to protamine platelet interaction and not to CPB itself.

Regardless of mechanisms involved, studies to date clearly reveal a significant functional platelet defect in most patients undergoing CPB. The magnitude of this defect would certainly be expected to compromise hemostasis during and after CPB. In addition, patients ingesting drugs known to interfere with platelet function would be expected to have more blood loss than those not ingesting these agents.

3. Vascular Defects

Little attention has been devoted to vascular defects during CPB. Recently, a syndrome of mild to moderate nonthrombocytopenic purpura accompanied by splenomegaly and atypical lymphocytosis following CPB has been reported by Behrendt and co-workers.[43] In this series, purpura was benign, self-limiting, and frequently only manifest after discharge from the hospital. Only one patient of seven suffered complications (glomerulonephritis of the type often seen with Henoch-Schonlein purpura) following development of purpura.

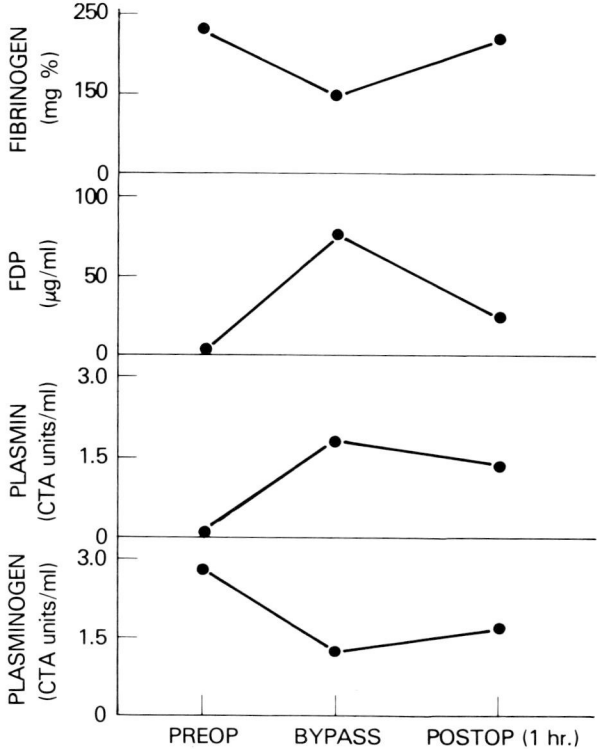

FIGURE 5. Fibrino(geno)lysis during cardiopulmonary bypass. (From Bick, R. L., Semin. Thromb. Hemostas., 3, 59, 1976. With permission).

In addition, a case of fatal purpura fulminans was reported following extracorporeal circulation for coronary artery bypass.[44] Massive purpura developed on the third postoperative day and was followed by development of progressive renal shutdown. High doses of steroids and low molecular weight dextran afforded no improvement, and the patient died of renal failure on the 18th postoperative day. These two reports suggest inflammatory vasculitis to be associated with CPB. The most benign forms are represented by purpura simplex. Rarely, purpura fulminans occurs. Aside from these two reports, no other mention of vascular defects associated with CPB has been made in the literature.

4. Isolated Coagulation Factor Defects

Numerous studies have examined and reported coagulation factor deficiencies during CPB. A wide variety of observations have been made and, like the finding of thrombocytopenia, may only reflect differences in surgical or pumping techniques, such as flow rate, priming solution, etc. Most studies have noted significant hypofibrinogenemia[45,46] that does not seem to be correlated with pump time. Some investigators[35,41] have found fibrinogen levels to be closely correlated with the degree of CPB fibrinolysis. Figure 5 depicts correlations noted between fibrinogen, plasminogen, plasmin, and FDP in patients undergoing CPB. Some authors[47] have concluded that hypofibrinogenemia occurs primarily as a consequence of DIC; others[35,41] have failed to find hypofibrinogenemia during CPB. It seems reasonable to conclude that hypofibrinogenemia, secondary to hyperfibrino(geno)lysis, is a frequent occurrence during CPB.

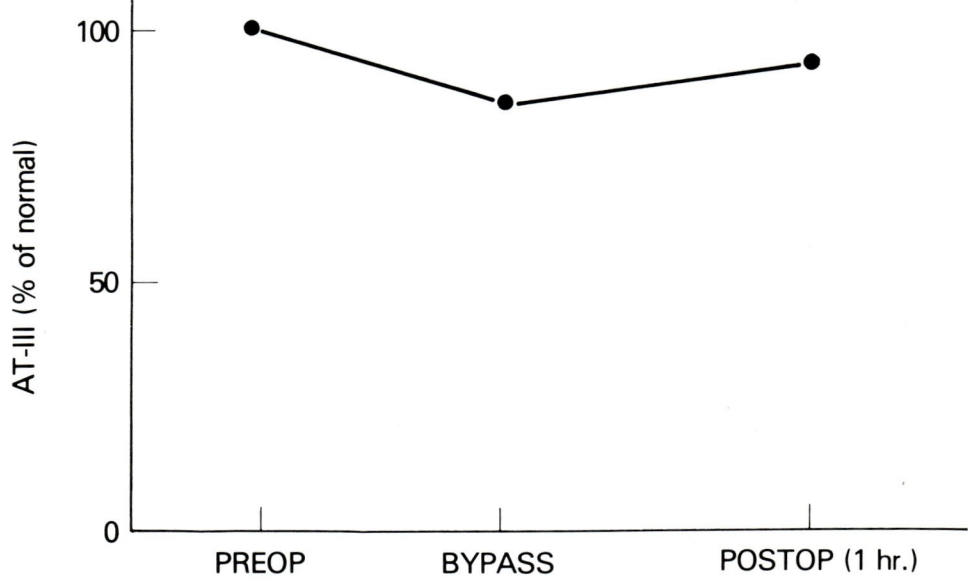

FIGURE 6. Antithrombin III (AT-III) levels (biologic activity) during cardiopulmonary bypass. (From Bick, R. L., *Semin. Thromb. Hemostas.*, 3, 59, 1976. With permission.)

Other coagulation factors most often found decreased and reported to play a role in CPB hemorrhage are Factors II, V, and VIII. As with hypofibrinogenemia, some authors[48] conclude these changes to be secondary to DIC, while others[49] think these decreases are secondary to a primary fibrino(geno)lytic syndrome. Others yet[50,51] have failed to find significant decrease in most coagulation factors, and some[52] have reported increased Factor VIII levels during CPB.

5. Disseminated Intravascular Coagulation

The question of DIC developing during and after CPB has led to confusion regarding altered hemostasis. Numerous early studies concluded DIC to be present during CPB, based on the observations that coagulation factors were decreased. The findings of fibrinogen, Factor VIII, or prothrombin complex factor deficiencies were often assumed to be secondary to DIC, without appropriate confirmatory tests being performed. Current evidence suggests that, in view of massive heparinization and the absence of significant or uniform thrombocytopenia, DIC is not associated with CPB.[35,41,53] Another finding in support of this is the normal or near normal AT-III levels during CPB (Figure 6). Preliminary evidence suggests that a decreased AT-III level is a reasonably good indicator of acute or chronic DIC.[54]

To summarize, although most early, and several recent, studies have detected primary hyperfibrino(geno)lysis in association with CPB, a few have concluded that DIC is present. These conclusions most likely derive from the marked superficial similarities between primary hyperfibrino(geno)lysis and DIC with secondary lysis, and from the difficulty in rendering a clear-cut differential diagnosis between these two states in the absence of sophisticated and complete coagulation studies.[55]

6. Primary Hyperfibrino(geno)lysis

Fibrinolytic activity is generally decreased or inhibited during and following most general surgical procedures. However, most studies, utilizing a variety of laboratory modalities, have found increased fibrinolysis during and after CPB. Many early studies of hemostasis during CPB assessed the extent of fibrinolysis with the euglobulin lysis time (ELT), thus the finding of fibrinolysis with CPB remained of unclear significance for a long period in view of recognized inadequacies of this technique.[56] More recent studies,[32,35,41] which have utilized more specific methods for assessing fibrinolysis, have confirmed earlier reports of a primary hyperfibrino(geno)lytic syndrome in the majority of patients undergoing CPB. Figure 5 depicts changes in the fibrinolytic system in patients undergoing CPB.

Because of early reports detecting primary hyperfibrino(geno)lysis during CPB, the empirical use of antifibrinolytic agents, usually aminocaproic acid (ACA), has become commonplace in spite of attendant hazards of this agent, which include hypokalemia, hypotension, ventricular arrhythmias, and DIC. Controlled studies with and without antifibrinolytic agents have failed to reveal any clear-cut differences in CPB hemorrhage.[57] Gomes and McGoon[58] and Tsuji and co-workers[50] have shown an increase in post-CPB hemorrhage with the empirical use of antifibrinolytics. While some investigators, finding primary hyperfibrino(geno)lysis during CPB, have concluded that this is inconsequential to CPB hemorrhage, others have thought this to be triggered only by specific events such as pyrogenicity of equipment, use of rheomacrodex, or induction of anesthesia. Since primary hyperfibrino(geno)lysis occurs in the majority of patients subjected to CPB, it seems more likely that activation by the fibrinolytic system may be occurring in the oxygenation mechanism or, alternatively, that pump-induced accelerated flow rates may activate the plasminogen-plasmin system or may alter endothelial plasminogen activator activity. In fact, the pathogenesis of fibrinolytic activation during CPB remains totally unclear (degree of fibrinolysis appears to be equal between bubble and membrane oxygenation systems).[59]

7. Other Defects

Heparin rebound has received significant attention as a potential cause of CPB hemorrhage. This was observed often in earlier studies, but with today's generally accepted doses of heparin and protamine, both heparin rebound and inadequate heparin neutralization are rarely, if ever, seen. In actual fact, heparin rebound, as well as inadequate heparin neutralization, have been poorly documented as actual causes of CPB hemorrhage. Likewise, protamine excess has been occasionally incriminated as a source of CPB hemorrhage. However, several carefully studied series have failed to note this phenomenon in a single patient undergoing CPB.[32,35,41] In addition, although protamine sulfate is a well-known in vitro anticoagulant,[60] it is unlikely that it causes in vivo hemorrhage.

Several authors have reported both coagulation defects and significant CPB hemorrhage to be associated with hypothermic perfusion.[61] Our experience[62] in studying hemostasis in dogs, comparing normothermic to hypothermic perfusion, has led to the same conclusions.

Many patients undergoing coronary artery bypass for coronary occlusive disease have been on warfarin. Verska and associates[63] have noted that although the prothrombin time had returned to normal prior to CPB, these patients demonstrated more hemorrhage than patients not warfarinized. One study[64] noted increased hemorrhage to be associated with a repeat CPB procedure. Other investigators,[58] however, have noted no increased hemorrhage to be associated with a second CPB procedure. Also, patients undergoing CPB for correction of cyanotic heart disease appear to have more severe derangements in hemostasis during perfusion than those with noncyanotic heart disease.[38]

8. Summary of Pathophysiology

It appears that overheparinization, heparin rebound, inadequate protamine neutralization, and protamine excess, though receiving attention as potential sources of CPB hemorrhage, in fact, have not been clearly documented as responsible triggers. Likewise, thrombocytopenia, although a potential source of hemorrhage, is an inconsistent finding during CPB and most likely arises as a consequence of differences in pumping technique among cardiovascular teams. The finding of isolated coagulation defects during CPB has added little to our understanding of altered hemostasis and most likely simply reflects isolated measurements of consequences of hyperfibrino(geno)lysis.

Although DIC has been thought by some to occur during CPB, most carefully done studies have failed to document this. The significant doses of heparin used during CPB, the absence of consistent thrombocytopenia, and the general correcting of hypofibrinogenemia, hypoplasminogenemia, and elevated FDP after heparin neutralization would all suggest that the presence of DIC during CPB is very unlikely. We have noted DIC in association with CPB only when another triggering event was provided, such as massive transfusions, hemolytic transfusion reaction, or sepsis.

Predisposing factors that do seem to be associated with enhanced CPB hemorrhage are (1) longer pump runs, (2) prior ingestion of warfarin drugs, and (3) cyanotic heart disease. More importantly, evidence suggests that the majority of patients undergoing CPB develop a primary hyperfibrino(geno)lytic syndrome. Although the exact triggering mechanism(s) for this syndrome remain unclear, the resultant secondary alterations in hemostasis would certainly create a potential for hemorrhage. In addition, virtually all patients undergoing CPB develop a severe platelet function defect. It is not clear if this defect is due to (1) coating of platelet surfaces by FDP, (2) membrane damage from the oxygenation mechanism, (3) platelet damage from fast flow rates, or (4) from other unrecognized mechanisms. Whatever the triggering mechanisms, it is quite clear that the most significant alterations in hemostasis associated with CPB are primary hyperfibrino(geno)lysis and defective platelet function. These two defects, alone or in combination, account for the majority of nonsurgical and nontechnical hemorrhage in patients undergoing CPB. Preliminary studies would suggest that the frequency and severity of functional platelet defects and primary hyperfibrino(geno)lysis is equal with membrane or bubble type oxygenators. However, thrombocytopenia appears to be less of a problem with the former type of oxygenation mechanism.[59]

C. Prevention

Since hemorrhage associated with CPB is usually catastrophic and often life threatening, caution must be emphasized in attending to differential diagnosis and rapid, efficacious therapy. Much attention must be given to prevention of CPB hemorrhage with respect to uncovering hereditary, acquired, or drug-induced bleeding diatheses before subjecting a patient to this procedure. The combination of an already existing bleeding diathesis, when coupled with alterations of hemostasis induced by CPB, may lead to disastrous results.

1. Historical Information

Many cases of CPB hemorrhage could be averted by simply obtaining an adequate hemostasis history. Ideally, this should be obtained before hospital admission in order to allow time for appropriate evaluation if a potential problem is uncovered.

Key questions that often suggest a bleeding diathesis are (1) does the patient suffer significant gingival bleeding with toothbrushing? (2) is there easy bruising or, more significantly, a history of spontaneous bruising? (3) has the patient experienced undue bleeding following dental extractions or prior surgical procedures? (4) is there a childhood history of epistaxis? and (5) is menstrual flow normal or excessive? These simple

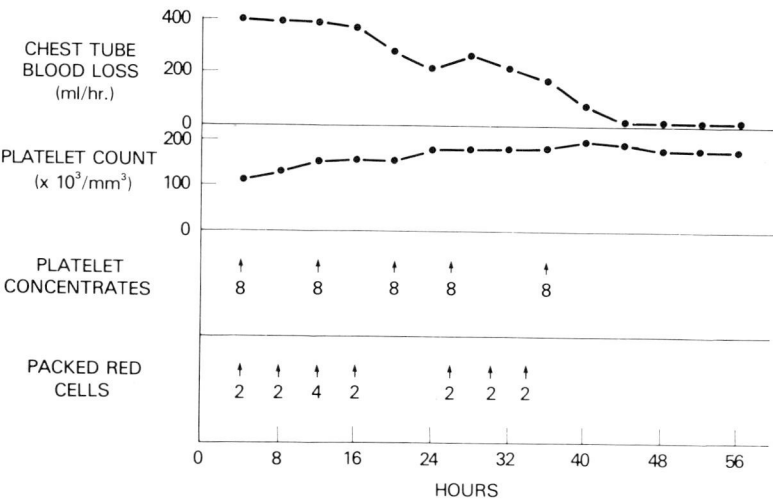

FIGURE 7. Postbypass hemorrhage in a patient injesting acetylsalicylic acid (600 mg BID) prior to surgery. (From Bick, R. L., *Semin. Thromb. Hemostas.*, 3, 59, 1976. With permission.)

questions certainly do not constitute a complete historical search for disorders of hemostasis, but a positive response is a good clue to the possibility of a bleeding diathesis. Obviously, all patients being subjected to CPB should also be questioned regarding hemoptysis, hematemesis, melena, hematochezia, and hematuria.

The family history should always include inquiry about bleeding tendencies in parents, siblings, and offspring. This may uncover a hereditary bleeding tendency that has remained silent because the hemostatic system has never been stressed by surgery or trauma. Often neglected is a detailed drug history. Many cases of CPB hemorrhage have been attributed to the ingestion of drugs known to interfere with hemostasis. Figure 7 demonstrates the sequence of events in a patient ingesting aspirin before CPB. Table 3 depicts post-CPB chest tube blood loss in a series of patients with and without a history of ingesting antiplatelet drugs prior to CPB. Many drugs interfere with hemostasis and, in many instances, the bleeding is mild in nature. However, when drug-induced defects are combined with hemostatic defects induced during CPB, hemorrhage may reach alarming proportions. Drugs may interfere with hemostasis by many mechanisms, but most commonly ingested drugs interfere with platelet function. Aspirin, aspirin-containing compounds, antihistamines, phenylbutazone, and papaverine-containing vasodialating drugs are the most common offenders in CPB patients.[65]

If the drug history is positive and CPB is *elective,* surgery should be cancelled for a full 14 days, since most drugs interfering with platelet function are generally effective for about 14 days, and this time period may be required for platelet function to return to normal. If the drug history is positive for antiplatelet agents and CPB is *emergent,* the patient should be given platelet concentrates (6 to 8 units for an adult), immediately prior to bypass and the same quantity immediately after leaving the operating room and then each morning for two postoperative days. This approach is vigorous, but certainly rewarding if life-threatening hemorrhage is avoided.

2. Physical Findings

The general appearance of the patient often provides hints of a bleeding tendency. All the hereditary and acquired connective tissue disorders are often associated with a significant vascular defect and the potential for surgical hemorrhage. In addition, most

TABLE 3

Blood Loss During Cardiopulmonary Bypass: Comparison of Patients with (+) and without (−) Ingestion of Antiplatelet Drugs Prior to Surgery

Patient	Chest tube drainage (ml/24 hr)	Total blood replacement (Units)	Antiplatelet drugs
1	895	3	+
2	1215	5	+
3	2700	10	+
4	1070	6	+
5	760	1	+
6	1170	5	+
7	2100	7	+
8	850	1	+
9	1050	6	+
10	1590	4	+
Average	1340	4.8	
11	270	2	−
12	600	2	−
13	490	3	−
14	640	3	−
15	525	3	−
16	240	2	−
17	390	2	−
18	480	3	−
19	560	2	−
20	640	3	−
Average	483	2.5	

of the hereditary collagen disorders are accompanied by poorly defined functional platelet defects. Clinical clues heralding the presence of collagen disorder are well known to most clinicians and include the body habitus of Marfan's syndrome, blue sclera, skeletal deformities, hyperextensible joints and skin, and nodular spider or pinpoint telangiectasia. The finding of one of these suggestive signs should promote a more complete investigation for the presence of collagen disease before CPB is attempted. Other disorders that may be associated with a vascular defect, therefore potential surgical bleeding, including Cushing's syndrome, malignant dysproteinemias, the allergic purpuras (Henoch-Schonlein), and hereditary hemorrhagic telangiectasia.

Most other subtle hints of an occult bleeding tendency are uncovered by careful observation of the mucous membranes and skin. The finding of mucosal petechiae, purpura, or significant telangiectasia should be searched for and explained, if present. Likewise, petechiae, purpura, significant ecchymoses, or telangiectasia of the skin or nail beds are often suggestive of a vascular defect, a functional platelet defect, or significant thrombocytopenia. Again, if any of these findings are present, they should be investigated and thoroughly explained before CPB is attempted. The usual physical findings of more common disorders associated with a significant hemorrhagic tendency, such as chronic liver disease, hypersplenism, chronic renal disease, rheumatoid arthritis, and systemic lupus, should also serve as an index of predisposition to hemorrhage. Prior laboratory screening will usually suggest the presence of any of these disorders if characteristic physical findings are absent.

If the personal history, family history, drug history, or physical examination is suggestive of a potential or real bleeding tendency, CPB should be postponed until the defect is ruled out, or fully delineated and a therapeutic plan carefully designed. In this regard, it should be emphasized that a bleeding disorder is rarely, if ever, a contraindication to performing CPB, provided the defect is first delineated, and a sound approach to correcting hemostasis during CPB and during the postoperative period is designed.

3. Pre-CPB Laboratory Screen

Any preoperative laboratory screen should generally represent simplicity and incur a minimum of expense to the patient, while providing adequate information. Usually, however, we tend to be too simple with respect to presurgical and, in particular pre-CPB, hemostasis screens. As with an adequate history and physical, one cannot be overcautious in screening for defects in hemostasis, since when preexisting defects are combined with those created by CPB, the resultant hemorrhage is often catastrophic.

The usually ordered biochemical survey, electrolytes, and CBC will detect those common acquired disorders often associated with a bleeding tendency, for example: chronic liver disease, chronic renal disease, and instances of hypersplenism or bone marrow failure. Most commonly, a pre-CPB hemostasis screen consists of a prothrombin time, an activated partial thromboplastin time, and a platelet count. While these tests will detect the majority of defects, they provide no information about vascular or platelet function and ignore fibrinolysis. Thus two additional procedures should be performed as part of the routine preoperative screen. A standardized template bleeding time, as described by Mielke and co-workers,[66] is performed on all patients. This provides a screen for adequate vascular and platelet function. It should be recalled that this should *not* be performed until adequate platelet numbers are noted by count or smear evaluation. In addition, a thrombin time is performed. The resultant clot is observed for 5 min after the test is run. A normal thrombin time and the absence of lysis after 5 min assures the absence of significant hypofibrinogenemia, dysfibrinogenemia, fibrinolysis, and/or FDP elevation. The addition of both these tests to the routine presurgical screen adds only minimal cost or laboratory time, while providing additional invaluable information not obtained from a prothrombin time, activated partial thromboplastin time, or platelet count. If hypothermic perfusion is to be performed, cryoglobulins should also be tested for. Table 4 depicts a routine pre-CPB screen and provides references for hemostasis tests.

D. Clinical and Laboratory Diagnosis

When bleeding occurs during or after bypass, it is obviously of extreme importance to define the defect as quickly as possible. As previously discussed, many instances of CPB hemorrhage are due to inadequate surgical technique, but alterations of hemostasis may also be responsible or may accentuate surgical CPB bleeding. The reasons for bleeding occurring during CPB are limited and are depicted in Table 5 in their order of occurrence.

The primary distinction to be made is between strictly surgical bleeding, defects in hemostasis, or a combination of the two. This distinction becomes more difficult and more important after the patient has left the operating room. During this period, a decision must be made regarding reexploration and the adequacy of hemostasis for reexploration. In distinguishing between surgical and nonsurgical bleeding, many physical findings are helpful. Is the bleeding localized or systemic? The noting of hematuria, petechiae/purpura, and oozing from intravenous sites in conjunction with increased chest tube blood loss usually means a hemostatic defect, while increased chest tube bleeding alone often signifies a surgical bleed. In addition, the surgeon will often note bleeding or oozing throughout the surgical field in instances of hemostatic dysfunction.

TABLE 4

Routine Precardiopulmonary Bypass Hemostasis Screen

Platelet count
Template bleeding time
Prothrombin time
Partial thromboplastin time (particulate activated)
Thrombin time[a]

[a] Observe for clot lysis at 5 min.

From Fekete, L. F. and Bick, R. L., *Semin. Thromb. Hemostas.*, 3, 83, 1976. With permission.

TABLE 5

Bleeding Syndromes Associated with Cardiopulmonary Bypass (In Descending Order of Probability)

Platelet function defects
    CPB induced
    Drug induced
Primary hyperfibrino(geno)lysis
Thrombocytopenia
Hyperheparinemia-heparin rebound (?)
Disseminated intravascular coagulation (?)

From Bick, R. L., *Semin. Thromb. Hemostas.*, 3, 59, 1976. With permission.

As soon as CPB hemorrhage is seen or suspected, the following laboratory tests are ordered:* thrombin time, reptilase time, fibrin/fibrinogen degradation products, peripheral blood smear, platelet count, and plasminogen/plasmin levels. A comparison of the thrombin time and reptilase time provide rapid information as to the status of heparin effect, protamine excess, FDP influence, and primary hyperfibrinolysis. The resultant clot from the thrombin time is always observed for 5 min for evidence of lysis, thus providing additional information regarding the presence of primary hyperfibrino(geno)lysis. Additional evidence for or against primary lysis is obtained by noting the FDP level. A smear and platelet count is invaluable to rapidly evaluate the potential of thrombocytopenic bleeding. The plasminogen and plasmin levels are time consuming and are not used for an immediate diagnosis, but are invaluable in making decisions regarding antifibrinolytic therapy at a later time.

If significant primary hyperfibrino(geno)lysis is present, the thrombin time and reptilase time will all be prolonged. In addition, FDP will be elevated, the thrombin time clot will lyse in 5 min, and plasminogen depletion and circulating plasmin will be noted. If, on the other hand, excess heparin is a problem, the reptilase time will be normal or near normal, the thrombin time will be prolonged, no significant clot lysis will be observed, and no significant FDP elevation is observed. Protamine excess, although not likely of clinical significance, is characterized by a slightly prolonged thrombin time, a slightly prolonged reptilase time, no significant FDP elevation, and no lysis of the thrombin time clot.

All patients undergoing CPB display some form of a functional platelet defect. When bleeding occurs, it is wise to assume the problem to be serious, and, although this might not represent the primary reason for hemorrhage, platelet dysfunction will be additive to any other defect, whether it be surgical or due to altered hemostasis.

The time period during which hemorrhage occurs, i.e., intraoperative, after heparin neutralization, or in the recovery room, appears to bare little relationship to the etiology of the primary hemostatic defect responsible for hemorrhage. Exceptions to this are thrombocytopenic bleeding, which usually occurs after the patient is in the recovery room, and drug-induced platelet defects, which usually are manifest as marked oozing as soon as the operative procedure is begun. Table 6 depicts a differential diagnostic screen for CPB hemorrhage using the above tests.

3. Management

When first seeing a patient with CPB hemorrhage, whether intra- or perioperative,

---

* Heparin assays[72] are now available for the rapid quantitation of free plasma heparin levels during and following CPB; these are simple to perform and rapidly assess efficacy of heparin reversal.

TABLE 6

Differential Diagnosis of Bleeding Syndromes Associated with Cardiopulmonary Bypass

	Functional platelet defect (always present)	Primary fibrino(geno)lysis	Thrombocytopenia	Heparin excess/ rebound	DIC?
Thrombin time	N[a]	L[b]	N	L	L
Thrombin time clot lysis	N	+[c]	N	N	+
Reptilase time	N	L	N	N	L
PSO$_4$-corrected thrombin time	N	L	N	SL	L
PSO$_4$-corrected thrombin time clot lysis	N	+	N	N	+
Fibrinogen degradation products	N	+	N	N	+
Plasmin	N	+	N	N	+
Plasminogen	N	D[d]	N	N	D
Soluble fibrin monomers (usually not required)	N	N	N	N	+

[a] N = normal/negative.
[b] L = prolonged (SL = slightly prolonged).
[c] + = positive.
[d] D = decreased.

of prime importance is (1) to note the type of bleeding (systemic vs. local), (2) to order a laboratory screen as outlined previously, and (3) to administer 6 to 8 units of platelet concentrates as quickly as possible. The administration of platelet concentrates while awaiting laboratory evaluation will often stop, or significantly blunt, most hemorrhages.

When bleeding begins immediately upon initiation of surgery, a functional platelet defect (usually drug induced) can be assumed to be present until further laboratory investigation can be accomplished. In this instance, the patient should be closed, if possible, and 6 to 8 units of platelet concentrate administered as fast as possible. If a functional platelet defect is found to be responsible for hemorrhage (with no laboratory evidence of significant fibrinolysis, hyperheparinemia, or protamine excess), 6 to 8 units of platelet concentrates should be repeated the evening after surgery and for two postoperative mornings. Thrombocytopenic CPB hemorrhage should be controlled in the same manner, although more than 8 units of platelet concentrates may be needed, as dictated by initial platelet count, amount of bleeding, and response to transfusions.

Hyperheparinemia and heparin rebound, if suspected to be a real clinical problem, are managed by delivering 25% of the initial calculated protamine dose. This is repeated every 30 min until bleeding ceases. Once again, it should be emphasized that hyperheparinemia and heparin rebound are not likely to be responsible for bleeding and should not be dwelled upon unless concrete laboratory evidence of hyperheparinemia is present, and evidence of primary lysis is clearly absent. Similarly, protamine excess is rarely, if ever, a clinical problem and should never require therapy.

Primary hyperfibrino(geno)lysis is commonly present and may or may not be responsible for hemorrhage. This syndrome should not be treated empirically, but antifibrinolytics should be considered if the patient has failed to respond to platelet concentrates and there is reasonable laboratory evidence for hyperfibrino(geno)lysis. For those performing plasmin-plasminogen assays, these results should be available by the time an adequate trial with platelet concentrates has passed. Primary hyperfibrino(geno)lytic bleeding is generally treated with aminocaproic acid (ACA) as an initial 5 to 10 g slow intravenous push, followed by 1 to 2 g/hr until bleeding ceases or slows to a nonthreatening level. ACA may be associated with ventricular arrhythmias, hypotension, hypokalemia, and disseminated intravascular thrombosis; thus it should be pushed slowly, and patients should be monitored carefully with regard to renal output, blood pressure, and electrolytes.

F. Summary

This section has provided a review of available literature regarding alterations of hemostasis associated with CPB. The primary pathology of altered hemostasis during CPB appears to be twofold: (1) a functional platelet defect of unclear etiology, which occurs in virtually all patients and (2) a primary hyperfibrino(geno)lytic defect, which occurs in the majority of patients. Significant thrombocytopenia does not appear to be a consistent problem and is probably a function of perfusion techniques. This may, however, be an important source of hemorrhage in some instances. Although hyperheparinemia, heparin rebound, and protamine excess have occasionally been incriminated as sources of hemorrhage during CPB, no well-documented cases appear in the literature. Likewise, although DIC gained popularity in early reports of CPB hemorrhage, it appears that this syndrome rarely, if ever, arises as a consequence of CPB alone. It can be seen, however, in CPB patients who are provided with a trigger such as shock, sepsis, or hemolytic transfusion reactions. It is likely that many reported alterations of hemostasis during CPB which were thought to represent DIC actually were due to hyperfibrino(geno)lysis.

The key to prevention of CPB hemorrhage rests simply on obtaining an adequate preoperative workup. Of extreme importance is an adequate history with respect to bleeding tendencies in both patient and family. Of equal importance is a careful history regarding the use of antiplatelet drugs. A careful physical examination, searching for clues of a real or potential bleeding diathesis, also can often prevent catastrophic cases of CPB hemorrhage. Lastly, an adequate presurgical laboratory screen must be performed. In addition to the usual prothrombin time, partial thromboplastin time, and platelet count, a thrombin time and standardized template bleeding time must be added.

The parameters recommended in this review will distinguish between surgical and nonsurgical bleeding if it occurs, and should, therefore, allow for a quick decision regarding necessity for reexploration and the adequacy of hemostasis. In addition, this screen will distinguish between difficulties with heparin, protamine, and the fibrinolytic system.

The vast majority of nonsurgical hemorrhage during CPB is due to a functional platelet defect, primary hyperfibrino(geno)lysis, or a combination of the two. The quick administration of platelet concentrates while awaiting laboratory evaluation will control or significantly blunt most CPB hemorrhages. If platelets fail to control bleeding and reasonable laboratory evidence of primary hyperfibrino(geno)lysis is present, antifibrinolytics should be then used.

CPB hemorrhage remains a very real problem in altering morbidity and mortality as well as taxing blood bank facilities. However, most instances of nonsurgical CPB hemorrhage are due to several well-defined defects in hemostasis, which should be readily controllable if approached in a logical manner and as a team effort among cardiac surgeons, pathologists, and hematologists.

V. HYPERFIBRINO(GENO)LYSIS IN MALIGNANCY

Solid tumors have been reported to be associated with a clinical hyperfibrino(geno)lytic syndrome. The spectrum of tumors involved is wide, but the most pronounced effect is seen in sarcomas. For the most part, the mechanism(s) by which this occurs remain poorly understood. In several instances, tissue extracts from biopsy specimens, when purified, have demonstrated the ability to either directly or indirectly activate the fibrinolytic system.[67] This has been noted especially with tissue homogenates from gastric carcinoma, sarcomas, and prostatic carcinoma.[68,69] The initiation of primary fibrinolysis or a continuous "thrombolytic state" may be of benefit in impeding fibrin formation and tumor metastases. Adriamycin®[70] and daunomycin[71] have been shown to activate fibrinolysis. Adriamycin® is a commonly used antineoplastic agent especially for breast carcinoma, and daunomycin is a mainstay form of therapy for the acute leukemias. Both agents are capable of inducing in vivo actvation of the fibrinolytic system, which is not secondary to DIC. The precise mechanism(s) of activation remains unclear. This fibrinolytic response may be of benefit to the patient with respect to tumor cell metastases and primary tumor growth, as these processes are thought to be facilitated by fibrin deposition. The subject of altered hemostasis in malignancy is discussed in detail in Chapters 11 and 12.

VI. SUMMARY

This chapter has defined the pathophysiology of primary hyperfibrino(geno)lytic syndromes and the clinical/laboratory diagnosis and management in chronic liver disease and cardiopulmonary bypass. The now recognized frequency and remarkable superficial similarities of this syndrome with DIC have rendered it imperative that the appropriate clinical setting be considered and appropriate laboratory modalities be carefully evaluated in order to achieve most effective management in case of hemorrhage.

REFERENCES

1. **Menon, I. S.**, A study of the possible correlation of euglobulin lysis time and dilute blood clot lysis time in the determination of fibrinolytic activity, *Lab. Pract.*, 17, 334, 1968.
2. **Kowalski, E., Kopec, M., and Niewiarowski, S.**, An evaluation of the euglobulin method for the determination of fibrinolysis, *J. Clin. Pathol.*, 12, 215, 1959.
3. **Astrup, T. and Mullertz, S.**, The fibrin plate method for estimating fibrinolytic actiity, *Arch. Biochem. Biophys.*, 50, 346, 1952.
4. **Bishop, R. C., Ekert, H., Gilchrist, G., Shanbrom, E., and Fekete, L. F.**, The preparation and evaluation of a standardized fibrin plate for the assessment of fibrinolytic activity, *Thromb. Diath. Haemorrh.*, 23, 202, 1970.
5. **Bruhn, H. D., Muller, L., and Duckert, F.**, Quantitative determination of plasminogen: a caseinolytic method, *Thromb. Diath. Haemorrh.*, 23, 191, 1970.
6. **Latallo, Z. S., Teisseyre, E., and Lopaciuk, S.**, Assessment of plasma fibrinolytic system with use of chromogenic substrate, *Haemostasis*, 7, 150, 1978.
7. **Menon, I. S.**, The role of the liver in fibrinolysis, *J. Indian Med. Assoc.*, 49, 474, 1967.
8. **Lechner, K., Niessner, H., and Thaler, E.**, Coagulation abnormalities in liver disease, *Semin. Thromb. Hemostas.*, 4, 40, 1977.
9. **Aledort, L. M.**, Clotting abnormalities in liver disease, *Prog. Liver Dis.*, 5, 350, 1976.
10. **Donaldson, G. W. K., Davies, S. R., Darg, S., and Richmond, J.**, Coagulation factors in chronic liver disease, *J. Clin. Pathol.*, 22, 109, 1969.
11. **Amir-Ahmadi, H., McGray, R. S., Martin, F., Mitch, W., Kantrowitz, P., and Zamcheck, N.**, Reassessment of massive upper gastrointestinal hemorrhage on the wards of the Boston City Hospital, *Surg. Clin. North Am.*, 49, 715, 1969.
12. **Gurewich, V.**, Guidelines for the management of anticoagulant therapy, *Semin. Thromb. Hemostasis.*, 2, 176, 1976.
13. **Densen, K. W. R.**, The levels of Factors II, VII, IX, and X by antibody neutralization techniques in the plasma of patients receiving phenindione therapy, *Br. J. Haematol.*, 20, 643, 1971.
14. **Stenflow, J.**, Vitamin K, prothrombin and gamma-carboxyglutamic acid, *N. Engl. J. Med.*, 296, 624, 1977.
15. **Green, G., Thompson, J. M., Poller, L., and Dymock, I. W.**, Abnormal fibrin monomer polymerization in liver disease, *Gut*, 16, 827, 1975.
16. **Woolf, I. L., Lane, D. A., Scully, M. F., Thomas, D. P., Kakkar, V. V., and Williams, R.**, Acquired dysfibrinogenemia in liver disease, *Digestion*, 14, 102, 1976.
17. **Lane, D. A., Scully, M. F., Thomas, D. P., Kakkar, V. V., and Williams, R.**, Acquired dysfibrinogenemia in acute and chronic liver disease, *Br. J. Haematol.*, 35, 301, 1977.
18. **Abildgaard, U., Fagerhol, M. K., and Egeberg, O.**, Comparison of progressive antithrombin activity and the concentrations of three thrombin inhibitors in human plasma, *Scand. J. Clin. Lab. Invest.*, 26, 349, 1970.
19. **Braunstein, K. M. and Evrenius, K.**, Minimal heparin cofactor activity in disseminated intravascular coagulation and cirrhosis, *Am. J. Clin. Pathol.*, 66, 48, 1976.
20. **Pises, P., Bick, R. L., and Siegal, B.**, Hyperfibrinolysis in cirrhosis, *Am. J. Gastroenterol.*, 60, 280, 1973.
21. **Purcell, G. and Phillips, L. L.**, Fibrinolytic activity in cirrhosis of the liver, *Surg. Gynecol. Obstet.*, 117, 139, 1963.
22. **Mosesson, M. W.**, Fibrinogen catabolic pathways, *Semin. Thromb. Hemostas.*, 1, 63, 1974.
23. **Kowalski, E., Kopec, M., and Wegrzynowics, L.**, Influence of fibrinogen degradation products on platelet aggregation, adhesiveness, and viscous metamorphosis, *Thromb. Diath. Haemorrh.*, 10, 406, 1963.
24. **Penny, R., Rosenberg, F. C., and Firkin, B. G.**, The splenic platelet pool, *Blood*, 17, 1, 1966.
25. **Thomas, D. P., Ream, V. J., and Stuart, R. K.**, Platelet aggregation in patients with cirrhosis of the liver, *N. Engl. J. Med.*, 276, 1344, 1967.

26. Kupfer, H. J. and Ewald, T., Statistical correlation of liver function tests with coagulation factor deficiencies in Laennec's cirrhosis, *Thromb. Diath. Haemorrh.*, 10, 317, 1964.
27. Bick, R. L., Platelet function studies, in *Current Concepts and Evaluations of Disorders of Hemostasis and Thrombosis,* Workshop Manual No. 548, American Society of Clinical Pathologists, Chicago, 1978.
28. Bick, R. L., Schmalhorst, W. R., and Shanbrom, E., Prothrombin complex concentrate: use in controlling the hemorrhagic diathesis of chronic liver disease, *Am. J. Dig. Dis.*, 20, 1, 1975.
29. Sandler, S. G., Rath, C. E., and Ruder, A., Prothrombin complex concentrate in acquired hypoprothrombinemia, *Ann. Intern. Med.*, 79, 485, 1973.
30. Beall, A. C., Yow, E. M., Bloodwell, R. D., Hallman, G., and Cooley, D., Open heart surgery without blood transfusion, *Arch. Surg. (Chicago)*, 94, 567, 1967.
31. Mammen, E. F., Natural protease inhibitors in extracorporeal circulation, *Ann. N.Y. Acad. Sci.*, 146, 754, 1968.
32. Bick, R. L., Arbegast, N. R., Crawford, L., Holfermann, M., Adams, T., and Schmalhorst, W. R., Hemostasis defects induced by cardiopulmonary bypass, *Vasc. Surg.*, 9, 228, 1975.
33. Porter, J. M. and Silver, D., Alterations in fibrinolysis and coagulation associated with cardiopulmonary bypass, *J. Thorac. Cardiovasc. Surg.*, 56, 869, 1968.
34. Blomback, K. M., Noren, I., and Senning, A., Coagulation disturbances during extracorporeal circulation and the postoperative period, *Acta Chir. Scand.*, 127, 433, 1964.
35. Bick, R. L., Alternations of hemostasis associated with cardiopulmonary bypass: pathophysiology, prevention, diagnosis, and management, *Semin. Thromb. Hemostas.*, 3, 59, 1976.
36. de Vries, S. E., von Creveld, S., Groen, P., Muller, E., and Wettermark, M., Studies on the coagulation of the blood in patients treated wth extracorporeal circulation, *Thromb. Diath. Haemorrh.*, 5, 426, 1961.
37. Miller, N., Popov-Cenic, S., Buttner, W., Kladetsky, R. G., and Egli, H., Studies of fibrinolytic and coagulation factors during open-heart surgery. II. Postoperative bleeding tendencies and changes in the coagulation system, *Thromb. Res.*, 7, 589, 1975.
38. Signori, E. E., Penner, J. A., and Kahn, D. R., Coagulation defects and bleeding in open heart surgery, *Ann. Thorac. Surg.*, 8, 521, 1969.
39. Holswade, G. R., Nachman, R. L., and Killip, T., Thrombocytopathies in patients with open heart surgery. Preoperative treatment with corticosteroids, *Arch. Surg. (Chicago)*, 94, 365, 1967.
40. Salzman, E. W., Blood platelets and extracorporeal circulation, *Transfusion, (Philadelphia)*, 3, 274, 1963.
41. Bick, R. L., Adams, T., and Schmalhorst, W. R., Bleeding times, platelet adhesion, and aspirin, *Am. J. Clin. Pathol.*, 65, 69, 1976.
42. Stass, S., Bishop, C., Fosberg, R., Hartley, M., and Cramer, A., Platelets as affected by cardiopulmonary bypass, *Trans. Am. Soc. Clin. Pathol.*, 1976, 35.
43. Behrendt, D. M., Epstein, S. E., and Morrow, A. G., Postperfusion nonthrombocytopenic purpura: an uncommon sequel of open heart surgery, *Am. J. Cardiol.*, 22, 637, 1968.
44. Bick, R. L., Comer, T. P., and Arbegast, N., Fatal purpura fulminans following total cardiopulmonary bypass, *J. Cardiovasc. Surg.*, 14, 569, 1973.
45. Tice, D. A. and Worth, M. H., Recognition and Treatment of postoperative bleeding associated with open heart surgery, *Ann. N.Y. Acad. Sci.*, 146, 745, 1968.
46. Wright, T. A., Darte, J., and Mustard, W. T., Postoperative bleeding after extracorporeal circulation, *Can. J. Surg.*, 2, 142, 1959.
47. Penick, G. D., Averette, H. E., Peters, R. M., and Brinkhous, K. M., The hemorrhagic syndrome complicating extracorporeal shunting of blood: a study of its pathogenesis, *Thromb. Diath. Haemorrh.*, 2, 212, 1958.
48. Kevy, S. V., Clinkman, R. M., and Brinkhous, K. M., The hemorrhagic syndrome complicating extracorporeal shunting of blood: a study of its pathogenesis, *Thromb. Diath. Haemorrh.*, 2, 218, 1958.
48. Kevy, S. V., Clinkman, R. M., Bernhard, W. F., Diamond, L., and Gross, R., The pathogenesis of the hemorrhagic defect in open-heart surgery, *Surg. Gynecol. Obstet.*, 123, 313, 1966.
49. Bick, R. L., Schmalhorst, W. R., and Arbegast, N. R., Alterations of hemostasis associated with cardiopulmonary bypass, *Thromb. Res.*, 8, 285, 1976.
50. Tsuji, H. R., Redington, J. V., Kay, J. H., and Goesswald, R. K., The study of fibrinolytic and coagulation factors during open heart surgery, *Ann. Thorac. Surg.*, 13, 87, 1972.
51. Bachmann, F., McKenna, R., Cole, E. R., and Maiafi, H. J., The hemostasis mechanism after open-heart surgery. I. Studies on plasma coagulation factors and fibrinolysis in 512 patients after extracorporeal circulation, *J. Thorac. Cardiovasc. Surg.*, 70, 76, 1975.
52. Woods, J. E., Kirklin, J. W., Owens, C. A., Thompson, J. H., and Taswell, H. F., The effects of bypass surgery on coagulation sensitive clotting factors, *Mayo Clin. Proc.*, 42, 724, 1967.

53. Bick, R. L., *Disseminated Intravascular Coagulation and Related Syndromes*, Manual No. 570, American Society of Clinical Pathologists, Chicago, 1978.
54. Bick, R. L., Dukes, M. L., Wilson, W. L., and Fekete, L. F., Antithrombin III (AT-III) as a diagnostic aid in disseminated intravascular coagulation, *Thromb. Res.*, 10, 721, 1977.
55. Fekete, L. F. and Bick, R. L., Laboratory modalities for assessing hemostasis during cardiopulmonary bypass, *Semin. Thromb. Hemostas.*, 3, 83, 1976.
56. Menon, I. S., A study of the possible correlation of euglobulin lysis time and dilute blood clot lysis time in the determination of fibrinolytic activity, *Lab. Prac.*, 17, 334, 1968.
57. Derman, U. M., Rand, P. W., and Barker, N., Fibrinolysis after cardiopulmonary bypass and its relationship to fibrinogen, *J. Thorac. Cardiovasc. Surg.*, 51, 223, 1966.
58. Gomes, M. M. and McGoon, D., Bleeding patterns after open heart surgery, *J. Thorac. Cardiovasc. Surg.*, 60, 87, 1970.
59. Bick, R. L. and Fekete, L. F., Personal observations.
60. Olledorff, P., The nature of the anticoagulant effect of heparin, protamine, polybrene, and toloidine blue, *Scand. J. Clin. Lab. Invest.*, 14, 267, 1962.
61. O'Neill, J. A., Ende, H., and Collins, H. A., A quantitative determination of perfusion fibrinolysis, *Surgery*, 60, 809, 1966.
62. Bick, R. L., Bishop, R. C., Warren, M., and Stemmer, E., Changes in fibrinolysis and fibrinolytic enzyxes during extracorporeal circulation, *Trans. Am. Soc. Hematol.*, 109, 1971.
63. Verska, J. J., Lonser, E. R., and Brewer, L. A., Predisposing factors and management of hemorrhage following open-heart surgery, *J. Cardiovasc. Surg.*, 13, 311, 1972.
64. Verska, J. J., Letter to editor, *Ann. Thorac. Surg.*, 13, 87, 1972.
65. Bick, R. L., Cardiopulmonary bypass hemorrhage: aggravation by preoperative ingestion of antiplatelet drugs, *Vasc. Surg.*, in press.
66. Mielke, C. N., Kaneshiro, M. M., Maher, L. A., Weiner, J., and Rapaport, S. I., The standardized normal ivy bleeding time and its prolongation by aspirin, *Blood*, 34, 204, 1969.
67. Clifton, E. E. and Grossi, C. E., Fibrinolytic activity of human tumors as measured by the fibrin plate technique, *Cancer (Philadelphia)*, 8, 1146, 1955
68. Omar, J. B., Saxena, H., and Mitel, H. S., Fibrinolytic activity in malignant disease, *J. Assoc. Physicians India*, 19, 293, 1971.
69. Soong, B. C. F. and Miller, J. P., Coagulation disorders in cancer: fibrinolysis and inhibitors, *Cancer (Philadelphia)*, 25, 867, 1970.
70. Bick, R. L., Fekete, L. F., and Wilson, W. L., Adriamycin® and fibrinolysis, *Thromb. Res.*, 8, 467, 1976.
71. Bick, R. L., Fekete, L. F., and Murano, G., Daunomycin and fibrinolysis, *Thromb. Res.*, 9, 201, 1976.
72. Bick, R. L., Heparin assay introduced, *JAMA*, 239, 10, 1978.

Chapter 10

ACQUIRED CIRCULATING ANTICOAGULANTS AND DEFECTIVE HEMOSTASIS IN MALIGNANT PARAPROTEIN DISORDERS

Rodger L. Bick

TABLE OF CONTENTS

I. Introduction 206

II. Acquired Inhibitors to Specific Coagulation Factors 206
    A. Fibrinogen 206
    B. Prothrombin (Factor II) 206
    C. Factor V 206
    D. Factor VII 206
    E. Factor IX 207
    F. Factor XI 207
    G. Factor XIII 207

III. Circulating anticoagulants associated with Systemic Lupus Erythematosus 208

IV. Defective Hemostasis in Malignant Paraprotein Disorders 208
    A. Introduction 208
    B. Thrombocytopenia 208
    C. Functional Platelet Defects 208
    D. Coagulation Protein Defects 209
    E. Other Defects 209
    F. Treatment of Hemorrhage in Malignant Paraprotein Disorders 209

V. Summary 210

References 210

I. INTRODUCTION

Acquired circulating anticoagulants (inhibitors) are generally uncommon causes of hemorrhage. They may be observed in a variety of diseases, as well as in normal individuals. Any coagulation factor may be affected, the most common being Factor VIII.

Acquired inhibitors may be divided into two types. The first type includes inhibitors that inactivate individual coagulation factors in a progressive, irreversible, time-dependent manner. The vast majority of these are immunoglobulins. Subtyping of these reveal the majority to be IgG_4 with a kappa light chain (IgG_4K). The second type of circulating inhibitor is characterized by being reversible (or partially reversible), immediate in action, representing a protein-protein interaction (complex formation) with either a specific coagulation factor or groups of factors. Current evidence suggests that the affected coagulation factor is not destroyed and may be recovered if the complex can be dissociated. When unexplained bleeding or when coagulation testing, especially the differential PTT, gives contradictory or confusing results, acquired inhibitors to the coagulation system should be suspected.

II. ACQUIRED INHIBITORS TO SPECIFIC COAGULATION FACTORS

A. Fibrinogen

Acquired inhibitors or antibodies to fibrinogen are extremely rare, with only four to five cases having been reported. In two instances, these have been noted in patients subsequent to transfusion. Acquired inhibitors to fibrin monomer and fibrin polymerization are not uncommon.[1]

B. Prothrombin (Factor II)

With the exception of paraprotein disorders, inhibitors to prothrombin have not been reported.

C. Factor V

Acquired inhibitors to coagulation Factor V have been reported and appear to be associated with streptomycin therapy.[2] In most instances, streptomycin therapy preceded the development of an inhibitor by about 2 weeks. In all cases studied thus far, the immunoglobulin has been an IgG and reacts rapidly with Factor V without the necessity for a prolonged incubation period to become manifest in vitro. In most cases, the acquired inhibitor has been transient and disappears several weeks after cessation of streptomycin therapy. The laboratory manifestations of acquired inhibitors to Factor V are a prolonged partial thromboplastin time, prolonged prothrombin time, a low Factor V level by specific factor assay, and a normal thrombin time.

D. Factor VIII

In classical hemophilia the overall incidence of acquired inhibitors to Factor VIII is approximately 10%.[3] Almost all of these occur in severe, CRM⁺* hemophiliacs. In all cases this is an irreversible, time-dependent reaction (often requiring 2 hr of in vitro incubation) that destroys Factor VIII activity. Interestingly, these inhibitors do not inhibit von Willebrand factor activity, as noted by the fact that they do not inhibit platelet retention in glass-bead columns or interfere with ristocetin-induced platelet aggregation. All studies to date indicate that the inhibitors are immunoglobulins of

---

* CRM⁺ = Cross-reacting material is present.

heavy chain subtype and kappa light chain (IgG$_4$K).[4] These inhibitors develop as the hemophiliac is exposed to plasma, cryoprecipitate, or commercial concentrates with equal incidence.[5] Once inhibitors form, they persist for long periods of time and, if they disappear, reappearance often occurs when the patient is reexposed to Factor VIII. The management of these patients may be quite difficult. Prednisone, Imuran®, and 6-mercaptopurine are of little value.[6] Cytoxan® or plasmapheresis appear to be questionably efficacious.[7] High titers of inhibitor can be managed with infusions of actived prothrombin complex concentrate, which presumably stops the bleeding by bypassing the necessity of Factor VIII in the coagulation sequence.[8,9]

Acquired inhibitors to Factor VIII have also been reported in numerous nonhemophiliac patients. In some postpartum women, these develop within a few months following a normal delivery.[10] Clinically, these patients present similarly to classical hemophiliacs. Bleeding, including intra-articular bleeds and hemarthroses, may be severe. Inhibitors to Factor VIII have also been reported in (1) collagen vascular diseases (most commonly rheumatoid arthritis, systemic lupus erythematosus, and temporal arteritis[11]), (2) myeloma and Walderstrom's macroglobulinemia, (3) ulcerative colitis, (4) regional enteritis, (5) pemphigus vulgaris, (6) psoriasis, (7) dermatitis herpetiformis, and (8) following exposure to drugs, usually penicillin, phenylbutazone, sulfas, and nitrofurazone.[12,13] In addition, acquired inhibitors to Factor VIII have been noted to occur in some normal individuals.[14] Unlike those in hemophilia, acquired inhibitors in these disorders usually respond to steroids or other immunosuppressive therapy.

Acquired inhibitors to von Willebrand factor have also been reported.[15] In several patients, associated autoimmune disorders have been present. A classical clinical picture of von Willebrand's disease develops with typical epistaxis, ecchymoses, easy and spontaneous bruisability, and moderate depression of procoagulant Factor VIII. In these patients, the acquired inhibitor to von Willebrand factor activity interferes with platelet retention in glass-bead columns and with ristocetin-induced platelet aggregation.

E. Factor IX

In hemophilia B (Christmas disease), the incidence of acquired inhibitors to Factor IX is approximately 5%.[16] Unlike the inhibitor found in hemophilia A, this inhibitor is rapid in its action and usually does not require in vitro incubation longer than 5 min for demonstration. In cases studied thus far, the inhibitor has been characterized as an IgG$_4$ with lambda light chains. Acquired inhibitors to Factor IX have also been reported in nonhemophilia B patients, usually associated with SLE, rheumatic fever, and a postpartum state.[17]

F. Factor XI

Acquired inhibitors to Factor XI have been reported in only one case of hemophilia C.[18] All other acquired inhibitors to Factor XI have been in patients with SLE.[19]

G. Factor XIII

Several cases of acquired inhibitors to Factor XIII (fibrin stabilizing factor) have been reported.[20] In most instances, development of the inhibitor has followed therapy with Isoniazid®. In most patients, the Isoniazid® had been used for several years before the inhibitor appeared. The specific type of immunoglobulin has not been defined; however, several studies have revealed that antibody activity appears to be directed against the alpha chain[21] of Factor XIII.

III. CIRCULATING ANTICOAGULANTS ASSOCIATED WITH SYSTEM LUPUS ERYTHEMATOUS

Acquired inhibitors to blood coagulation factors have been described in several autoimmune disorders, most commonly systemic lupus erythematosus (SLE). A specific "lupus anticoagulant" has been identified and may precede the disease by several years. The presence of lupus anticoagulant is characterized by a prolonged partial thromboplastin time (PTT), a prolonged prothrombin time, prolongation of the PTT done on a mixture of normal plasma plus patients' plasma, and a normal thrombin time and bleeding time.[22] It remains unclear as to where this anticoagulant functions in the clotting sequence. Most of the evidence suggests that the activity is directed against prothrombin or a combination of the prothrombin complex factors. The inhibitor appears in approximately 6% of patients with SLE, and in many there is an associated deficiency of prothrombin. In those cases studied, the anticoagulant does not lead to a significant bleeding diathesis unless other associated coagulation defects are also present. Inhibitory activity correlates closely with disease activity and responds to immunosuppressive therapy. Other specific inhibitors to coagulation factors may also develop in SLE or any other of the collagen vascular diseases. The factors most commonly effected are Factors VIII, IX, XI, and XIII, as previously discussed.

IV. DEFECTIVE HEMOSTASIS IN MALIGNANT PARAPROTEIN DISORDERS

A. Introduction

Defects in hemostasis associated with malignant paraprotein disorders are well known, as these commonly lead to significant hemorrhage and/or thrombosis with subsequent difficulties in managing afflicted patients. The actual incidence of hemorrhage varies somewhat, depending upon the particular disease. About 15% of patients with IgG myeloma experience hemorrhage, while those with IgA myeloma have a 40% incidence of hemorrhage. Patients with Waldenstrom's macroglobulinemia have a greater than 60% incidence of hemorrhage.[23]

There are numerous reasons for hemorrhage in patients with malignant paraprotein disorders. Most commonly, abnormalities of hemostasis are a manifestation of circulating paraprotein. In addition, uremia and the attendant abnormal platelet function (thought to be due to circulating guanidosuccinic acid) account for significant hemorrhage. Many patients develop liver disease, with resultant decreased systhesis of the prothrombin complex factors, abnormal fibrinogens, abnormal fibrinolytic activity, and other coagulation defects. Disseminated intravascular coagulation has been reported in myeloma and may account for significant hemorrhage in selected patients.[24]

B. Thrombocytopenia

Thrombocytopenia is very commonly seen in multiple myeloma, but often is not pronounced enough to account for significant clinical bleeding. It can occur via several mechanisms, primarily through the development of hypersplenism, liver disease, radiation and/or chemotherapy, and marrow replacement.[25]

C. Functional Platelet Defects

Abnormalities of platelet function are more common causes of hemorrhage in malignant paraprotein disorders than is thrombocytopenia. Many patients with multiple myeloma demonstrate a prolonged template bleeding time that correlates reasonably well with clinical bleeding. However, some patients will have normal bleeding times even with marked defects in platelet function. Platelet adhesion correlates well with clinical bleeding. Abnormalities of platelet function in multiple myeloma have not been clearly defined, but are thought to be due to coating of platelet membrane surfaces by paraprotein.[26] Abnormal platelet adhesion is seen in greater than 50% of patients with myeloma and does not correlate well with the type of protein.[27] However, there appears to be some correlation with the quantity of paraprotein circulating. Abnormal platelet factor 3 release is usually normal in patients with myeloma and associated abnormal platelet adhesion and/or aggregation. It is thought that platelet membrane coating by paraprotein is not an antigen-antibody reaction, rather a protein-protein interaction.

Platelet aggregation is often abnormal in multiple myeloma. However, this modality correlates poorly with clinical bleeding and template bleeding times.[28] About 70% of myeloma patients have abnormal aggregation; epinephrine-induced aggregation is abnormal in about 90%, ADP induced-aggregation is abnormal in about 60%, and collagen-induced aggregation is abnormal in 60% of patients.[27] It appears that the most sensitive indicator of abnormal platelet aggregation in myeloma is epinephrine-induced platelet aggregation. It is of interest to note that some individuals demonstrating both abnormal platelet aggregation and adhesion have normal template bleeding times and the absence of clinical bleeding.[28]

In addition to the above, there are, of course, other causes of abnormal platelet function in myeloma, including uremia, liver disease, and elevated fibrin-fibrinogen degradation products. Also, malignant paraproteins may coat the vascular wall and thus interfere with in vivo collagen-induced platelet aggregation. However, this is not proven and remains of unclear significance with respect to clinical bleeding.

D. Coagulation Protein Defects

Malignant paraproteins are known to interfere with a number of coagulation proteins. The most publicized alteration of the coagulation system is that of the specific inhibition of Factors II, V, VII, VIII, or X. In actuality, this phenomenon is rare and the least common cause of hemorrhage. When specific inhibition of blood coagulation factors by paraprotein is present, IgG is usually directed against Factor II, Factor VII, Factor X, or thrombin, while IgA and IgM paraprotein is usually directed against Factor VIII or Factor V activity.*[29,30] The most common inhibition occurs where paraprotein selectively attaches to fibrin monomer and impedes polymerization. It is unclear if paraprotein coats the intact fibrinogen molecule or fibrin monomer after generation from fibrinogen. It has been proposed that the F(ab) fragment is the primary site of attachment to fibrin monomer. The noting of an abnormal thrombin time and/or reptilase time (which occurs in greater than 50% of patients) is a good indication of inhibition of fibrin monomer polymerization in paraprotein disorders and correlates well with clinical bleeding.[28]

E. Other Defects

Chronic low-grade disseminated intravascular coagulation is uncommonly present in patients with myeloma. Enhanced fibrino(geno)lytic activity is more commonly observed. This is manifested by elevated FDP, circulating plasmin, and the absence of soluble fibrin monomers. The mechanism by which this occurs is unclear.

F. Treatment of Hemorrhage in Malignant Paraprotein Disorders

Therapy of hemorrhage in patients with myeloma presents difficult management

---

* We have yet to see a specific coagulation factor inhibition problem in a large population of patients with malignant paraprotein disorders.

problems. The exact alteration of hemostasis must be clearly defined and then attempts made to deliver specific therapy. The alterations of hemostasis associated with hypersplenism, uremia, etc. are usually best controlled by treating the paraprotein disorder itself. This also applies to paraprotein inhibition of platelet function or the coagulation proteins. Often these defects will correct with decreases in the myeloma cell population induced by cytotoxic therapy. When bleeding becomes of marked significance and rapid control is imperative, plasmapheresis has proven quite effective as a means for rapidly lowering the paraprotein concentration and restoring normal hemostasis.[31]

V. SUMMARY

This chapter has summarized some of the rare acquired circulating anticoagulants. It should be recalled, however, that anticoagulants associated with hemophilia and SLE are not uncommon. In addition, the alterations of hemostasis associated with malignant paraprotein disorders must be appreciated in their complexity in order to rationally define the defect in a given patient and thus deliver appropriate therapy.

REFERENCES

1. **Kowalski, E.,** Fibrinogen derivatives and their biologic activities, *Thromb. Diath. Haemorrh.,* 10, 406, 1963.
2. **Feinstein, P. I., Rapaport, S. I., McGehee, W. G., and Patch, M. J.,** Factor V anticoagulants: clinical, biochemical, and immunological observations, *J. Clin. Invest.,* 49, 1578, 1970.
3. **Strauss, H. S.,** Acquired circulating anticoagulant in hemophilia A, *N. Engl. J. Med.,* 281, 866, 1969.
4. **Anderson, B. R. and Terry, W. D.,** Gamma G4-globulin antibody causing inhibition of clotting Factor VIII, *Nature (London),* 217, 174, 1968.
5. **Biggs, R.,** Jaundice and antibodies directed against Factors VIII and IX in patients treated for hemophilia or Christmas disease in the United Kingdom, *Br. J. Haematol.,* 26, 313, 1974.
6. **Lechner, K., Ludwig, E., Niessner, H., Thaler, E., and Deutsch, E.,** Immunosuppressive Treatment of Patients with Inhibitors of Blood Coagulation, in Proc. 3rd Congr. Int. Soc. Thromb. Haemostasis, Washington, D. C., 1972, 118.
7. **Stein, R. S.,** Hemophilia: cyclophosphamide and Factor VIII concentrate, *Ann. Intern. Med.,* 79, 84, 1973.
8. **Fekete, L. F., Holst, S. L., Peetoom, F., and de Veber, L. L.,** "Auto" Factor IX concentrate: a new therapeutic approach to treatment of hemophilia in patients with inhibitors, 14th Int. Congr. Hematol., Sao Paulo, Brazil, July 16 to 21, 1972, Abstr. 279.
9. **Kurczynski, E. M. and Penner, J. A.,** Activated prothrombin complex concentrate for patients with Factor VIII inhibitors, *N. Engl. J. Med.,* 291, 164, 1974.
10. **Greenwood, R. J. and Rabin, S. L.,** Hemophilia-like postpartum bleeding, *Obstet. Gynecol.,* 30, 262, 1967.
11. **Sise, H. S., Garther, J., Desforges, J., and Becker, R.,** Spontaneous circulating anticoagulant (antifactor VIII), *Am. J. Med.,* 32, 964, 1962.
12. **Margolius, A., Jackson, D. P., and Ratnoff, O. D.,** Circulating anticoagulants: a study of 40 cases and a review of the literature, *Medicine (Baltimore),* 40, 145, 1961.
13. **Shapiro, S. S. and Hultin, M.,** Acquired inhibitors to the blood coagulation factors, *Semin. Thromb. Hemostas.,* 1, 336, 1975.
14. **Biggs, R., Denson, K. W. E., and Nossel, H. L.,** A patient with an unusual circulating anticoagulant, *Thromb. Diath. Haemorrh.,* 12, 1, 1964.
15. **Ingram, G. I. C., Kingstone, P. J., Leslie, J., and Bowie, E. J. W.,** Four cases of acquired von Willebrand's syndrome, *Br. J. Haematol.,* 21, 189, 1971.
16. **Roberts, H. R.,** Acquired inhibitors in hemophilia B, *Thromb. Diath. Haemorrh.,* 45, 217, 1971.
17. **Castro, O., Farber, L. R., and Clyne, L. P.,** Circulating anticoagulants against Factors IX and V in systemic lupus erythematosis, *Ann. Intern. Med.,* 77, 543, 1972.

18. **Josephson, A. M. and Lisker, R.**, Demonstration of a circulating anticoagulant in plasma thromboplastin antecedent deficiency, *J. Clin. Invest.*, 37, 148, 1958.
19. **Cronberg, S. and Nilsson, I, M.**, Circulating anticoagulant against Factors XI and XII together with massive spontaneous platelet aggregation, *Scand. J. Haematol.*, 10, 309, 1973.
20. **Lewis, J. H.**, Hemorrhagic disease associated with inhibitors of fibrin cross-linkage, *Ann. N.Y. Acad. Sci.*, 202, 213, 1972.
21. **Lorand, L., Maldonado, N., Fradera, J., Atencio, A. C., Robertson, B., and Urayama, T.**, Hemorrhagic syndrome of autoimmune origin with a specific inhibitor against fibrin stabilizing factor (Factor XIII), *Br. J. Haematol.*, 23, 17, 1972.
22. **Schleider, M. A., Nachman, R. L., Jaffe, E. A., and Coleman, M.**, A clinical study of the lupus anticoagulant, *Blood*, 48, 499, 1976.
23. **Perkins, H. A., Mackenzie, M. R., and Fudenberg, H. H.**, Hemostatic defects in dysproteinemias, *Blood*, 35, 695, 1970.
24. **Mohler, E. R., Kennedy, J. H., and Brakman, P.**, Blood coagulation and fibrinolysis in multiple myeloma, *Am. J. Med. Sci.*, 253, 325, 1967.
25. **Nordenson, H. G.**, Myelomatosis: a clinical review of 310 cases, *Acta Med. Scand.*, 179, 178, 1966.
26. **Bick, R. L.**, Alterations of hemostasis associated with malignancy: etiology, pathophysiology, diagnosis and management, *Semin. Thromb. Hemostas.*, 5, 1, 1978.
27. **Bick, R. L.**, Treatment of bleeding and thrombosis in the patient with malignancy, in *Management of the Patient with Cancer*, Nealon, T. Ed., W. B. Saunders, Philadelphia, 1976, 48.
28. **Bick, R. L., Klein, C. A., Fekete, L. F., and Wilson, W. L.**, Alterations of hemostasis associated with malignant paraprotein disorders, *Trans. Am. Soc. Hematol.*, 63, 1976.
29. **Castaldi, P. A. and Penny, R.**, A macroglobulin with inhibitory activity against coagulation Factor VIII, *Blood*, 35, 370, 1970.
30. **Lackner, H.**, Hemostatis abnormalities associated with dysproteinemias, *Semin. Hematol.*, 10, 125, 1973.
31. **Godal, H. C. and Borchgrevink, C. F.**, The effect of plasmapheresis on the hemostatic function in patients with macroglobulinemia of Waldenstrom and multiple myeloma, *Scand. J. Clin. Lab. Invest.*, 17, 135, 1965.

Chapter 11

ALTERATIONS OF HEMOSTASIS ASSOCIATED WITH MALIGNANCY

Rodger L. Bick

TABLE OF CONTENTS

I.	Introduction	214
II.	Hypercoagulability and Thrombosis	214
	A. Pathophysiology	214
	B. Management of Thrombosis	216
III.	Hemorrhage	217
IV.	Platelets and Bleeding	219
	A. Thrombocytopenia	219
	B. Platelet Function Defects	220
V.	Effects of Chemotherapy on Hemostasis	221
VI.	Summary	221
References		222

I. INTRODUCTION

Alterations of hemostasis in cancer patients have long been recognized. Trousseau, in 1865, was the first to note this association,[1] and Morrison[2] initiated the first major study of blood changes in malignancy in 1932. The problems of altered hemostasis in malignancy remain extremely complex, present major clinical challenges, and many instances of bleeding or thrombosis in these diseases remain unexplained. Changes in hemostasis secondary to malignancy are certainly multifaceted, and the development of clinical bleeding or thrombosis represents a sum total clinical expression of numerous hemostatic alterations.

II. HYPERCOAGULABILITY AND THROMBOSIS

A. Pathophysiology

The first described hemostatic abnormality in malignancy was that of hypercoagulability and thrombosis, and the first large study of blood changes in cancer revealed accelerated bleeding times in over 60% of patients.[1,2] Since these classic descriptions, many investigators have reported hypercoagulability and thrombosis in association with all types of malignancy.[3-11] Many have found elevated clotting factors. Those commonly found elevated and thus implicated in causing hypercoagulability have been Factors I, V, VIII, IX, and XI.[9,10,12-14] In addition, most patients are noted to have shortened partial thromboplastin times, prothrombin times, and accelerated silicone clotting times.[9,13-16] Although we assume these parameters to be indicative of hypercoagulability, there is no actual correlation with the development of clinical thrombosis.[17,18]

Increased fibrinogen and platelet turnover (decreased survival) occurs in malignancy.[19] In addition, increased levels of FDP, cryofibrinogens, and fibrin monomer are seen in many patients with malignancy.[10,19-21] These findings suggest that many patients with cancer have a low-grade intravascular clotting process. The shortened survival of fibrinogen, platelets, and other coagulation proteins is followed by an overcompensated increase in coagulation factors and fibrinolytic enzymes, although these latter proteins may be decreased in the myeloproliferative disorders.[22] These changes are accompanied by a decrease in major coagulation inhibitors, the Antithrombin III (AT-III) fraction of plasma.[6,23] This sequence of changes alters the balance between coagulation, clot lysis, and clotting inhibition, rendering the patient highly sensitive to minor changes in the hemostatic system, which may predispose to localized intravascular coagulation (thrombosis) or disseminated intravascular coagulation (hemorrhage). Thrombus formation is the more common of the two expressions of intravascular coagulation, and may approach 50%, in cancer patients.[24] In some instances, the degree of alteration in coagulation factors has been correlated with amount of tumor and patient survival. Some coagulation abnormalities tend to normalize following treatment of malignancy; this is noted following surgery, radiation therapy, or chemotherapy.[8,9,10]

The mechanism(s) by which malignant tissue initiates localized or disseminated intravascular coagulation (DIC) is poorly understood. However, when compared to normal tissue, tumor tissue is capable of initiating the clotting process, and many tumor specimens are commonly associated with surrounding fibrin formation. In addition, malignant tissue has the ability to initiate fibrin formation without appropriate subsequent activation of the fibrinolytic system.[25,26] Many types of malignant tissue produce thromboplastin-like activity and, presumably, release this activity either locally or systemically, thus initiating the clotting process. The amount released probably dictates whether localized intravascular coagulation (thrombus) or DIC (hemorrhage) will occur.[27,28] Low levels of AT-III will allow this process to start more easily and to proceed without normal inhibition once under way.[9]

Mucinous adenocarcinomas are the tumors most commonly associated with thrombus formation. In this malignancy, the sialic acid moiety of the secreted mucin has been shown capable of initiating coagulation by the apparent nonenzymatic activation of Factor X.[13,14] In pancreatic carcinoma, the release of systemic trypsin is thought to trigger intravascular clotting. Thrombosis is seen more commonly with carcinoma of the body and tail rather than the head, since carcinoma of the head of the pancreas is associated with ductal obstruction and minimal trypsin release. Carcinoma of the body or tail is associated with morphologically disrupted, but functionally intact surrounding tissue and large amounts of trypsin release; thus more common thrombus formation.[6,29]

DIC is the coagulopathy of adenocarcinoma of the prostate.[30,31] However, malignant prostatic tissue has the ability to activate not only the coagulation, but also the fibrinolytic system. Therefore, in this instance, it appears that both DIC and inordinately excessive fibrinolysis from both primary activation and secondary to DIC occurs. This coagulopathy will usually manifest as bleeding rather than thrombosis, demonstrating the wide variety of expression in intravascular coagulation. Therapy of prostatic carcinoma is often followed by correction of coagulation and fibrinolytic parameters. This is noted particularly with administration of estrogens, whereas testosterone has been noted to enhance coagulation abnormalities.[20,32,33] A recent study has shown that many patients with prostatic carcinoma have preoperative evidence of DIC (elevated FDP and presence of soluble fibrin monomer), and these findings correlate with postsurgical blood loss.[34] This is noted, but to a lesser extent, in benign prostatic disease as well.

Hypercoagulability in cancer patients may also arise from platelet abnormalities. The role of platelets in contributing to thrombosis in malignancy was suspected long ago, and the first large study of this problem was by Moolten and associates in 1949.[35] These studies revealed abnormal increases in platelet numbers and abnormal morphology, lysis, and adhesion to glass wool. Good correlation between platelet adhesiveness and the development of thrombosis was noted. The increased platelet adhesion was better correlated with thrombosis than was thrombocytosis. Increased platelet adhesion as measured by short bleeding times, accelerated thromboplastin generation, shortened prothrombin consumption, and increased adhesion to glass has been found in numerous subsequent studies and appears to be uniform in a wide variety of solid tumors.[8-10] It is not clear if these alterations are primary disturbances caused by the malignancy or if they are due to primary coagulation changes that "prime" platelets for adhesion or aggregation. Thrombocytosis is well documented in malignancy and, most commonly, is associated with carcinoma of the pancreas, lung, gastrointestinal tract, ovary, and breast. Patients undergoing bone marrow suppressive therapy will have less thrombocytosis than those not being so treated.[2,9,10,36] The most pronounced instances of thrombocytosis are usually noted in the myeloproliferative disorders.[37]

As outlined above, there are various mechanisms enabling malignant tissue to induce changes in coagulation factors and platelets to create a hypercoagulable state. This intravascular coagulation may be mild and detected only by abnormal tests of hemostasis, which we interpret as hypercoagulability. It may proceed to thrombosis, or, in extreme cases, may be manifest as DIC and hemorrhage. The malignancies most commonly associated with thrombosis are depicted in Table 1. The overall incidence of thrombosis in malignancy is about 15%, but may be higher in specific tumors, such as in the pancreas, where it exceeds 50%.[3,6] The patient with cancer is much more

TABLE 1

Malignancies Most Commonly Associated with Thrombosis

Pancreas
Stomach
Lung
Colon
Ovaries
Gallbladder
Myeloproliferative disorders
Malignant paraproteinemias

likely to develop postoperative thrombophlebitis than is the patient without cancer. In carcinoma of the gastrointestinal tract, the rate of postoperative thrombosis may approach 40%.[4,13,14,38]

B. Management of Thrombosis

Antitumor therapy is associated with some correction of abnormal hemostasis. This is especially noted in prostatic carcinoma. The use of anticoagulants (warfarin and heparin) and antiplatelet drugs (acetylsalicylic acid and dipyridamole) has been associated with some correction of altered coagulation factors and normalization of fibrinogen and platelet survival.[10,19,32] In spite of these findings, however, cancer patients are notoriously resistant to anticoagulant therapy,[39,40] and thrombosis often persists. In addition, warfarin and heparin are associated with significant bleeding problems,[18,19] perhaps owing to large amounts of necrotic tumor surface. Many patients with malignancy have decreased AT-III levels, thus the response to heparin will be less than optimal. This is especially true in patients with liver metastases, as is shown in Table 2.

Our experience with antiplatelet drugs in cancer patients, on the other hand, has been good. We commonly use acetylsalicylic acid(ASA), 600 mg twice a day with 20 ml of liquid antacid, in patients with thromboses. We find this to be effective for immediate prophylaxis of extension of thrombi, as well as for long-term prophylactic therapy in cases of recurrent thromboses. If the patient has extensive thromboses or develops new thromboses while on ASA, dipyridamole at a dose of 50 mg four times a day is added to this regimen. The use of ASA preoperatively or immediately postoperatively seems effective for prophylaxis in those patients with tumors known to be associated with a high rate of postoperative thrombosis.[18]

Bleeding complications are not noted to be associated with antiplatelet therapy, even in patients with recent bowel surgery, but it is important to use a liquid antacid with ASA. ASA exerts an effect by inhibiting acetylcholine esterase, thus blocking vascular constriction, and by inhibiting the platelet release reaction.[41,42] To demonstrate the efficacy of ASA, one should note at least a 2 min prolongation of the base line template bleeding time about 2 hr after giving ASA.[43] The effect of ASA may last for 4 to 10 days after the last dose; this must be considered in the event of bleeding or planned surgery. Bleeding from antiplatelet therapy can be controlled with the use of platelet concentrates. When the patient with malignancy suffers life-threatening thrombosis and has adequate levels of AT-III, our approach is to use mini-heparin, as this has been found to be equally as efficacious as medical doses of heparin and does not seem to lead to bleeding from tumor surfaces as readily as medical doses of heparin.[18]

TABLE 2

Antithrombin III Levels in Malignancy: Effect of Liver Metastases[a]

Patient	AT-III (%)	Liver involved	Malignancy
1	33	+	Breast
2	75	+	Hodgkin's
3	80	+	Breast
4	58	+	Breast
5	76	+	Ovary
6	83	+	Colon
7	71	+	Breast
8	92	+	Colon
9	160	+	Carcinoid
10	160	+	Colon
11	120	−	Hodgkin's
12	92	−	Breast
13	121	−	Lung
14	117	−	Lung
15	112	−	Breast
16	92	−	Ovary
17	104	−	Pancreas
18	140	−	Breast
19	104	−	Breast
20	150	−	Breast

[a] Author's observations.

III. HEMORRHAGE

As discussed previously, intravascular coagulation is present in many patients with malignancy and manifests varying clinical expressions, the most extreme form being disseminated intravascular coagulation (DIC) and catastrophic hemorrhage. DIC in cancer patients may be *acute* or *chronic*.[31] The *chronic* form is slightly more common and manifests clinically by mild to moderate bleeding, usually of the integument or mucous membranes. Easy and spontaneous bruisability, petechiae, purpura, ecchymoses, gingival bleeding, and minor gastrointestinal bleeding are the usual manifestations.

In contrast, *acute* DIC is characterized by explosive, catastrophic hemorrhage, with bleeding usually occurring from at least three unrelated sites at once. The most commonly noted abnormalities are petechiae, purpura, and ecchymoses, seen in conjunction with significant gastrointestinal or genitourinary hemorrhage. In addition, most patients will manifest oozing at intravenous sites or sites of invasive procedures. Although these are the common bleeding manifestations, more life-threatening bleeding, such as intracranial and intraperitoneal and massive hemoptysis may also occur. This form of DIC has been reported in association with almost all types of solid tumor and is most commonly seen with carcinoma of the lung, gallbladder, stomach, colon, breast, and ovary, and in malignant melanoma.[9,13,14,44-47] It is especially common in carcinoma of the prostate.[20,30,31,48-52] In these latter disorders, initiation of chemotherapy has been associated with triggering or accelerating DIC,[10,47,53,54] due to release of thromboplastin-like or clot-promoting material from necrosing tumor cells. In acute promyelocytic leukemia, low-dose heparin given before starting cytotoxic drugs may protect against this development.[54]

In addition to malignancy itself, other common complications in cancer patients may also cause DIC. These include sepsis, initiation of radiotherapy, microangiopathic

TABLE 3

Malignancies Most Commonly Associated with DIC

Acute promyelocytic leukemia
Lung
Gallbladder
Stomach
Colon
Breast
Ovary
Melanoma
Prostate

TABLE 4

Sequential Therapy of DIC in Malignancy

1. Treat the malignancy
    Chemotherapy
    Radiotherapy
    Surgery
2. Stop the clotting process
    Mini-heparin
    Heparin
    AT-III[a] concentrates
    Antiplatelet agents (chronic DIC)
3. Component replacement therapy, if indicated
    Platelet concentrates
    Clotting factors
    Fibrinogen
    AT-III[a] concentrates
4. Inhibit residual fibrinolysis
    ACA[b] only if necessary: 5 g slow IVP, followed by
    2 g q 2 hr × 24 hr

[a] AT-III = Antithrombin III.
[b] ACA = Aminocaproic acid.

hemolytic anemia, hemolytic transfusion reactions, and transfusion of large amounts of banked whole blood.[24,55]

The malignancies most commonly associated with DIC and hemorrhage are listed in Table 3. The pathophysiology and diagnosis of DIC are discussed in Chapter 8.

Therapy of DIC in the cancer patient represents a major clinical challenge. Table 4 outlines the approach. Efficacious therapy is multiphasic and must be approached in a sequential manner. The first and most important modality is to treat the malignancy, since this is providing the trigger for intravascular coagulation. Therapy may be surgical, radiotherapeutic, or chemotherapeutic, as the clinical situation warrants. Treatment of the trigger (tumor) is often associated with cessation or significant improvement of DIC. Until attempts at antineoplastic therapy are initiated, subsequent therapy of bleeding is often unsuccessful. If significant bleeding continues after reasonable efforts to control the malignancy, anticoagulant therapy must be considered. For the patient with malignancy and *acute* DIC, one starts with mini-heparin therapy at 2500 to 5000 units subcutaneously every 8 to 12 hr, as severity of hemorrhage dictates. In patients with *chronic* DIC and bothersome, but not significant hemorrhage, antiplatelet agents, especially ASA and dipyridamole, as previously described, will usually stop the intravascular clotting process. The medical management of DIC, including an approach to the patient with malignancy, is thoroughly discussed in Chapter 8.

Cancer patients may also develop bleeding from other coagulation factor abnormalities. These are somewhat less common and are usually associated with less serious hemorrhage. Patients with liver metastases may acquire deficiencies of the prothrombin complex (vitamin K-dependent) factors.[9,56] When this results in bleeding, vitamin K is usually ineffective, and the hemorrhage must be controlled with fresh frozen plasma, fresh whole blood, or prothrombin complex concentrates. However, before using these modalities, DIC must be excluded.

Factor XIII deficiency or dysfunction is common in malignancy and is most pronounced in patients with liver metastases.[46,57] Factor XIII is associated with albumin, and cancer patients with hypoalbuminemia are often Factor XIII deficient, although usually not to a clinically significant degree. The deficiency may or may not cause hemorrhage; more commonly, impaired clot formation and poor wound healing will be noted. When Factor XIII deficiency is suspected to cause or to contribute to hemorrhage, it can be managed by transfusions with fresh frozen plasma 5 ml/kg every 6 to 8 days.[58]

Patients with liver metastases will often have low levels of prekallikrein (Fletcher factor) and Factor XII, but this is of questionable clinical significance. Of particular significance is the development of a dysfibrinogenemia with either primary hepatoma, or metastases to the liver. Structural abnormalities in fibrinogen/fibrin monomer polymerization are seen in these patients and may lead to hemorrhage.

Acquired circulating anticoagulants may occur with a wide variety of tumors; however, these have been isolated findings and have an unclear relationship to actual hemorrhage. Most are heparinoid in nature and are found in association with lung tumors. Some, inhibiting the contact phase of coagulation or acting as antithrombins, have been noted in association with breast carcinoma.[59] Circulating anticoagulants in the form of FDP may assume paramount clinical importance in cancer patients with intravascular coagulation; their mode of action has been previously discussed in Chapter 8. Circulating anticoagulants also may assume major importance in the malignant paraprotein disorders.[60]

Primary hyperfibrino(geno)lysis has been noted in malignancy.[20,33,46,61] In this disorder, hemorrhage is caused by plasmin degradation of fibrinogen, Factors V and VIII, and the creation of circulating FDP.

Many malignant tissues are capable of spontaneous fibrinolytic activity and fibrinolytic enzyme activation. This is seen in breast, thyroid, colon, and stomach cancer, but the greatest activity seems to be in sarcoma.[61] Kwaan et al.[62] have noted a decrease in tumor fibrinolytic activity in patients with liver metastases and ascribe this phenomenon to increased levels of fibrinolytic inhibitors. Primary hyperfibrino(geno)lytic hemorrhage is treated with agents that inhibit the fibrinolytic enzyme system (Chapter 9).

IV. PLATELETS AND BLEEDING

A. Thrombocytopenia

Thrombocytopenia is unquestionably the most common cause of bleeding in patients with both solid tumors and hematologic malignancies.[19] Thrombocytopenia is commonly the result of marrow suppression by radiation therapy or chemotherapy. Alkylating agents are clearly the worst offenders in this regard.[63,64] Thrombocytopenia also commonly results from marrow involvement by tumor and, in general, correlates well with the degree of marrow invasion.[9,10,19] Marrow metastases should be suspected and carefully searched for when unexplained thrombocytopenia develops. This is accomplished by examination of a marrow aspirate or biopsy. Biopsy is much more reliable than aspirate in evaluating marrow involvement.[65-69]

In addition to marrow suppressive therapy and marrow metastases, cancer patients may also develop other types of thrombocytopenia. When splenomegaly develops as part of the malignant process, hypersplenism and subsequent thrombocytopenia may ensue.[70] Development of splenic metastases is more common than generally recognized, especially in carcinoma of the lung, breast, prostate, colon, and stomach.[71,72] If clinically feasible, splenectomy may be of benefit in hypersplenic situations. An infusion of epinephrine may be helpful in predicting the response to this procedure.

When thrombocytopenia from decreased marrow production or increased splenic sequestration becomes significant, platelet concentrates provide the mainstay of management. Platelet counts below 10,000 per cubic millimeter are commonly associated with spontaneous and serious hemorrhage, whereas platelet counts above 30,000 per cubic millimeter are not, unless the patient is challenged with traumatic or surgical stress.[73] It is general practice to infuse platelet concentrates in most situations in which the platelet count is less than 10,000 per cubic millimeter and the patient develops signs of bleeding, or when surgery or other invasive procedures are contemplated. Platelet concentrates are now readily available in most community hospitals and provide the most efficient modality of platelet replacement therapy. An ideal platelet concentrate contains approximately 1.25×10^{11} platelets, and, in general, one unit of platelet concentrate will elevate the platelet count by about 5000 to 7000 per cubic millimeter in an adult and by about 10,000 to 12,000 per cubic millimeter in an infant. In practice, 6 to 8 U of platelet packs are usually administered to the severely thrombocytopenic adult every time the platelet count falls below 10,000 per cubic millimeter. Appropriately decreased numbers are used for children and infants.[74] If long-term platelet transfusions are contemplated and appropriate facilities are available, HL-A compatible platelets should be used.

Autoimmune thrombocytopenia (ITP) occasionally occurs in patients with solid tumors, but is more common in lymphoreticular malignancies.[75] When this occurs, the approach to management should be that generally used for this disorder, utilizing steroids, and possibly splenectomy, if indicated. In cases of ITP that remain refractory to usual forms of therapy, the use of intravenous vincristine has been found potentially useful.[76,77] Another type of increased platelet destruction that is occasionally associated with malignancy is thrombotic thrombocytopenia purpura (TTP).[78] This rare syndrome is usually fatal when it develops in the cancer patient, but may respond to heparin, dextrans, steroids, or antiplatelet drugs.[79-82]

B. Platelet Function Defects

Abnormalities of platelet function are commonly found in association with both solid tumors and hematologic malignancies. Because of relatively frequent intravascular coagulation and resulting elevated FDP noted in cancer patients, the coating of platelet surfaces by these fragments probably constitutes the most common cause of abnormal platelet function (Chapters 8 and 9). However, additional platelet abnormalities are also frequently noted. These include decreased Platelet Factor 3, decreased platelet aggregation to adenosine diphosphate (ADP), decreased adhesion, and other presumptive evidence of faulty platelet function as measured by prolonged thromboplastin generation, prolonged bleeding times, positive tourniquet tests, and poor clot retraction.[10,48,60,83] It remains unclear if these defects develop secondary to the malignancy itself, if they come about from partial release of platelet contents after contact with malignant tissue, or if they develop in response to activated clotting factors. The malignant paraprotein disorders are associated with platelet function abnormalities that develop from coating of platelet surfaces by immunoglobulins[84] (Chapter 10). Consistent platelet aggregation abnormalities are found in the myeloproliferative disorders[37] and in preleukemia.[83] The exact significance of these numerous functional platelet defects in contributing to hemorrhage in cancer patients remains unclear. However, they appear to correlate better with the development of hemorrhage than does the platelet count.[48,83] At the very least, these defects must be presumed to aggravate bleeding in patients who already have compromised hemostasis or thrombocytopenia.

Clinical clues to the existence of a functional platelet defect include the noting of easy or spontaneous bruisability, gingival bleeding with toothbrushing, and other minor forms of mucosal bleeding in the face of a normal platelet count. In addition, a prolonged template bleeding time and abnormal platelet adhesion to glass-bead columns (all in the face of a normal platelet count) are good laboratory indications of abnormal platelet function.[85]

Unless secondary to intravascular coagulation, bleeding due to or aggravated by a functional platelet abnormality requires platelet replacement therapy. This requires platelet concentrates and should be approached in the same manner as outlined for thrombocytopenia. In addition, the patient should be strongly cautioned regarding the use of common drugs known to interfere with platelet function (aspirin, diphenhydramine, papaverine vasodilators, phenylbutazone, and dipyridamole).

V. EFFECTS OF CHEMOTHERAPY ON HEMOSTASIS

Chemotherapy may alter hemostasis by a variety of mechanisms. The most common and significant of these have been previously discussed and include the thrombocytopenia so commonly associated with marrow-suppressive cytotoxic drugs and the initiation or enhancement of DIC by cytotoxic drugs in both solid tumors and acute promyelocytic leukemia. Antineoplastic agents that may interfere with hemostasis are listed in Table 5.

L-Asparaginase therapy is commonly associated with signifiant hypofibrinogenemia, which is an almost universal complication of this agent. Although earlier investigations attributed this phenomenon to decreased fibrinogen synthesis,[86] more recent studies have shown this to be a consequence of a functionally abnormal fibrinogen.[87] This is thought to arise from reactions between L-asparaginase and asparagine residues of the fibrinogen molecule.[88] Mithramycin therapy is associated with hemorrhage in greater than 50% of patients receiving this drug. Although this agent causes thrombocytopenia, hemorrhage is thought more likely to be the result of impaired platelet function, hyperfibrinolysis, and decreased levels of Factors II, V, VIII, and X.[89] In the face of these findings, the triggering of DIC by mithramycin seems reasonable. Actinomycin D has also been associated with significant hemorrhage. This occurs from vitamin K antagonism by this drug and the resulting defective synthesis of Factors II, VII, IX, and X.[90] Melphalan may cause a significant defect in the platelet release reaction and may interfere with fibrin monomer polymerization. The use of Adiamycin® and daunomycin have been associated with primary activation of the fibrinolytic system and subsequent clinical hemorrhage.[91,92]

VI. SUMMARY

The patient with disseminated malignancy suffers many alterations of hemostasis. Hemorrhage or, less commonly, thrombosis are not infrequently the final clinical event in many individuals. Patients with malignancy present a major clinical challenge in this day of new oncological awareness and more aggresive care. Thus it is important to realize that these alterations of hemostasis must be approached in a logical manner with respect to diagnosis, as well as efficacious therapy. By far the most common alteration of hemostasis is that of hemorrhage associated with thrombocytopenia,

TABLE 5

Antineoplastics that May Alter Hemostasis

Agent	Mechanism
ActinomycinD	Vitamin-K antagonist
L-Asparaginase	Dys/hypofibrinogenemia
Melphalan	Platelet dysfunction, dysfibrinogenemia
Mithramycin	Thrombocytopenia, disseminated intravascular coagulation
Adriamycin®	Primary fibrino(geno)lysis
Daunomycin	Primary fibrino(geno)lysis

either drug induced or from marrow invasion. However, hemorrhage due to disseminated intravascular coagulation is also a problem. In addition, many antineoplastic drugs, as well as radiotherapy, may lead to hemorrhage. Thrombosis in the patient with malignancy is usually a consequence of disseminated intravascular coagulation manifest as an intravascular thrombotic, rather than an intravascular generalized proteolytic event. When approaching the patient with malignancy and either hemorrhage or thrombosis, all of the potential defects in hemostasis must be taken into account, defined from the laboratory standpoint, and treated in as precise a manner as possible.

REFERENCES

1. **Trousseau, A.,** Phlegmasia alba dolens in *Clinical Medicale de l'Hotel de Paris,* Vol. 3, 2nd ed., Balliere, Paris, 1865.
2. **Morrison, M.,** An analysis of the blood picture in 100 cases of malignancy, *J. Lab. Clin. Med.,* 17, 1071, 1932.
3. **Sproul, E. F.,** Carcinoma and venous thrombosis, *Am. J. Cancer,* 34, 566, 1938.
4. **Edwards, E. A.,** Migrating thrombophlebitis associated with carcinoma, *N. Engl. J. Med.,* 240, 1031, 1949.
5. **Fisch, C., Jones, A. W., and Gambill, W. D.,** Acute thrombophlebitis associated with carcinoma of the stomach, *Gastroenterology,* 18, 290, 1951.
6. **Innerfield, I., Anrist, A., and Benjamin, J. W.,** Plasma antithrombin patterns in disturbances of the pancreas, *Gastroenterology,* 19, 843, 1951.
7. **Perlow, S. and Daniels, J. L.,** Venous thrombosis and obscure visceral carcinoma, *Arch. Intern. Med.,* 97, 184, 1956.
8. **Amundsen, M. A., Spittel, J. A., Jr., and Thompson, J. H., Jr.,** Hypercoagulability associated with malignant disease and with the postoperative state, *Ann. Intern. Med.,* 58, 608, 1963.
9. **Miller, S. P., Sanchez-Avalos, J., and Stefanski, T.,** Coagulation disorders in cancer. I. Clinical and laboratory studies, *Cancer (Philadelphia),* 20, 1452, 1967.
10. **Davis, R. B., Theologides, A., and Kennedy, B. J.,** Comparative studies of blood coagulation and platelet aggregation in patients with cancer and nonmalignant disease, *Ann. Intern. Med.,* 71, 67, 1969.
11. **Kremer, W. B. and Laszlo, J.,** Hematologic effects of cancer, in *Cancer Medicine,* Holland, J. F. and Frei, E., Eds., Lea & Febiger, Philadelphia, 1973, 1865.
12. **Fumarola, D. and del Buono, G.,** The blood coagulation pattern in malignancies, *Prog. Med. Napoli,* 14, 327, 1958.
13. **Pineo, G. F., Regoeczi, E., and Hatton, M. W. C.,** The activation of coagulation by extracts of mucus: a possible pathway of intravascular coagulation accompanying adenocarcinomas, *J. Lab. Clin. Med.,* 82, 255, 1973.
14. **Pineo, G. F., Brain, M. C., and Gallus, A. S.,** Tumors, mucus production, and hypercoagulability, *Ann. N.Y. Acad. Sci.,* 230, 262, 1974.

15. **Waterbury, L. S. and Hampton, J. W.**, Hypercoagulability with malignancy, *Angiology*, 18, 197, 1967.
16. **Miller, S. P. and Davison, T.**, Defibrination syndrome in cancer: treatment with heparin, *N.Y. State J. Med.*, 67, 452, 1967.
17. **Merskey, C.**, Altered blood coagulability in patients with malignant tumors, *Ann. N.Y. Acad. Sci.*, 230, 289, 1974.
18. **Bick, R. L.**, Treatment of bleeding and thrombosis in the patient with cancer, in *Care of the Cancer Patient*, Nealon T., Ed., W. B. Saunders, Philadelphia, 1976, chap. 5.
19. **Slichter, S. J. and Harker, L. A.**, Hemostasis in malignancy, *Ann. N.Y. Acad. Sci.*, 230, 252, 1974.
20. **Phillips, L. L., Skrodelis, V., and Furey, C. A.**, The fibrinolytic enzyme system in prostatic cancer, *Cancer (Philadelphia)*, 12, 721, 1959.
21. **Astedt, B., Svanberg, L., and Nelsson, I. M.**, Cancer, FDP and radiotherapy, *Br. Med. J.*, 2, 47, 1972.
22. **Bick, R. L. and Adams, T.**, Fibrinolytic abnormalties in the myeloproliferative disorders, *Clin. Res.*, 21, 264, 1973.
23. **Bick, R. L., Dukes, M. L., Wilson, W. L., and Fekete, L. F.**, Antithrombin-III as a diagnostic aid in disseminated intravascular coagulation, *Thromb. Res.*, 10, 721, 1977.
24. **Pick, S. D. and Reiguam, C. W.**, Disseminated intravascular coagulation in cancer patients: supportive evidence, *Cancer (Philadelphia)*, 31, 1114, 1973.
25. **O'Meara, R. A. Q.**, Coagulation properties of cancers, *Ir. J. Med. Sci.*, 394, 474, 1958.
26. **Boggust, W. A., O'Brien, D. J., O'Meara, R. A. Q., and Thernes, R. D.**, The coagulative factors of normal human and human cancer tissue, *Ir. J. Med. Sci.*, 6, 131, 1963.
27. **Al-Mondhiry, H.**, Disseminated intravascular coagulation: experience in a major cancer center, *Thromb. Diath. Haemorrh.*, 34, 181, 1975.
28. **Rohner, R. F., Prior, J. T., and Sipple, J. H.**, Mucinous malignancies, venous thrombosis, and terminal endocarditis with emboli: a syndrome, *Cancer (Philadelphia)*, 19, 1805, 1966.
29. **Gore, I.**, Thrombosis and pancreatic carcinoma, *Am. J. Pathol.*, 29, 1093, 1953.
30. **Rapaport, S. I. and Chapman, C. G.**, Coexistent hypercoagulability and acute hypofibrinogenemia in a patient with prostatic carcinoma, *Am. J. Med.*, 27, 144, 1959.
31. **Owen, C. A., Jr., Oels, H. C., and Bowie, E. J. W.**, Chronic intravascular coagulation (ICF) syndrome, *Thromb. Diath. Haemorrh. Suppl.*, 36, 197, 1969.
32. **Brown, R. C., Campbell, D. C., and Thompson, J. H.**, Increased fibrinolysin with malignant disease, *Arch. Intern. Med.*, 109, 129, 1962.
33. **Omar, J. B., Saxena, H., and Mital, H. S.**, Fibrinolytic activity in malignant neoplastic disease, *J. Assoc. Physicians India*, 19, 293, 1971.
34. **Mertins, B. F., Green, L F., Bowie, E. J. W., Elveback, L. R., and Owen, C. A.**, Fibrinolytic split products and ethanol gelation test in preoperative evaluation of patients with prostatic disease, *Mayo Clin. Proc.*, 49, 624, 1974.
35. **Mootlten, S. E., Vroman, L., and Vroman, G. M. S.**, Role of blood platelets in thromboembolism, *Arch. Intern. Med.*, 84, 667, 1949.
36. **Levin, J. and Conley, C. L.**, Thrombocytosis associated with malignant disease, *Arch. Intern. Med.*, 114, 487, 1964.
37. **Adams, T., Schultz, L., and Goldberg, L.**, Platelet function abnormalities in myeloproliferative disorders, *Scan. J. Haematol.*, 13, 215, 1974.
38. **Kakkar, V. V., Howe, C. T., and Nicolaides, A. N.**, Deep vein thrombosis of the leg: is there a "high risk group"? *Am. J. Surg.*, 120, 527, 1970.
39. **Fischer, M. M. and Hochberg, L. A.**, Recurrent thrombophlebitis in obscure malignant tumor of the lung, *JAMA*, 147, 1213, 1951.
40. **Lieberman, J. S., Borrero, J., and Urdaneta, E.**, Thrombophlebitis and cancer, *JAMA*, 177, 542, 1961.
41. **Quick, A. J.**, *Bleeding Problems in Clinical Medicine*, W. B. Saunders, Philadelphia, 1970, 14.
42. **Mustard, J. F. and Packham, M. A.**, Factors influencing platelet function: adhesion, release, and aggregation, *Pharmacol. Rev.*, 22, 97, 1970.
43. **Mielke, C. H., Kaneshiro, M. M., and Maher, I. A.**, The standardized normal bleeding time and its prolongation by aspirin, *Blood*, 34, 104, 1969.
44. **Biben, R. L. and Tyan, M. L.**, Hemorrhagic diathesis in carcinoma of the stomach: a case report, *Ann. Intern. Med.*, 17, 917, 1958.
45. **Didisheim, P., Bowie, E. J., and Owen, C. A., Jr.**, Intravascular coagulation fibrinolysis (ICF) syndrome and malignancy: historical review and report of two cases with metastatic carcinoid and with acute myomoncytic leukemia, *Thromb. Diath. Haemorrh. Suppl.*, 36, 215, 1969.
46. **Soong, B. C. P. and Miller, S. P.**, Coagulation disorders in cancer: fibrinolysis and inhibitors, *Cancer (Philadelphia)*, 25, 867, 1970.

47. **Goodnight, S. H., Jr.,** Bleeding and intravascular clotting in malignancy: a review, *Ann. N.Y. Acad. Sci.,* 230, 271, 1974.
48. **Perry, S.,** Coagulation defects in leukemia, *J. Lab. Clin. Med.,* 50, 229, 1957.
49. **Rosenthal, R. L.,** Acute promyelocytic leukemia associated with hypofibrinogenemia, *Blood,* 21, 495, 1963.
50. **Didisheim, P., Trombold, J. S., and Vandervort, R. L. E.,** Acute promyelocytic leukemia with fibrinogen and Factor V deficiencies, *Blood,* 23, 717, 1964.
51. **Rand, J. J., Maloney, W. C., and Kise, H. S.,** Coagulation defects in acute promyelocytic leukemia, *Arch. Intern. Med.,* 123, 39, 1969.
52. **Polliack, A.,** Acute promyelocytic leukemia with disseminated intravascular coagulation, *Am. J. Clin. Pathol.,* 56, 155, 1971.
53. **Leavey, R. A., Kahn, S. B., and Brodsky, I.,** Disseminated intravascular coagulation: a complication of chemotherapy in acute myelomonocytic leukemia, *Cancer (Philadelphia),* 26, 142, 1970.
54. **Gralnick, H. R. and Tan, J. K.,** Acute promyelocytic leukemia, *Hum. Pathol.,* 5, 661, 1974.
55. **Bick, R. L. and Adams, T.,** Disseminated intravascular coagulation: etiology, pathophysiology, diagnosis and treatment, *Med. Counterpoint,* 6, 38, 1974.
56. **Frick, P. G.,** Acute hemorrhagic syndrome with hypofibrinogememia in metastatic cancer, *Acta Haematol.,* 16, 11, 1956.
57. **Nussbaum, M. and Morse, B. S.,** Plasma fibrin stabilizing factor activity in various diseases, *Blood,* 23, 669, 1964.
58. **Ikkala, E.,** Transfusion therapy in congenital deficiencies of plasma factor XIII, *Ann. N.Y. Acad. Sci.,* 202, 200, 1972.
59. **Margoliusa, A., Jr., Jackson, D. P., and Ratnoff, O. D.,** Circulating anticoagulants: a study of 40 cases and a review of the literature, *Medicine (Baltimore),* 40, 145, 1961.
60. **Sanchez-Avalos, J., Soong, B. C. F., and Miller, S. P.,** Coagulation disorders in cancer. II. Multiple myeloma, *Cancer (Philadelphia),* 23, 1388, 1969.
61. **Cliffton, E. E. and Grossi, C. E.,** Fibrinolytic activity of human tumors as measured by the fibrin-plate method, *Cancer (Philadelphia),* 8, 1146, 1955.
62. **Kwaan, H. C., Lo, R., and McFadzean, A. J. S.,** Antifibrinolytic activity in primary carcinoma of the liver, *Clin. Sci.,* 18, 251, 1959.
63. **Livingston, R. B. and Carter, S. K.,** *Single Agents in Cancer Chemotherapy,* Plenum Press, New York, 1970.
64. **Rubin, P. and Casarett, G. W.,** *Clinical Radiation Pathology,* W. B. Saunders, Philadelphia, 1968, 778.
65. **Lanier, P. F.,** Sternal marrow in patients with metastatic cancer, *Arch. Intern. Med.,* 84, 891, 1949.
66. **Johnsson, U. and Rundles, R. W.,** Tumor metastases in bone marrow, *Blood,* 6, 16, 1951.
67. **Berkheiser, S. W.,** The incidence of malignant cells in routine bone marrow examination, *Cancer (Philadelphia)* 8, 958, 1955.
68. **Hansen, H. H., Muggia, F. M., and Selawry, O. S.,** Bone marrow examination in 100 consecutive patients with bronchogenic carcinoma, *Lancet,* 1, 443, 1971.
69. **Jamshidi, K. and Swaim, W. R.,** Bone marrow biopsy with unaltered architecture: a new biopsy device, *J. Lab. Clin. Med.,* 77, 335, 1971.
70. **Harker, L. A. and Finch, C. A.,** Thrombokinetics in man, *J. Clin. Invest.,* 48, 963, 1969.
71. **Marymount, J. H. and Gross, S.,** Patterns of metastatic cancer in the spleen, *Am. J. Clin. Pathol.,* 40, 58, 1963.
72. **Miale, J. B.,** *Laboratory Medicine Hematology,* C. V. Mosby, St. Louis, 1972, 53.
73. **Gardner, G. F.,** Platelet transfusion, in *Platelets: Production Function, Transfusion, and Storage,* Baldini, M. G. and Elbe, S., Eds., Grune & Stratton, New York, 1974, 393.
74. **Huestis, D. W., Bove, J. R., and Busch, S.,** *Practical Blood Transfusion,* Little, Brown, Boston, 1969.
75. **Cocking, J. B.,** Thrombocytopenic purpura with bronchiogenic carcinoma, *Postgrad. Med. J.,* 42, 521, 1966.
76. **Marmont, A. M., Damasio, E. E., and Gori, E.,** Vinblastine sulphate in idiopathic thrombocytopenic purpura, *Lancet,* 2, 94, 1971.
77. **Ahn, Y. S., Harrington, W. J., and Seelman, R. C.,** Vincristine therapy of idiopathic and secondary thrombocytopenias, *N. Engl. J. Med.,* 291, 376, 1974.
78. **Brooks, J. and Konwaler, B. E.,** Thrombotic thrombocytopenic purpura: association with metastatic gastric carcinoma and a possible autoimmune disorder, *Calif. Med.,* 102, 222, 1965.
79. **Lerner, R. G., Rapaport, S. I., and Meltzer, J.,** Thrombotic thrombocytopenic purpura: serial clotting studies, relations to the generalized Shwartzman reaction and remission after adrenal steroid and dextran therapy, *Ann. Intern. Med.,* 66, 1180, 1967.

80. **Steinberg, A. D., Green, W. T., Jr., and Talal, N.,** Thrombotic thrombocytopenic purpura complicating Sjogren's syndrome, *JAMA*, 215, 757, 1971.
81. **Dekker, A., O'Brien, M. E., and Cammarata, R. J.,** The association of thrombotic thrombocytopenic purpura with systemic lupus erythematosus: a report of two cases with successful treatment of one, *Am. J. Med. Sci.*, 267, 243, 1974.
82. **Rossi, E. C., Redondo, D., and Borges, W. H.,** Thrombotic thrombocytopenic purpura, *JAMA*, 228, 1141, 1974.
83. **Friedman, I. A., Schwartz, S. O., and Leithold, S. L.,** Platelet function defects with bleeding, *Arch. Intern. Med.*, 113, 177, 1964.
84. **Lackner, H.,** Hemostatic abnormalities associated with dysproteinemias, *Sem. Hematol.*, 10, 125, 1973.
85. **Bick, R. L. and Shanbrom, E.,** A systematic approach to the diagnosis of bleeding disorders, *Med. Counterpoint*, 4, 27, 1972.
86. **Bettigole, R. E., Himelstein, E. S., Oettgen, H. F., and Clifford, D. O.,** Hypofibrinogenenia due to L-asparaginase: studies of fibrinogen survival using autologus L-fibrinogen, *Blood*, 35, 195, 1970.
87. **Brodsky, I., Kahn, S. B., Vash, G., Ross, E. M., and Petkov, G.,** Fibrinogen survial with (^{75}Se) selenomethionine during L-asparaginase therapy, *Br. J. Haematol.*, 20, 447, 1971.
88. **Brodsky, I. and Conroy, J. F.,** The effects of chemotherapy of hemostasis, *Cancer Chemother. Rep.*, 2, 85, 1972.
89. **Monto, R. W., Talley, R. W., and Caldwell, M. J.,** Observations of the mechanisms of hemorrhagic toxicity in mithramycin therapy, Cancer Res., 29, 697, 1969.
90. **Olson, R. E.,** Vitamin K-induced prothrombin formation antagonism by actinomycin D, *Science*, 145, 926, 1964.
91. **Bick, R. L., Fekete, L., and Wilson, W. L.,** Adriamycin® and fibrinolysis, *Thromb. Res.*, 8, 467, 1976.
92. **Bick, R. L., Fekete, L., Murano, G., and Wilson, W. L.,** Daunomycin and fibrinolysis, *Thromb. Res.*, 9, 201, 1976.

Chapter 12

MALIGNANCY AND ANTICOAGULATION

William L. Wilson

TABLE OF CONTENTS

I.	Introduction	228
II.	Procoagulants or Fibrinolytics	228
III.	Animal Experiments	228
IV.	Observations in Humans	230
V.	Anticoagulation in Cancer	231
VI.	Summary	231
References		232

I. INTRODUCTION

The effect of coagulation on the development of metastases in the clinical course of patients is at this time poorly understood because of conflicting information. It is well known that certain patients with cancer will have episodes of thrombophlebitis, and, in fact, this may appear before any obvious evidence of malignancy is detectable. In contradistinction, other patients with malignancy will exhibit a subclinical or clinical disseminated intravascular coagulation. These facts, coupled with the observation that a tumor cell can lodge in a fibrin network and penetrate the vascular wall, thereby initiating a metastatic deposit, constitute clearcut accounts of the relationship between coagulation and metastases. Enough data are available to initiate clinical studies involving the use of anticoagulant or fibrinolytic agents in cancer patients.

II. PROCOAGULANTS OR FIBRINOLYTICS

Boggust et al.[1] have studied procoagulants of normal human tissues, as well as human cancerous tissues. These studies indicate that water soluble, heat labile factors in the tumor tissue will promote fibrin formation, thereby indicating that the cells have "thromboplastic" activity. Other workers[2] have demonstrated that cancer cells in tissue culture show a very definite fibrinolytic activity. Salsbury et al.[3] studied excised human tumors and demonstrated that of 28 tumors, 24 showed fibrinolytic activity on fibrin plates. Nineteen of these patients had enhanced fibrinolytic activity in the blood, and circulating malignant cells were present in 18. Four tumor tissue samples showed no evidence of fibrinolytic activity on fibrin plates, but one had fibrinolytic activity in the blood. None of these four patients had any evidence of circulating tumor cells.

Cliffton and Grossi[4] studied a variety of malignant tumors. In breast carcinoma, they found that this tissue would initiate fibrinolysis; however, 11 of 60 tumors examined caused clot lysis without activating plasminogen. They also observed that (1) squamous cell carcinomas do not have significant activator properties, (2) adenocarcinomas of the GI tract activate through the plasminogen-plasmin system, and (3) sarcomas appear to have a high degree of inherent fibrinolytic activity not related to plasmin formation. Therefore, we are left with the situation that tumor cells have both procoagulant and fibrinolytic activity, and the correlation of the two appears difficult in view of the original observations that tumor cells promote fibrin deposition and implantation, resulting in the development of metastases.

III. ANIMAL EXPERIMENTS

Studies done in mice have suggested that either inhibition of coagulation or increasing fibrinolytic activity may have a definite effect on whether or not metastases develop. Cliffton and Agostino[5] studied a series of rats that were treated with heparin or warfarin prior to the injection of Walker 256 carcinoma cells. Results indicated a definite decrease in pulmonary metastases. They later studied the effect of ε-aminocaproic acid (EACA) and Bayer A-128 (as fibrinolytic inhibitors). When these compounds were administered prior to the injection of Walker 256 carcinoma cells, a significant increase in pulmonary metastases was noted. This effect was not counteracted by simultaneous heparin administration. The authors proposed that the cancer cells were rapidly fixed in the capillaries by fibrin or cell "stickiness".

Ryan et al.[6] reported on a series of mice treated with Coumadin®. They were C3H/HeN mice with mammary carcinoma and C57/3L/6N mice with anaplastic sarcoma T241 of Lewis. The mice were started on Coumadin® the second day after transplantation. The prothrombin times were increased between 2.1 and 3.3 times the normal value. Histologic examination showed a statistically significant decrease in the number of pulmonary metastases.

Fisher and Fisher[7] initially reported that heparinization of rats for a period of 4 to 7 days following tumor injections of Walker 256 carcinoma significantly decreased the instance of hepatic metastases. Heparinization at the time of tumor cell injection also caused a significant decrease in the metastases. If the animals were heparinized 4 hr before tumor cell injection and maintained for 4 to 7 days, the incidence of metastases was even lower and, the longer the period (7 days), more significant. They also reported that plasmin injection decreased metastases. This effect was more significant if the plasmin was injected 15 min prior to the tumor injection. However, the same investigators, in a study utilizing the uptake of ^{51}Cr-labeled tumor cells in various organs of rats and rabbits,[8] concluded that heparin, fibrinolysis, and EACA actually had no effect on the development of metastases. Unfortunately, histological studies were not done to confirm that the ^{51}Cr was present on a viable cell.

Boeryd,[9] using CBA mice with methylcholanthrene-induced rhabdomyosarcoma (MCG-1), observed that heparinization decreased pulmonary metastases and increased hepatic metastases, whereas EACA increased the total mass of pulmonary metastases and decreased hepatic metastases. Kudrjashov et al.[10] studied a variety of animals including mice with sarcoma-180, mice with Ehrlich's sarcoma, rats with sarcoma-45, and a dog with a mammary carcinoma. They utilized heparin in one series, a trypsin-activated "fibrinolysin" preparation in another series, and "thrombolytin", which is a combination of heparin and trypsin, in a third series. They also utilized a compound identified as "Aminasin", which is both a sympathetic and parasympathetic blocking agent. Aminasin alone caused regression of tumors. When this was given in conjunction with "fibrinolysin" and "thrombolytin" it caused a decomposition of the tumors, and, in a number of instances, the tumors were completely necrotic with substantial connective tissue infiltration. The use of three agents simultaneously diminished the number of metastases and had a very definite direct antitumor effect in mice and rats, as well as in the dog with spontaneous mammary carcinoma. The dog eventually died of the tumor, but repeat biopsies of various masses did exhibit the changes mentioned.

Regelson,[11] who has studied heparin, heparinoids, and synthetic polyanions extensively, feels that their effect extends considerably beyond anticoagulation. He has observed that they have a regulatory effect on cell growth by affecting a variety of enzymes, surface action, and histone displacement. He also proposes that these compounds play a role in the immunological state of the host, provided the host is not immunosuppressed.

Thornes[12] has reported on effects other than the anticoagulant action of warfarin. He proposes that prolonged administration (over 7 days) paralyses the cell membrane. Withdrawal of warfarin and the administration of vitamin K restores the cell membrane function. This may be correlated with the observation that warfarin is a powerful inhibitor of oxidative phosphorylation, resulting in the loss of readily available high-energy phosphate.[13]

Millar and Ketcham[14] reviewed a large series of studies and concluded that the protective effect of anticoagulation (heparin and warfarin) was dependent on the route of administration, the type of tumor, and the tumor cell load that was given. Tumor loads of 10^3 to 10^5 cells in anticoagulated animals were inhibited from implanting in the first capillary bed encountered (pulmonary for vena cava injection and hepatic for portal vein injection). When tumor loads of 10^5 to 10^6 cells were injected, there was no demonstrable protection with the anticoagulation. They also noted that certain tumors, even when circulating cells could be demonstrated, develop extrapulmonary metastases.

IV. OBSERVATIONS IN HUMANS

It has been known for some time that thrombophlebitis is associated with carcinoma of the pancreas. Gore[15] has observed that carcinoma of the body and the tail of the pancreas is associated with a continuous release of trypsin-like substance into the circulation, resulting in a decrease in multiple coagulation factors. The same is true for metastatic tumors, as well as primary tumors, in the body and tail of the pancreas. The tumor growing in a disrupted glandular bed may lead to a low-grade intravascular coagulopathy, as well as thrombosis.

Fisher et al.[16] have reported four cases of recurrent thrombophlebitis in patients on anticoagulants, all of whom, at a later date, developed lung carcinoma as their primary disease. This was not suspected at the time of the initial episodes of thromboses. Rohner et al.[17] have reported on a series of patients with nonbacterial thrombotic endocarditis. Unfortunately, most of these were diagnosed postmortem, as they all had the sysmptoms of endocarditis, but all had multiple negative blood cultures. This syndrome is seen primarily in patients with mucous-producing carcinomas that include carcinoma of the stomach and lung, as well as pancreas, and also in patients with anaplastic tumors. Cowan and Haut,[18] reporting on patients with acute leukemia, found that the platelet surface reactivity and release mechanism appear to be defective, since bleeding was not related to the platelet count.

Numerous studies on coagulation factors in patients with cancer have been done by Levin and Connelly.[19] A high incidence of thrombocytosis, with platelet counts over 400,000 were noted. They also demonstrated that marrow involvement was not affected, but was noted to occur. This observation has been substantiated by a number of other investigators. Comparative studies on patients with cancer and nonmalignant diseases have revealed accelerated partial thromboplastin times (PTT), as well as increased fibrin(ogen) degradation products (FDP) in patients with cancer. Miller et al.,[20] in a population of 50 patients, found very complex disturbances in hemostasis, mainly, an increase in a number of specific factors, including Factor V, Factor VIII, fibrinogen, platelets, etc. Antithrombin III levels were not significantly altered. They proposed that the most sensitive indicator of hypercoagulability is a siliconized glass clotting time and a recalcification time.

Several studies have demonstrated an increase in fibrinolytic activity. Kwaan et al.[21] demonstrated increased fibrinolytic activity in patients with cirrhosis that was spontaneous. The cirrhotic patients who then developed hepatocellular carcinoma, developed an activity that inhibited the fibrinolytic system. These patients also had fibrinogen levels higher than normal controls. This is in contrast to the work of Salsbury et al.[3] who demonstrated a low fibrinogen and a short euglobulin lysis time in 11 of 30 patients with malignancy. In another series of 36 patients (all exhibiting circulating malignant cells), short euglobulin lysis times were noted, with 32 of the patients exhibiting significant fibrinolytic activity.

Soong and Miller[22] reported nine (of ten) patients with carcinoma having elevated FDP and increased fibrinolytic activity, but only two had clinical episodes of bleeding; both had metastatic carcinoma of the prostate. These same investigators demonstrated the presence of a urokinase inhibitor and felt that this inhibitor was significantly elevated in some patients with cancer. Innerfield et al.[23] studied plasma antithrombin profiles in diseases of the pancreas. They found an increase in plasma "antithrombin" in carcinoma of the head of the pancreas with jaundice and a decrease in plasma "antithrombin" in extensive carcinoma of the pancreas. At that time, techniques differentiating the various antithrombins were not available.

V. ANTICOAGULATION IN CANCER

Clinical studies with regard to anticoagulation in cancer are scarce. Of interest is a series of cardiac patients studied by Michaels.[24] All were receiving anticoagulant therapy, primarily warfarin, for myocardial disease. In reviewing this large series, the author observed the expected number of cancers, but a marked decrease in the expected number of deaths and/or the expected number of patients developing metastatic disease. Elias[25] has reported on the use of large doses of heparin (30,000 to 40,000 units) in patients with lung carcinoma. In this series, patients who had failed to respond to chemotherapy, when treated with heparin for approximately 1 week prior to reinstitution of chemotherapy, responded with a very dramatic antitumor effect.

The most significant report on the use of anticoagulants in malignancy is that of Thornes.[29] A controlled study was done on 128 patients with one of the following malignancies: lymphosarcoma, (non-Hodgkins), carcinoma of the ovary, or carcinoma of the breast. The patients had untreated disseminated cancer and were comparably staged. All had the same chemotherapy, except that alternate patients were placed on warfarin. The prothombin time was increased to one and a half to two times the normal value. All patients were regularly followed by the same physician. The end point of the study was mortality. The warfarin-treated group had a 2 year survival of 40.6% as compared to 17.8% for the control group. It was interesting that, in the breast carcinoma patients on warfarin, a reduction in the dose of cytotoxic agents was possible.

An adjuvant study is currently in progress on patients undergoing curative resections for carcinoma of the colon. A total of 45 of the planned 50 patients have been entered. The patients are randomized at the time of surgery to receive either a saline infusion or a streptokinase infusion over 30 min immediately following resection of the tumor. The study has not been in progress long enough to obtain 5 year survivals, but the results at the time indicated a corrected 5 year survival of 75% for the streptokinase-treated group, as compared to a corrected 5 year survival of 40% for the control group.

That a single dose of streptokinase could induce such a change in survival is difficult to understand. However, the effect of streptokinase on the immune system may provide more information. In the streptokinase-treated patients, the lymphocyte counts fell 32%, as compared to 50% in the control group.

Warfarin has not been used for the clinical trials because of its reported depression of delayed skin hypersensitivity.[30] The finding that fibrinolysis enhances the cellular immune mechanism[31] would make such therapy a more logical choice as an adjuvant in "curative surgery".

VI. SUMMARY

To date, studies demonstrate that (1) tumor cells have both thromboplastic as well as fibrinolytic activity, (2) tumor cells do enmesh in fibrin networks, promoting implantation, platelet aggregation, and thrombus formation and, (3) tumor cells circulate ents with malignancy, but most, apparently do no implant. Various combinations of hemostatic defects occur in cancer patients, including (1) thrombocytosis, (2) increase in Factors V, VIII, and fibrinogen, and (3) increase in fibrinolytic activity. If one relies on the earlier studies in mice and rats, it appears that the institution of anticoagulant (heparin or warfarin) or fibrinolytic therapy reduces the incidence of metastases. This is also observed in humans, as noted by Michaels.[24] The work of Elias[25] appears extremely interesting; however, there have been no reports corraborating his observations.

Recent work has shown that, in vivo, there is a marked increase in fibrinolytic activity with both Adriamycin® and daunomycin[26-28] This property, in itself, may have some bearing on the antineoplastic activity of Adriamycin® and other derivatives of this antibiotic. With the advent of mini-heparin, it would appear that a clinical prospective study with heparinization prior to surgery might be of interest, particularly in postmenopausal breast cancer patients with positive nodes. In this group, Alkeran® does not increase survival, and, possibly, the same is true for the use of Cytoxan®, methotrexate, and 5-fluorouracil, although the results on the latter are not definitive at the present time.

The use of fibrinolytic agents, such as urokinase or streptokinase, with chemotherapy would also be an interesting area to explore. However, each patient would have to be individually screened for urokinase or streptokinase inhibitors.

REFERENCES

1. **Boggust, W. A., O'Brien, D. J., O'Meara, R. A. Q., and Thornes, R. D.,** The coagulative factors of normal human and human cancer tissue, *Ir. J. Med. Sci.*, 6, 131, 1963.
2. **Seeger, R. C., Rayner, S. A., Banerjee, A., Chung, H., Laug, W. E., Neustein, H. B., and Benedict, W. F.,** Morphology, growth, chromosomal pattern, and fibrinolytic activity of two new human neuroblastoma cell lines, *Cancer Res.*, 37, 1364, 1977.
3. **Salsbury, A. J., White, C., Tsolakidis, P., McKinna, J. A., and Griffiths, J. D.,** Fibrinolysis and circulating malignant cells, *Surg. Gynecol. Obstet.*, 136, 733, 1973.
4. **Cliffton, E. E. and Grossi, C. E.,** Fibrinolytic activity of human tumors as measured by the fibrin-plate method, *Cancer (Philadelphia)*, 8, 1146, 1955.
5. **Cliffton, E. E. and Agostino, D.,** Effect of inhibitors of fibrinolytic enzymes on development of pulmonary metastases, *J. Natl. Cancer Inst.*, 33, 753, 1964.
6. **Ryan, J. J., Ketcham, A. S., and Wexler, H.,** Reduced incidence of spontaneous metastases with long-term Coumadin® therapy, *Ann. Surg.*, 168, 163, 1968.
7. **Fisher, B. and Fisher, E. R.,** Experimental studies of factors which influence hepatic metastases. VIII: Effect of anticoagulants, *Surgery*, 50, 240, 1961.
8. **Fisher, B. and Fisher, E. R.,** Anticoagulants and tumor cell lodgement, *Cancer Res.*, 27, 421, 1967.
9. **Boeryd, B.,** Action of heparin and plasminogen inhibitor (EACA) on metastatic tumor spread in a isologous system, *Acta Pathol. Microbiol. Scand.*, 65, 395, 1965.
10. **Krudrjashov, B. A., Kalishevskaya, T. M., and Kolomina, S. M.,** Blood anticoagulating system and malignant tumors, *Nature (London)*, 222, 548, 1969.
11. **Regelson, W.,** The antimitotic activity of polyanions: heparin and heparinoids, *J. Med.*, 5, 50, 1974.
12. **Thornes, R. D.,** Oral anticoagulant therapy of human cancer, *J. Med.*, 5, 83, 1974.
13. **Martius, C. and Nitz-Litzow, D.,** Sum wirkungsmechanismus des Vitamin K, *Biochem. Z.*, 327, 1, 1955.
14. **Millar, R. C. and Ketcham, A. S.,** The effect of heparin and warfarin on primary and metastatic tumors, *J. Med.*, 5, 23, 1974.
15. **Gore, I.,** Thrombosis and pancreatic carcinoma, *Am. J. Pathol.*, 29, 1093, 1953.
16. **Fisher, M. M. Hochberg, L. A., and Wilensky, N. D.,** Recurrent thrombophlebitis in obscure malignant tumor of the lung, *JAMA*, 147, 1213, 1951.
17. **Rohner, R. F., Prior, J. T., and Sipple, J. H.,** Mucinous malignancies, venous thrombosis and terminal endocarditis with emboli, *Cancer (Philadelphia)*, 19, 1805, 1966.
18. **Cowan, D. H. and Haut, M. J.,** Platelet function in acute leukemia, *J. Lab. Clin. Med.*, 79, 893, 1972.
19. **Levin, J. and Conley, C. L.,** Thrombocytosis associated with malignant disease, *Arch. Intern. Med.*, 114, 497, 1964.
20. **Miller, S. P., Sanchez-Avalos, J., Stefanski, T., and Zuckerman, L.,** Coagulation disorders in cancer. I. Clinical and laboratory studies, *Cancer (Philadelphia)*, 20, 1452, 1967.
21. **Kwaan, H. C., Lo, R., and McFadzean, A. J. S.,** Antifibrinolytic activity in primary carcinoma of the liver, *Clin. Sci.*, 18, 251, 1959.

22. **Soong, B. C. F. and Miller, S. P.**, Coagulation disorders in cancer. III. Fibrinolysis and inhibitors, *Cancer (Philadelphia)*, 25, 867, 1970.
23. **Innerfield, I., Angrist, A., and Benjamin, J. W.**, Plasma antithrombin patterns in disturbances of the pancreas, *Gastroenterology*, 19, 843, 1951.
24. **Michaels, L.**, Cancer incidence and mortality in patients having anticoagulant therapy, *Lancet*, 2, 832, 1964.
25. **Elias, G. E.**, Heparin anticoagulation as adjuvant to chemotherapy in carcinoma of the lung, *J. Med.*, 5, 114, 1974.
26. **Bick, R. L., Klein, C. A., Fekete, L. F., and Wilson, W. L.**, Alterations of hemostasis associated with malignant paraprotein disorders, *Trans. Am. Soc. Hematol.*, 163, 1976.
27. **Bick, R. L., Fekete, L. F., and Wilson, W. L.**, Adriamycin® and fibrinolysis, *Thromb. Res.*, 8, 467, 1976.
28. **Bick, R. L., Murano, G., Fekete, L. F., and Wilson, W. L.**, Daunomycin and fibrinolysis, *Thromb. Res.*, 9, 201, 1976.
29. **Thornes, R. D.**, Adjuvant therapy of cancer via the cellular immune mechanism or fibrin by induced fibrinolysis and oral anticoagulants, *Cancer (Philadelphia)*, 35, 91, 1975.
30. **Cohen, S., Benacerraf, B., McCluskey, T., and Ovary, Z.**, Effect of anticoagulants on delayed hypersensitivity reactions *J. Immunol.*, 98, 351, 1966.
31. **Thornes, R. D., Smyth, H., Browne, O., and Holland, P. D. J.**, BCG and Protease I in malignant melanoma, *Lancet*, 1, 1386, 1973.

Hypercoagulability, Thrombosis, and Therapy

Chapter 13

HYPERCOAGULABILITY AND THROMBOSIS

Rodger L. Bick

TABLE OF CONTENTS

I.	Introduction	238
II.	Changes in Blood Flow	238
III.	Changes in the Circulating Blood	238
IV.	Changes in the Vessel Wall	240
V.	Laboratory Diagnosis of Thrombosis Hypercoagulability	241
VI.	Summary	242
References		242

I. INTRODUCTION

Hypercoagulability and thrombosis are poorly understood. Despite "sophistication" in the blood coagulation laboratory and in clinical hemostasis, the etiology of hypercoagulability and thrombosis remains undefined in most instances. At the present time, no satisfactory laboratory modalities exist for the assessment of hypercoagulability, and those available for confirmation of thrombosis are less than ideal. Furthermore, present modalities of hemostasis testing in the laboratory do not allow any conclusions to be made regarding etiology. Therapy, likewise, has been largely empirical. This is to be expected, since we are just beginning to understand etiological aspects and to develop reasonably accurate diagnostic tools for the assessment of these disorders. In general, there are three primary factors in thrombus formation. These are (1) changes in the *blood flow*, (2) changes in the *circulating blood*, and (3) changes in the *vessel wall*.

II. CHANGES IN BLOOD FLOW

With respect to changes in the blood flow, very little is known regarding venous stasis and the initiation of thrombus formation. The most popular theory as to why altered blood flow leads to thrombus formation is that advanced by Hume and co-workers.[1] This hypothesis proposes that during the period of stasis, especially in venous valve pockets, there is activation of Factors XII, XI, and IX. Because of activation of these early "contact activation" factors, there is generation of Factor X_a, which in turn generates thrombin activity, which then propagates thrombus formation via two mechanisms: fibrin formation, and induction of platelet aggregation with a subsequent release of platelet factor 3 and ADP. This then cascades into more platelet aggregation and more blood coagulation. There is no proof, however, that this accounts for most instances of stasis and thrombosis; it is quite possible also that this hypothesis is only one of many potential alterations in coagulation and platelet function that lead to thrombus formation in the face of systemic stasis.

III. CHANGES IN THE CIRCULATING BLOOD

Changes in the circulating blood, both before and after thrombosis, are well defined; however, the meaning of many of these changes remains unclear. Some of these changes are especially difficult to assess because they have been measured after the fact (thrombosis). Table 1 depicts changes in the circulating blood that could, theoretically, lead to hypercoagulability and/or thrombosis.

Increased platelet adhesibility, as measured by a variety of techniques, has been noted in association with various disorders.[2,3] In general, increased platelet adhesion is noted in patients with *acute* thrombosis.[4] However, this has usually been assessed after the fact. It is significant that platelet adhesion is most often normal in patients with aged arterial thrombi, suggesting that platelet adhesion defects play no role in the etiology of these disorders. It has been well documented that increased platelet adhesion is seen in many patients with recurrent deep vein thrombophlebitis.[5] However, again, this has usually been assessed after thrombosis has occurred. The postoperative state is known to be associated with an increased incidence of thrombosis, and in a general surgical postoperative population, increased platelet adhesion can usually be measured.[6] Likewise, in the postpartum state, the risk of thrombosis is increased, and in many postpartum females increased platelet adhesion can be demonstrated. Increased platelet adhesion is noted in many patients with malignancy (Chapter 11).

TABLE 1

Changes in the Circulating Blood Which May Lead to Hypercoagulability and/or Thrombosis (Hemostatic System)

Increased platelet adhesion
Increased coagulation factors
Decreased coagulation inhibitors
Decreased fibrinolytic activity
Increased fibrinolytic inhibitors
Increased lipids

Interestingly, studies have now shown increased platelet adhesion in patients with diabetes mellitus;[7] of course, this disorder is often fraught with thrombus formation. It has also been reported that increased platelet adhesion is noted in many individuals with atherosclerosis.

It remains controversial, however, as to whether any correlation exists between increased platelet adhesion and the incidence of actual clinical thrombosis. The only conclusion that may be drawn is that this change is probably an important predisposing factor in thrombosis, especially when coupled with other changes in coagulation. Evidence that increased platelet adhesion actually *causes* clinical thrombosis is still lacking.[8]

Changes in circulating coagulation factors have also been well documented in both thrombosis and situations leading to thrombosis. Increased coagulation factors are often noted postoperatively, as well as in the postpartum period, in patients suffering fractures or trauma, in ulcerative colitis, in malignancy, in acute thrombosis, and in recurrent deep vein thrombophlebitis.[9-11] Like the finding of increased platelet adhesion, however, many increases in coagulation factors that have been described have been measured after the fact, and the significance of this finding remains unclear. The coagulation factors most commonly increased in the above-mentioned disorders are fibrinogen, Factor VIII, Factor V, and Factor VII, and many investigators have measured "increased thromboplastin generation".[12]

It must be emphasized, however, that there is very poor correlation between any individual increased clotting factor and the development of clinical thrombosis. Factor VIII and fibrinogen are the coagulation factors most often noted to be increased and are found to be increased in pregnancy, chronic inflammation, malignancy, postoperatively, and in intravascular hemolysis. All of these situations are associated with an increased incidence of thrombosis.

Decreased coagulation inhibitors are noted in many disorders associated with thrombus formation — specifically, the major physiological anticoagulant Antithrombin III (heparin cofactor, Factor X_a inhibitor). All are familiar with hereditary thrombophilia in which there is a hereditary decrease in Antithrombin III (AT-III). These patients usually begin to suffer widespread and life-threatening deep vein thrombosis in their teenage years.[13] In most disorders associated with acute thrombosis, AT-III has been found to be decreased. However, this has usually been measured after the fact, and it is unclear as to whether this has played an etiological role or is simply due to consumption in the clotting process.[14] Several reports have confirmed a decrease in AT-III following acute myocardial infarction.[15,16] In general, postoperative patients have decreased levels of AT-III, but the significance of this remains unclear.[17] Numerous investigators have shown clearcut decreases in AT-III in women using oral contraceptives; this is thought to be of etiological significance in thrombus formation in these individuals.[18,19] Interestingly, AT-III levels are reported as normal in most instances of recurrent deep vein thrombophlebitis.

Decreased fibrinolytic activity and decreased fibrinolytic activator activity, at least in theory, predisposes to thrombus formation. It should be recalled that plasminogen, the precursor of plasmin, is synthesized in the liver; however, it appears that the majority of physiologically important plasminogen activator activity is from vascular endothelium.[20] Hypoactivity and predisposition to thrombus formation can arise from either decreased plasminogen levels, decreased plasminogen activator activity, or increased fibrinolytic inhibitor activity. Decreased fibrinolytic activity has been noted in acute myocardial infarction,[21] as well as in patients with generalized atherosclerosis.[22] In this latter condition, this may be due to intimal damage and the loss of fibrinolytic activator activity.

Decreased fibrinolytic activity is present in diabetes[23] and in acute pulmonary embolism; in the latter, whether this is of etiological significance or simply due to consumption remains unclear. In general, decreased fibrinolytic activity is noted in recurrent deep vein thrombophlebitis, as well as in most patients in the postoperative state.[24]

Increased inhibitors of fibrinolytic activity are noted in numerous disorders. The primary inhibitors of fibrinolytic activity are alpha-2-macroglobulin, alpha-1-antitrypsin, and alpha-2-antiplasmin. The former two are found to be increased in pulmonary fibrosis, malignancy, infections, acute myocardial infarction, and in thromboembolism.[25] In addition, alpha-2-macroglobulin and alpha-1-antitrypsin are increased in the postoperative state as well as in pregnancy, diabetes, and in users of oral contraceptives.

Inhibitors of the fibrinolytic system are normal in most individuals with recurrent deep vein thrombophlebitis. As with other changes in the circulating blood, the finding of increased inhibitors of fibrinolytic activity (alpha-2-macroglobulin and alpha-1-antitrypsin) has usually been noted after the fact, and it remains speculative as to whether this plays an actual etiological role or whether it is due to an "acute phase reaction".[26]

Many disorders are associated with increased fibrinolytic activator inhibition as measured by a variety of techniques, most commonly the heated fibrin plate. There is inhibition of fibrinolytic activator activity in the postoperative state, in infections, and in general inflammatory disorders.[27] However, there is no detectable inhibition against fibrinolytic activator activity in patients suffering acute thrombosis.

It can only be concluded that, in general, reactive processes are associated with thrombosis and *hypo*fibrinolysis, the latter coming about through several mechanisms: (1) decreased plasminogen, (2) decreased plasminogen activator activity, (3) increased fibrinolytic inhibitors, and (4) increased plasminogen activator inhibition. The significance of these findings remains completely unclear, as it is not known whether many of these changes were present prior to thrombus formation and thus potentially etiological or whether they simply developed as a consequence of thrombosis.

It has been suggested that increased lipids predispose to thrombus formation.[28] However, this subject is controversial and fraught with much conflicting evidence.

IV. CHANGES IN THE VESSEL WALL

Changes in the vessel wall are probably the most common etiologic factors in arterial thrombus formation.[29,30] These changes can come about via numerous mechanisms. Collagen can be exposed by local injury to the vessel as well as by inflammatory vascular changes. Exposed collagen has the capacity to initiate platelet aggregation, as well as activate the blood coagulation system through the generation of Factor XII_a.[31] In addition, decreased fibrinolytic activator activity is expected, and indeed found, in many vascular disorders. It is significant that there is much less plasminogen activator activity in the lower extremities as compared to the upper extremities, and this may account for, or at least contribute to, the higher incidence of thrombosis in the lower extremities.[32] Decreased fibrinolytic activator activity is found in approximately 75% of patients who have recurrent deep vein thrombophlebitis, and this is often ascribed to primary vascular damage. The significance of this, however, remains unclear.

V. LABORATORY DIAGNOSIS OF THROMBOSIS AND HYPERCOAGULABILITY

The laboratory diagnosis of thrombosis and hypercoagulability is in its infancy. Despite recent advances in the coagulation laboratory, there are nevertheless very few tools that will either confirm a hypercoagulable state or confirm thrombosis. The findings of increased fibrin(ogen) degradation products only allow for conclusions that fibrinolysis is occurring, presumably secondary to thrombus formation. The measurement of plasminogen and plasmin often gives meaningful data; depleted plasminogen is suggestive of thrombus formation or may be of etiological significance in thrombus formation. In addition, the finding of circulating plasmin is highly suggestive of fibrinolysis secondary to thrombosis. A shortened kaolin-activated PTT (less than 25 sec) may have significance in detecting patients who are hypercoagulable.[33] Accelerated silicone and glass clotting times or accelerated thrombin time or reptilase time may also be indicative of hypercoagulability or recent thrombus formation. Paracoagulation reactions utilizing either protamine sulfate or ethanol gelation are both indicative of the presence of soluble fibrin monomer (Chapter 8), the presence of which is strongly suggestive of either disseminated intravascular coagulation or significant thrombus formation. The role of soluble fibrin monomer in hypercoagulability before thrombus occurs, however, is unclear. The measurement of AT-III levels may be of significance in detecting patients who are hypercoagulable. This is especially necessary to rule out hereditary thrombophilia in young patients who suffer recurrent deep vein thrombophlebitis and who have a strong family history.

A recent advance in the diagnosis of both thrombosis and hypercoagulability has been the development of fibrinogen chromatography.[34,35] Much useful data have come from this modality, and it is quite likely that this will become a highly applicable and readily available clinical tool within the next several years. The procedure has now been automated to the point that it can be done in several hours; however, the equipment required is still quite expensive. Fibrinogen chromatography, used clinically, is able to detect several fibrinogen subspecies:

1. Fibrin monomer (molecular weight of approximately 320,000) is fibrinogen minus fibrinopeptide-A and fibrinopeptide-B, i.e., it represents fibrinogen that has been acted upon by thrombin.
2. Fibrinogen dimer has a molecular weight of approximately 650,000 and represents one intact fibrinogen molecule complexed with one fibrin monomer.
3. Fibrinogen polymer (molecular weight of approximately 400,000 up to one million) represents fibrinogen complexed with various fibrin/fibrinogen fragments.
4. Fibrinogen first derivative (molecular weight of 267,000) represents the fibrinogen molecule that has been cleaved at the COOH end of the A-alpha chain by plasmin.

The applicability of fibrinogen chromatography becomes evident when looking at those disorders that are characterized by the presence of fibrinogen dimer and fibri-

TABLE 2

States Characterized by Increased Fibrinogen Dimer and Polymer

Deep vein thrombophlebitis
Oral contraceptive users
Pulmonary emboli
Cerebrovascular thrombosis
Myocardial infarction

nogen polymer. Table 2 depicts states characterized by increased fibrinogen dimer and polymer. In addition, fibrinogen chromatography may play an important role in monitoring patients with thrombus formation.

In general, thrombosis is characterized by an increase in fibrinogen-fibrin complexes of molecular weight of 450,000 or greater, and, when these fragments are found, one may be sure that thrombosis has occurred. As the thrombus resolves, secondary to fibrinolysis, the following will be noted: (1) a decrease in fibrinogen-fibrin complexes, (2) an increase in FDP, and (3) an increase in fibrinogen first derivative. One study has shown fibrinogen chromatography to be of significance in the prognosis of acute myocardial infarction. In this study, an increase in fibrinogen dimer was considered to be abnormal if it accounted for more than 20% of the total fibrinogen present.[36] About 50% of patients had abnormal fibrinogen patterns for approximately 3 days, which then normalized; 30% had fibrinogen dimer that persisted for longer than 10 days; 20% had no abnormality in fibrinogen patterns. Those 30% of patients with abnormal patterns that persisted for longer than 10 days tended to fair most poorly. It is interesting to note that the addition of heparin and/or warfarin during the post myocardial infarction course did *not* alter the fibrinogen chromatographic profiles.

VI. SUMMARY

This chapter has summarized known alterations of hemostasis in the hypercoagulable patient and in the patient undergoing thrombus formation. It remains unclear as to whether these alterations are of etiologic significance or are manifestations (consequences) of already present, and perhaps clinically undetectable, thrombus formation. At present, common laboratory modalities do not allow for a differentiation between "cause and effect". Hopefully, in the near future, *practical* techniques that detect fibrin(ogen) derivatives and fibrinopeptides will be developed for (1) diagnosing thrombosis, (2) monitoring the patient who has suffered a thrombosis, and (3) detecting a predesposition to thrombosis.

REFERENCES

1. **Hume, M., Sevitt, S., and Thomas, D. P.,** *Venous Thrombosis and Pulmonary Embolism,* Harvard University Press, Cambridge, 1970.
2. **Hellem, A. J.,** Platelet adhesiveness, *Ser. Haematol.,* 1, 99, 1968.
3. **Hume, M. and Chan, Y. K.,** Examination of the blood in the presence of venous thrombosis, *JAMA,* 200, 747, 1967.
4. **Bobek, K., and Kepelak, V.,** Laboratory diagnosis of venous thrombosis, *Acta Med. Scand.,* 160, 121, 1958.

5. Isacson, S. and Nilsson, I. M., Coagulation and platelet adhesiveness in recurrent "idiopathic" venous thrombosis and thrombophlebitis, *Acta Chir. Scand.*, 138, 263, 1972.
6. Emmons, P. R. and Mitchell, J. R. A., Post-operative changes in platelet-clumping activity, *Lancet*, 1, 71, 1965.
7. Hellum, A. J., Adenosine diphosphate induced platelet adhesiveness in diabetes mellitus with complications, *Acta Med. Scand.*, 190, 291, 1971.
8. Becker, J., The relation of platelet adhesiveness to post-operative venous thrombosis of the legs, *Acta Chir. Scand.*, 138, 781, 1972.
9. Davidson, E. and Tomlin, S., The levels of the plasma coagulation factors after trauma and childbirth, *J. Clin. Pathol.*, 16, 112, 1963.
10. Nicolaides, A. N. and Irving, D., Clinical factors and the risk of deep venous thrombosis, in *Thromboembolism: Etiology, Advances in Prevention and Management*, Nicolaides, A. N., Ed., University Park Press, Baltimore, 1975, 193.
11. Nilsson, I. M., Thrombosis and treatment of thrombosis, in *Hemorrhagic and Thrombotic Diseases*, Nilsson, I. M., Ed., John Wiley & Sons, New York, 1974, 163.
12. Davis, R. B., Theologides, A., and Kennedy, B. J., Comparative studies of blood coagulation and platelet aggregation in patients with cancer and non-malignant disease, *Ann. Intern. Med.*, 71, 67, 1969.
13. Egeberg, O., Thrombophilia caused by inheritable deficiency of blood antithrombin, *Scand. J. Clin. Lab. Invest.*, 17, 92, 1965.
14. Bick, R. L., Dukes, M. L., and Fekete, L. F., AT-III as a diagnostic aid in disseminated intravascular coagulation, *Thromb. Res.*, 10, 721, 1977.
15. von Kaulla, E. and von Kaulla, K. N., Antithrombin-III and diseases, *Am. J. Clin. Pathol.*, 48, 69, 1967.
16. Yue, R. H., Gertler, M. M., Starr, T., and Koutrouby, R., Alteration of plasma antithrombin-III levels in ischemic heart disease, *Thromb. Haemostas.*, 35, 598, 1976.
17. Bergstrom, K. and Lahnborg, G., The effect of major surgery, low doses of heparin and thromboembolism on plasma antithrombin. Comparison of immediate thrombin inhibiting capacity and the antithrombin-III content, *Thromb. Res.*, 6, 223, 1975.
18. Conrad, J., Samama, M., and Soloman, Y., Antithrombin-III and the estrogen content of combined estro-progesterone contraceptives, *Lancet*, 1, 1148, 1972.
19. Fagerhol, M. K., Abildgaard, R., Bergsjo, P., and Jacobson, J. N., Oral contraceptives and low antithrombin-III concentration, *Lancet*, 1, 1175, 1970.
20. Verstraete, M., The place of long-term stimulation of the endogenous fibrinolytic system: present achievements and clinical perspectives, in *Progress in Chemical Fibrinolysis and Thrombolysis*, Vol. 1, Davidson, J. F., Samama, M. M., and Desnoyers, P. C., Eds., Raven Press, New York, 1975, 289.
21. Bick, R. L., Bishop, R. C., and Shanbrom, E., Fibrinolytic activity in acute myocardial infarction, *Am. J. Clin. Pathol.*, 57, 359, 1972.
22. Naims, S., Goldstein, R., and Proger, S., Studies of coagulation and fibrinolysis of arterial and venous blood in normal subjects and patients with atherosclerosis, *Circulation*, 27, 904, 1963.
23. Almer, L. D., Pandolfi, M., and Osterlin, S., The fibrinolytic system in patients with diabetes mellitus with special reference to diabetic retinopathy, *Opthalmologica*, 170, 353, 1975.
24. Mansfield, A. O., Alterations in fibrinolysis associated with surgery and venous thrombosis, *Br. J. Surg.*, 59, 754, 1972.
25. Ganrot, P. O., Studies on serum protease inhibitors with special reference to α-2 macroglobulin, *Acta Univ. Lund. Sect. 2*, 2, 2, 1967.
26. Fischer, C. L. and Gill, L. W., Acute phase proteins, in *Serum Protein Abnormalities*, Ritzmann, S. E. and Daniels, J. C., Eds., Little, Brown, Boston, 1975, 331.
27. Hedner, U. and Nilsson, L. M., Urokinase inhibitors in serum in a clinical series, *Acta Med. Scan.*, 189, 185, 1971.
28. Wessler, S., Factors in the initiation of deep venous thrombosis, in *Thromboembolism: Etiology, Advances in Prevention and Management*, Nicolaides, A. N., Ed., University Park Press, Baltimore, 1975, 9.
29. Spaet, T. H. and Erichson, R. B., The Vascular Wall in the Pathogenesis of Thrombosis, in *Proc. 2nd Int. Conf. Thromb., Basel*, 1965, 67.
30. Stemerman, M. B., Vascular intimal components: precursors of thrombosis, *Prog. Hemostasis Thromb.*, 2, 1, 1974.
31. Wilner, G. D., Nossel, H. L., and Le Roy, E. C., Activation of Hageman factor by collagen, *J. Clin. Invest.*, 47, 2608, 1968.
32. Nilsson, I. M. and Pandolfi, M., Fibrinolytic response of the vascular wall, *Thromb. Diath. Haemorrh.*, 40, 231, 1970.

33. **Bick, R. L. and Fekete, L. F.**, personal observations.
34. **Fletcher, A. P. and Alkjaersig, N.**, Blood hypercoagulability, intravascular coagulation, and thrombosis: new diagnostic concepts, *Thromb. Diath. Haemorrh.*, 45, 389, 171.
35. **Alkjaersig, N., Roy, L., and Fletcher, A. P.**, Analysis of gel exclusion chromatography data by chromatographic plate theory analysis: application to plasma fibrinogen chromatography, *Thromb. Res.*, 3, 525, 1973.
36. **Fletcher, A. P. and Alkjaersig, N.**, Laboratory diagnosis of intravascular coagulation, in *Recent Advances in Thrombosis,* Poller, L., Ed., Churchill Livingstone, London, 1973, 87.

Chapter 14

ANTICOAGULANT AND ANTIPLATELET THERAPY

Rodger L. Bick

TABLE OF CONTENTS

I.	Introduction	246
II.	Oral Anticoagulants	246
	A. Mechanisms of Action	246
	B. Clinical Aspects	246
	C. Laboratory Monitoring	248
	D. Clinical Trials and Indications	248
III.	Heparin and "Mini-Dose" Heparin	249
	A. Mechanisms of Action	249
	B. Clinical Aspects	250
	C. Laboratory Monitoring	251
	D. Clinical Trials and Indications	252
IV.	Antiplatelet Agents	252
	A. Mechanisms of Action	253
	B. Clinical Aspects	254
	C. Laboratory Monitoring	254
	D. Clinical Trials and Indications	255
V.	Summary	256

References 256

I. INTRODUCTION

Anticoagulant therapy is in a state of revolution, with many new techniques and dosages of various anticoagulant and antiplatelet agents being subjected to numerous multicentered, double-blind prospective randomized trials. At the same time, many earlier and more traditional thoughts regarding anticoagulant therapy are having to be abandoned because of results of recent work. In addition, the results may be markedly different, depending upon the particular method used as an end point of a clinical trial, i.e., whether it be clinical thrombosis, ^{125}I-fibrinogen scanning, Doppler ultrasound, impedence plethysmography, or thromboscintograms. The modalities useful for the diagnosis of thrombotic disease are listed in Table 1. The advantages and disadvantages of these techniques are listed in Table 2.

In attempting to choose an appropriate anticoagulant or antiplatelet agent, as well as an appropriate dose, one should *always* keep in mind the fact that anticoagulant or antiplatelet agents, in any form, function *only prophylactically*, preventing further thrombus propagation, thrombosis, or thromboembolism. The initiation of anticoagulant or antiplatelet therapy does not ameliorate the existing disease. It is with this very important concept in mind that anticoagulant therapy will be reviewed. For the most part, this discussion will be limited to indications and doses suggested by prospective randomized double-blind clinical trials.

II. ORAL ANTICOAGULANTS

The oral anticoagulants are of two types, the coumarins and the indanedione derivatives. Both are vitamin K antagonists (VKAs). Subgroups of VKAs will not be discussed.

A. Mechanisms of Action

All of the VKAs interfere with the normal synthesis of the prothrombin complex factors: Factors II, VII, IX, and X. Current evidence suggests that the function of vitamin K is to attach calcium-binding prosthetic groups postribosomally on the amino terminal regions of these four prothrombin complex factors.[1,2] The calcium-binding prosthetic groups have been identified as gamma-carboxyglutamic acid.[3] In the absence of vitamin K, i.e., in patients undergoing any type of VKA therapy, Factors II, VII, IX, and X are synthesized, but are incomplete, lacking the specific calcium-binding sites, and thus unable to function as procoagulants. However, they are present in plasma in normal immunological concentrations (Chapter 3).

B. Clinical Aspects

In general, 100% of VKAs are absorbed from the gastrointestinal tract and are bound to plasma albumin. The onset of action is between 8 and 12 hr, with a maximum effect occurring in approximately 36 hr. The duration of action as an anticoagulant is approximately 72 hr.[4] It should be noted that Factor VII activity decreases most rapidly and best correlates with the prothrombin time determination. However, Factor IX and Factor X depression best correlates with both the anticoagulant effect, as well as the undesirable and serious side effect of hemorrhage.[5] VKAs do cross the placenta and should not be used in pregnant women.

Loading doses of VKAs were used in the past, but are no longer indicated. A loading dose simply serves to accelerate the abnormal synthesis of Factor VII, not Factors II, IX, and X.[6] Again, it is to be recalled that Factor VII best correlates with the prothrombin time determination, but correlates least with clinical effectiveness or pro-

TABLE 1

Methods for Diagnosis of Deep Venous Thrombosis

Clinical examination
^{125}I-Fibrinogen scans
Doppler ultrasonography
Impedence plethysmography
Venograms
Thromboscintograms

TABLE 2

Advantages and Disadvantages of Various Methods Used for the Diagnosis of Deep Venous Thrombosis

Method	Reliability	Clinical usefulness	Comments
^{125}I-Fibrinogen test	High, except for lesions above groin area	Extremely valuable for evaluating recurrent thrombophlebitis; Follow the migration of thrombosis	Time consuming; risk of hepatitis; false positive result from hematoma; no value above the inguinal ligament
Doppler ultrasound	High, except for lesions below the knee	In experienced centers, recommended for diagnosing initial thrombophlebitis	Results affected by collateral circulation and venous recanalization
Venography	High, except for soleal sinuses	Confirmation of diagnosis unable to be established by other noninvasive techniques	Painful and time consuming; allergic reactions
Impedence plethysmography	Low	Repeatedly normal tests probably exclude major deep vein thrombosis	Lack of reproducibility; numerous false positive and negative results
Thromboscintograms	High	Highly valuable for evaluating recurrent thrombophlebitis	Advantage is that pulmonary ventilation/perfusion scan for pulmonary embolus can be simultaneously performed

pensity to hemorrhage. VKAs are fraught with side effects, the most frequently encountered being hemorrhage, most commonly from the genitourinary tract. However, any site, including vital organs, is subject to serious hemorrhage,[7] which is quite usual in the patient treated with VKAs in the presence of the usual contraindications to anticoagulant therapy, e.g., malignant hypertension, ingestion of agents known to interfere with hemostasis, peptic ulcer disease, or a defect in hemostasis. This is often not the case with patients receiving heparin. An additional side effect, although rare, is "rebound thrombosis", which occurs primarily after cessation (for bleeding complications) of therapy.[8] An extremely rare idiosyncratic reaction, which can be quite serious, is that of a small vessel vasculitis that gives rise to skin necrosis and a violatious rash. The clinical and pathological features of this have been well described.[9,10]

C. Laboratory Monitoring

During recent years much new information has appeared in the literature, providing guidelines for adequate monitoring of oral anticoagulant therapy. However, many laboratories are still not adopting newer techniques. It has been documented that reporting prothrombin times in "percent activity" has little or no meaning. This can be readily appreciated in view of the described mechanism of action of VKAs and by asking the question: percent activity of what: Factor II, Factor VII, Factor IX, or Factor X? In addition, it has been shown that comparing percent activity has no meaning when using two different reagents, two different coagulation instruments, or when two different technicians perform the assay. However, the reporting of a prothrombin time as a "prothrombin index"* has been shown to be reasonably comparable between two laboratories, two technicians, two different reagents, and two different instruments. Thus most studies have advocated the use of a prothrombin index rather than percent activity.[11-13] In general, an adequate therapeutic range is defined as a prothrombin time, which is 1.5 to 2.5 times the base line value, thus the prothrombin index is 1.5 to 2.5. Hemorrhage rarely occurs if the prothrombin index is less than 2.5 to 3.0.

When changing therapy from heparin to VKA, the regimen is quite simple and well established. Some overlap is needed since there is a delayed onset of action with VKAs in the heparinized patients. Exact adjustment of a prothrombin index must be empirical. The usual procedure is to start a heparinized patient on VKAs at 10 to 15 mg/day for 2 to 3 days and to cease heparin therapy when the prothrombin index is greater than 1.5. It should be recalled that 0.75 units of heparin per milliliter prolongs the prothrombin time.

There are many drugs that interact with VKAs. Many of these potentiate the activity and others interfere with the activity of VKAs. In addition, VKAs may enhance the action of other drugs. The most common drugs interacting with VKAs are depicted in Table 3. More complete lists have been published.[14,15]

D. Clinical Trials and Indications

In the past, VKAs have been used widely in patients with acute myocardial infarction (MI). The only rationale for their use in these individuals is to: (1) prevent venous thrombosis and thromboembolism while at bed rest and (2) prevent reinfarction. Several early reports showed significant differences between mortality, reinfarction rate, thromboembolic disease following MI, and recurrent MI in patients treated with VKAs vs. those not treated.[16] However, recent prospective trials have failed to show any significant difference in mortality, reinfarction rate, or thromboembolic complications.[17]

Many uncontrolled trials encompassing a variety of thrombotic and thromboembolic disorders (including patients considered at "high risk" for thromboembolic disease) have been conducted. Unfortunately, it is impossible to draw any conclusions from these studies, since they have been retrospective, uncontrolled, nonrandomized, and no uniform dose used. Numerous randomized prospective trials (although not double-blind) have been conducted. Most of these studies addressed a variety of disorders, including pulmonary embolization, recurrent deep vein thrombophlebitis, and transient cerebral ischemic attacks. Results indicate a trend in decreased mortality in many

---

* A prothrombin index is obtained by dividing the control time into the patient's time.

TABLE 3

Drug Interactions with Vitamin K Antagonists (VKA)

Drugs that may potentiate VKA effect	Drugs that may inhibit VKA effect	Drugs whose action may be enhanced by VKA
Anabolic steroids	Barbiturates	Diphenylhydantoin
Broad spectrum antibiotics	Corticosteroids	Chlorpropamide
Chloral hydrate	Cholestyramine	Tolbutamide
Chloramphenicol	Etchlorvynol	
Clofibrate	Glutethimide	
Disulfiram	Griseofulvin	
Ethacrynic acid	Haloperidol	
Glucagon	Meprobamate	
Mefenamic acid	Oral contraceptives	
Methlyphenidate	Rifampin	
Quinine		
Quinidine		
Vitamin E		

"high risk" patients and, to a lesser extent, a trend in decreased pulmonary embolization, recurrent deep vein thrombophlebitis, and thromboembolic disease, depending on the end point used.[18-21]

It can only be concluded that the efficacy of VKAs in thromboembolic disease is questionable. In addition, the contraindications, expense in monitoring, and the risk of hemorrhage is now leading many physicians to rely more heavily on heparin for immediate prophylaxis and antiplatelet agents for long-term prophylaxis of patients at high risk for thrombosis.

III. HEPARIN AND "MINI-DOSE" HEPARIN

A. Mechanisms of Action

As discussed in Chapter 3, Antithrombin III (heparin cofactor) functions as the major modulator of thrombin and other serine protease-activity. Heparin accelerates the activity of Antithrombin III (AT-III) by several orders of magnitude. This is recognized as the primary mechanism by which heparin functions as an anticoagulant. To understand the mechanism of action of heparin and the rationale for the use of medical dose heparin and "mini-dose" heparin therapy, several kinetic studies need to be considered. The elegant studies of Yin[22] have shown that, in the absence of heparin, 2 μg of AT-III will inhibit 1 unit of Factor X_a. In the presence of heparin, at a concentration of 0.01 unit/mℓ, 1 μg of AT-III will inhibit 15 units of Factor X_a. Since 1 unit of Factor X_a can generate 50 units of thrombin, 1 μg of AT-III is able to inhibit the eventual generation of 750 units of thrombin. These kinetics are depicted in Tables 4 and 5. The rationale for mini-dose heparin therapy is to deliver small doses of heparin that will inhibit the generation of Factor X_a in situations associated with hypercoagulability. In addition, it should be considered that mini-dose heparin therapy might also be efficacious in any thrombotic disorder, since once Factor X_a generation has been inhibited, the generation of thrombin is no longer possible. Thus medical dose heparin therapy, conceivably may become absolete and subcutaneous or intravenous mini-dose heparin therapy may become the modality of choice in the prophylaxis of many thrombotic disorders.

TABLE 4

Heparin and AT-III Activity

Without heparin
  2 μg AT-III inhibits 1 unit Factor X_a
With Heparin (0.01 unit/ml)
  1 μg AT-III inhibits 15 units Factor X_a
Therefore, at 0.01 unit/ml, heparin accelerates AT-III activity × 30

TABLE 5

Kinetics of Heparin and AT-III (The Basis of Heparin and "Mini-Dose" Heparin Therapy)

1 unit Factor X_a generates 50 units thrombin
1 μg AT-III inhibits 15 units Factor X_a (in the presence of heparin at 0.01 unit/ml)
Therefore, 1 μg AT-III, in the presence of heparin, is able to potentially inhibit the generation of 750 units of thrombin

B. Clinical Aspects

Heparin can be administered by several routes, depending upon the desired effect. The most commonly used has been intravenous infusion. This has the advantage of an immediate onset of action. It requires constant infusion. Clinical data obtained by Estes and Paulin[23] have shown that if intravenous pushes are to be given, heparin must be given at 1.5 hr intervals to maintain a constant "therapeutic" blood level. Figure 1 depicts these data. Another popular route of heparin administration is subcutaneous injection, which is delivered as mini-dose heparin.

In general, medical dose heparin is administered in a dose of 20,000 to 30,000 units/24 hr by constant infusion. This provides a plasma heparin level of between 2.5 to 5 units/ml. When administered subcutaneously, the usual heparin level is between 0.1 and 1 unit/ml. Subcutaneous mini-dose heparin, in general, is delivered at 2500 to 5000 unit every 6 to 12 hr. It need not be given only in the anterior abdominal wall; in fact, alternating injection sites in any subcutaneous tissue is desirable and more comfortable for the patient. Heparin administered intramuscularly is not recommended, since it can quite often lead to serious intramuscular hematomas. European trials[24] have shown that heparin by inhalation will also provide a very adequate plasma heparin level that appears to be efficacious in thrombotic or thromboembolic disease. During cardiopulmonary bypass surgery, heparin is often used at doses that provide a 10- to 100-fold therapeutic plasma concentration.[25]

It should be noted that no laboratory test, including the activated partial thromboplastin time, activated clotting time, whole blood recalcification time, or thrombin time offer any predictability of hemorrhage. Spontaneous bleeding is rare with heparin therapy. The majority of bleeds are seen in situations in which there is a general contraindication to anticoagulant therapy, such as peptic ulcer disease, malignant hypertension, a defect in hemostasis, or the simultaneous ingestion of antiplatelet agents. Occasionally, hematuria is seen in elderly females;[26] however, this side effect is not a contraindication for continued therapy. An idiosyncratic reaction of thrombocytopenia due to heparin-induced in vivo platelet aggregation was considered extremely rare until a recent study suggested that it is not as uncommon as previously thought.[27] An additional complication of heparin therapy in the past has been osteoporosis.[28]

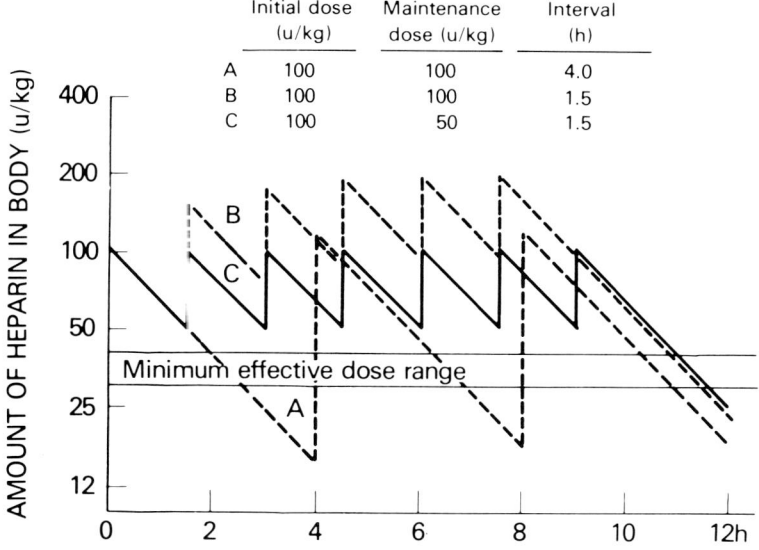

FIGURE 1. Half-life (T ½) of heparin administered as intermittent intravenous push. (From Estes, J. W. and Paulin, P. F., *Thromb. Diath. Haemorrh.*, 33, 26, 1975. With permission.)

However, this occurs only when heparin is used for a period of greater than 6 months and at 10,000 units/day minimum dose. This dosage regimen is rarely used anymore, and thus osteoporosis is rarely, if ever, seen. Heparin, unlike VKAs, does *not* cross the placenta and may be used in pregnant women. About 80% of heparin is degraded by the liver and 20% by the kidney; thus in liver or kidney failure, appropriate adjustments in dosage should be made, especially when using medical doses.

C. Laboratory Monitoring

It has been demonstrated by numerous investigators that the activated partial thromboplastin time, as well as other general screening tests of hemostasis, do *not* correlate with plasma heparin concentration.[29,30] This is quite understandable, since the efficacy of heparin therapy depends upon the heparin/AT-III/thrombin and other serine proteases/fibrinogen axis (COAX)*, and no test measures all these factors simultaneously. With the Lee-White clotting time, an adequate dose of heparin is empirically defined as a clotting time that is 1.5 to 2.5 times the base line value. This modality has several disadvantages. The test must be done at the bedside immediately after the blood is drawn, it is highly questionable in reliability, and offers no information about overdose. At approximately 45 min the test becomes influenced by liquid-air surface interactions, and the result bears little relation to plasma contents.

The activated partial thromboplastin time was developed as a screening test for hemophilia and was never intended to be used for monitoring heparin therapy.[31] Numerous studies have shown that there is no correlation between an activated partial thromboplastin time and plasma heparin concentration.[29-31] This is understandable, since the test depends upon the COAX described above, and much of the variability may be attributed to varying concentrations of AT-III in thrombotic disorders.[32] At about 100 sec, the test becomes dependent on reagents used rather than the patient's plasma con-

---

* Coagulant-anticoagulant axis (COAX).

stituents; thus adjustments of heparin dosages based upon times of greater than 100 sec is meaningless. In addition, only citrated blood can be used. An adequate time has been empirically defined as 1.5 to 2.5 times the base line value. Likewise, the thrombin time also has disadvantages in monitoring heparin therapy; it is too sensitive. The clotting time becomes prolonged-infinite with small to moderate doses of heparin.

In summary, no test offers predictability of "overdose"* and hemorrhage from heparinization. However, all of the aforementioned tests, including the activated clotting time, will allow one to conclude that the patient *has* responded to heparin therapy. There are two laboratory modalities that may prove helpful. Plasma heparin concentrations, including "mini-dose" can be easily determined by a heparin assay.[33] In addition, biological AT-III levels can be determined. This allows one to predict heparin efficacy.[34] When administering intravenous heparin, the author's method is to obtain an activated partial thromboplastin time approximately 30 to 60 min after initiation of therapy. If the test becomes prolonged, it can then be concluded that adequate amounts of AT-III are present to allow heparin to be efficacious. There are only two reasons for a heparin therapy failure. First, AT-III levels may be too low for heparin to be effective. Secondly, an existing thrombus may dislodge and embolize; this is often interpreted as a "new" thrombus by the clinician who then assumes inefficacy of heparin. In the former instance, clotting tests will *not* be appropriately prolonged; in the latter, they *will* be prolonged.

D. Clinical Trials and Indications

Numerous double-blind prospective randomized trials have been performed utilizing heparin and mini-dose heparin. In general, the results of these trials have shown that both medical doses of heparin as well as mini-dose heparin are efficacious in the *prophylaxis* of thrombotic or thromboembolic disease, whether it be pulmonary embolism, other thromboembolic disease, recurrent deep vein thrombophlebitis, or postsurgical deep vein thrombophlebitis.[35-37] It appears that mini-dose heparin therapy is as efficacious prophylactically for any of the above-mentioned disorders, as medical dose heparin therapy. In addition, mini-dose heparin therapy seems to be equally efficacious as medical doses of heparin in disseminated intravascular coagulation, a state characterized by massive serine protease (activated clotting factors) generation.[38] The results (recently summarized[35]) utilizing mini-dose heparin therapy for the prophylaxis of postsurgical deep vein thrombophlebitis in general elective surgery, malignant prostatic surgery, surgery for malignant disease, and hip surgery are depicted in Tables 6, 7, 8, and 9.[35]

IV. ANTIPLATELET AGENTS

Numerous antiplatelet agents have been used in both prospective as well as older retrospective trials to assess efficacy in affording prophylaxis for thrombotic or thromboembolic disease. Only the three most commonly used agents will be discussed in this chapter. They are aspirin, dipyridamole, and sulfinpyrazone. Interpreting data obtained in these clinical trials is extremely difficult, because in some studies only one agent was used; in other studies antiplatelet agents in combination with warfarin or heparin were used; a few trials evaluated combinations of antiplatelet agents. An additional variable complicating the evaluations is the wide variety of "hypercoagulable" states studied. This discussion addresses the results obtained in some prospective randomized trials, as well as the author's personal clinical experience.

---

* What is an overdose of heparin?

TABLE 6

Low-Dose Heparin Prophylaxis in Elective General Surgery — Randomized Studies[a]

Study	Heparin regimen		Frequency of thrombosis	
	Preoperative dose	Postoperative dose	Treated (%)	Untreated (%)
1	10,000 u	2500 u 5000 u	15	41
2	5000 u	5000 u	8	42
3	5000 u	5000 u	8	42
4	5000 u	5000 u	1	24
5	5000 u	5000 u	2	16
6	5000 u	5000 u	4	29
7	5000 u	5000 u	5	20
8	2500 u	5000 u	12	37
9	5000 u	5000 u	7	44
10	5000 u	5000 u	4	16
11	5000 u	5000 u	6	5
12	5000 u	5000 u	13	36
13	5000 u	5000 u	8	25

[a] Modified from 35.

TABLE 7

Low-Dose Heparin Prophylaxis in Prostatic Surgery[a]

Study	Frequency of thrombosis	
	Treated (%)	Untreated (%)
1	57	80
2	0	100
3	16	—
4	0	28
5	33	34
6	9	29
7	24	20

[a] Modifed from 35.

TABLE 8

Low-Dose Heparin Prophylaxis in Surgery for Malignant Disease[a]

Study	Frequency of thrombosis	
	Treated (%)	Untreated (%)
1	7	53
2	8	
3	18	59
4	5	59
5	9	22
6	30	53

[a] Modified from 35.

A. Mechanisms of Action

The antiplatelet action of aspirin (ASA) is attributed to its ability to inhibit the synthesis of prostaglandins.[39] Specifically, it is known to inhibit cyclo-oxygenase, thereby decreasing the production of thromboxane A_2— a compound that promotes platelet aggregability (Chapters 1, 2, and 6). Dipyridamole is reported to inhibit cyclic AMP phosphodiesterase, thus increasing cyclic AMP in the platelet, thereby increasing phosphorylated receptor protein, which increases calcium binding and, like aspirin, decreases platelet aggregability and platelet adhesiveness.[40] Much less is known about sulfinpyrazone. It appears to have an action similar to that of aspirin.*

---

* Interestingly, if aspirin inhibits cyclo-oxygenase, one would assume that while inhibiting aggregation in a patient through decreased synthesis of thromboxane A_2 it could theoretically make one equally hypercoagulable by inhibiting the synthesis of prostacyclin. It may be that aspirin works as an antithrombotic agent by preferentially inhibiting the intraplatelet biosynthetic pathway.

TABLE 9

Low-Dose Heparin Prophylaxis in Patients Having Hip Surgery[a]

Study	Preoperative dose	Postoperative dose	Frequency of thrombosis	
			Treated (%)	Untreated (%)
1	5000 u	5000 u	11	50
2	5000 u	5000 u	46	54
3	5000 u	5000 u	7	48
4	5000 u	5000 u	33	42
5	5000 u	5000 u	5	37

[a] Modified from 35.

B. Clinical Aspects

In general, any combination of two of the above antiplatelet agents is required for most effective prophylaxis against thrombotic or thromboembolic disease.[41] The usual dose for aspirin is 600 mg given orally twice a day with 30 cc of liquid antacid. An ideal plasma level, without severe toxicity, is between 4 to 10 mg/dl.[42] Above 10 mg/dl patients commonly develop gastric intolerance, manifest by nausea and emesis, which are the common side effects of aspirin therapy. In addition, many patients complain of tinnitus. The usual dose for dipyridamole is 50 mg administered orally four times a day and the usual dose for sulfinpyrazone is 200 mg administered orally three times a day. In the author's experience, a combination of two antiplatelet agents is required to obtain a most effective clinical response. The usual side effects of dipyridamole therapy are headaches, dizziness, nausea, flushing, and syncope. In addition, mild gastrointestinal distress, similar to that seen with aspirin may be noted during therapy. Like aspirin and dipyridamole, the most common side effects of sylfinpyrazone are upper gastrointestinal disturbances manifest by nausea and emesis. Sulfinpyrazone will aggrevate or reactivate peptic ulcer disease. Usually a patient on antiplatelet therapy, especially on a combination of two agents, will often admit to easy and spontaneous bruising, as well as mild mucosal membrane bleeding usually manifest as gingival bleeding with toothbrushing and periodic melena. These are accepted side effects of antiplatelet therapy for prophylaxis of serious thrombotic or thromboembolic disease. It should be further noted that the effects of these agents lasts a full 7 to 10 days. Thus if a patient is ingesting these agents and is involved in trauma or requires emergency surgery, platelet concentrates may be indicated.

C. Laboratory Monitoring

No laboratory monitoring of antiplatelet therapy is necessary. However, should one wish to document a clinical response, a template bleeding time, and an "aspirin tolerance test" can be performed to document the efficacy of therapy.[43] The aspirin tolerance test is equally applicable to sulfinpyrazone and dipyridamole. In practice, a baseline template bleeding time is repeated approximately 1 to 2 weeks after starting a patient on antiplatelet therapy. In addition, platelet aggregation as well as adhesion studies may be performed. Classically, aspirin causes blunted collagen and ristocetin-induced aggregation and eradicates the second wave of epinephrine-induced aggregation.[44]

Platelet adhesion is not immediately impaired, but may be impaired 24 to 48 hr after the initiation of therapy.[43,45] Dipyridamole and sulfinpyrazone both blunt aggregation curves, as well as interfere with platelet adhesion studies done by the Bowie technique.[46]

D. Clinical Trials and Indications

Like other forms of anticoagulant therapy, antiplatelet therapy is in a remarkable state of flux, with numerous double-blind prospective randomized trials being conducted. The results of these trials should, in the future, dictate more clear-cut indications for antiplatelet therapy.

Alterations in platelet reactivity have been observed in patients with existing deep vein thrombosis.[47-49] This leads to the obvious suggestion that antiplatelet therapy may be indicated in thrombotic and thromboembolic disease. The antiplatelet drug that has attracted the most attention is aspirin. The advantages are obvious: it is a very inexpensive anticoagulant and relatively free from side effects. There have been numerous clinical trials using aspirin for a wide variety of disorders. However, there has been a lack of standardized dosage, and, in many instances, aspirin has been used in combination with another antiplatelet agent, warfarin, or heparin. Aspirin has been clearly shown to decrease the incidence of deep vein thrombophlebitis and pulmonary emboli in patients with hip fractures, as well as in patients undergoing total hip replacement.[51,52] There have been two retrospective studies in a large patient population, the results of which reveal a decrease in the incidence of acute myocardial infarction.[53,54] In addition, aspirin has been shown to decrease thromboembolic disease associated with prosthetic heart valves.[55] Another study has shown a favorable response with aspirin in decreasing recurrent myocardial infarction. However, the results did not reach statistical significance.[56] Several double-blind prospective studies have shown aspirin to be effective as a single agent for the prophylaxis of deep vein thrombophlebitis and pulmonary emboli in postoperative patients.[57]

Dipyridamole has been studied, like aspirin, in combination with other antiplatelet agents, as a single agent, and in combination with warfarin or heparin. In one study, it alone decreased the rate of renal allograft rejection in patients with transplants.[58] Another study has shown that dipyridamole, as a single agent, will normalize platelet survival in patients with prosthetic heart valves.[59] This same study showed that aspirin was without a similar effect and that sulfinpyrazone was as effective as dipyridamole. Other studies have shown that dipyridamole plus aspirin significantly decrease the incidence of deep vein thrombophlebitis and pulmonary emboli postoperatively, but dipyridamole was ineffective as a single agent.[60] In several studies, sulfinpyrazone, as a single agent, has been shown to be effective in decreasing the incidence of transient cerebral ischemic attacks,[61] thromboembolism in patients with rheumatic heart disease,[62] recurrent deep vein thrombophlebitis,[63,64] and shunt thrombosis.[65]

The above studies account for the majority of recent double-blind prospective trials with antiplatelet agents. Hopefully, future studies using combination therapy in a prospective double-blind controlled manner will allow for more clear-cut indications. It is the author's experience that a combination of two of the above three antiplatelet agents is very effective in decreasing incidents of recurrent deep vein thrombophlebitis, deep vein thrombosis, and pulmonary emboli. However, the author's clinical hemostasis practice and clinical experience is somewhat biased, as most patient's placed on combined antiplatelet therapy have been individuals with recurrent thrombotic or thromboembolic disease who have failed to respond to warfarin therapy. The vast majority of these patients do *not* rethrombose on a combination of any two of the three aforementioned antiplatelet agents.

V. SUMMARY

This chapter summarizes current kinetic knowledge, apparent indications, and the results of major clinical trials using anticoagulant and antiplatelet therapy. Since many studies have been retrospective in nature, some without uniform dosages, and a wide variety of disorders studied, efficacy, at the present time, with respect to warfarin therapy, heparin vs. mini-heparin therapy, and antiplatelet therapy remains questionable. Current ongoing double-blind prospective trials should provide more clear-cut answers.

REFERENCES

1. **Denson, K. W. E.**, The levels of Factors II, VII, IX, and X by antibody neutralization techniques in the plasma of patients receiving phenindione therapy, *Br. J. Haematol.*, 20, 643, 1971.
2. **Pereira, M. and Couri, D.**, Studies on the site of action of dicumarol on prothrombin synthesis, *Biochem. Biophys. Acta*, 237, 348, 1971.
3. **Stenflo, J.**, Vitamin K, prothrombin, and gamma-carboxyglutamic acid, *N. Engl. J. Med.*, 296, 624, 1977.
4. **Quick, A. J.**, Hypoprothrombinemic states, in *Hemorrhagic Disease and Thrombosis*, Quick, A. J., Ed., Lea & Febiger, Philadelphia, 1966, 60.
5. **Loeliger, E. A., von der Esch, B., Mattern, M. J., and den Bracander, A. S. H.**, Behaviour of Factors II, VII, IX, and X during long-term treatment with coumarin, *Thromb. Diath. Haemorrh.*, 9, 74, 1963.
6. **Keykin, D.**, Warfarin therapy, *N. Engl. J. Med.*, 287, 691, 1970.
7. **O'Reilly, R. A.**, The pharmacodynamics of the oral anticoagulant drugs, *Prog. Hemostas. Thromb.*, 2, 175, 1974.
8. **Marshall, J.**, Rebound phenomenon after anticoagulant therapy in cerebrovascular disease, *Circulation*, 28, 329, 1962.
9. **Nalbandian, R. M., Mader, I. J., Barrett, S. L., Pearce, J. F., and Rupp, E. C.**, Petechiae, ecchymoses, and necrosis of skin induced by coumarin congeners, *JAMA*, 192, 107, 1965.
10. **Nalbandian, R. M., Beller, F. K., Kamp, A. K., Henry, R. L., and Wolf, P. L.**, Coumarin necrosis of skin treated successfully with heparin, *Obstet. Gynecol.*, 38, 395, 1971.
11. **Zucker, S., Brosills, E., and Cooper, G. R.**, One-stage prothrombin time survey, *Am. J. Clin. Pathol.*, 53, 340, 1970.
12. Editorial, Control of anticoagulants, *Br. Med. J.*, 1, 126, 1969.
13. Report of the working party on anticoagulant therapy in coronary thrombosis to the medical research council, *Br. Med. J.*, 1, 335, 1969.
14. **Udall, J. A.**, Recent advances in anticoagulant therapy, *Gen. Pract.*, 11, 116, 1969.
15. **Sigell, L. T. and Flessa, H. C.**, Drug interactions with anticoagulants, *JAMA*, 214, 2035, 1970.
16. **Ebert, R. V.**, Long-term anticoagulant therapy after myocardial infarction: final report of the veterans administration cooperative study, *JAMA*, 207, 2263, 1969.
17. **Ebert, R. V.**, Anticoagulants in acute myocardial infarction: results of a cooperative clinical trial, *JAMA*, 225, 724, 1973.
18. **Barker, H. W., Cromer, H. E., Hurn, M., and Waugh, J. M.**, The use of dicumarol in the prevention of postoperative thrombosis and embolism with special reference to dosage and safe administration, *Surgery*, 17, 207, 1945.
19. **Pyorala, T. and Lampinen, V.**, Preoperative anticoagulant treatment in gynecologic surgery, *Acta Obstet. Gynecol.*, 49, 215, 1970.
20. **Gallus, A. S. and Hirsh, J.**, Treatment of venous thromboembolic disease, *Semin. Thromb. Hemostas.*, 2, 291, 1976.
21. **Wessler, S.**, Anticoagulant therapy — 1974, *JAMA*, 228, 757, 1974.
22. **Yin, E. T.**, Effect of heparin on the neutralization of Factor X_a and thrombin by the plasma alpha-2-globulin inhibitor, *Thromb. Diath. Haemorrh.*, 33, 43, 1975.
22. **Estes, J. W. and Paulin, P. F.**, Pharmacokinetics of heparin: distribution and elimination, *Thromb. Diath. Haemorrh.*, 33, 26, 1975.

24. Jaques, L. B., Mahndoo, J., and Kavanagh, L. W., Intrapulmonary heparin — a new procedure for anticoagulant therapy, *Lancet*, 2, 1157, 1976.
25. Bick, R. L., Schmalhorst, W. R., and Arbegast, N. R., Alterations of hemostasis associated with cardiopulmonary bypass, *Thromb. Res.*, 8, 205, 1976.
26. Moser, R. H., Disorders produced by anticoagulants, *Clin. Pharmacol. Ther.*, 9, 388, 1968.
27. Bell, W. R., Tomasulo, P. A., Alving, B. M., and Duffy, T. P., Thrombocytopenia occurring during the administration of heparin; a prospective study in 52 patients, *Ann. Intern. Med.*, 85, 155, 1976.
28. Griffith, G. C., Nichols, G. and Asher, J. D., Heparin osteoporosis, *JAMA*, 193, 91, 1965.
29. Teiem, A. N. and Abildgaard, R., On the value of the activated partial thromboplastin time in monitoring heparin therapy, *Thromb. Haemostas.*, 35, 592, 1976.
30. Shapiro, G. A., Huntzinger, S. W., and Wilson, J. E., Variation among commercial activated partial thromboplastin time reagents in response to heparin therapy, *Am. J. Clin. Pathol.*, 67, 477, 1977.
31. Triplett, D. A., Harms, C. S., and Koepke, J. A., The effect of heparin on the activated partial thromboplastin time, *Am. J. Clin. Pathol. (Suppl.)*, 70, 556, 1978.
32. Bick, R. L., Editorial note: varying AT-III levels in thrombotic disorders, *Semin. Thromb. Hemostas.*, 4, 357, 1978.
33. Fekete, L. F. and Bick, R. L., Laboratory modalities for assessing hemostasis during cardiopulmonary bypass, *Semin. Thromb Hemostas.*, 3, 83, 1976.
34. Bick, R. L., Kovacs, I., and Fekete, L. F., A new two-stage functional assay for antithrombin-III (heparin cofactor), *Thromb Res.*, 8, 745, 1976.
35. Gallus, A. S. and Hirsh, J., Prevention of venous thromboembolism, *Semin. Thromb. Hemostas.*, 2, 232, 1976.
36. Jacques, L. B. and Mahadoo, J. M., Pharmacodynamics and clinical effectiveness of heparin, *Semin. Thromb. Hemostas.*, 4, 298, 1978.
37. Kakkar, V. V., Spindler, J., Flute, P. T., Corrigan, T., Fossard, D. P., and Crellin, R. Q., Efficacy of low-doses of heparin in prevention of thrombosis after major surgery: a double-blind randomized trial, *Lancet*, 2, 101, 1972.
38. Bick, R. L., Disseminated intravascular coagulation and related syndromes: etiology, pathophysiology, diagnosis and management, *Am. J. Hematol.*, 5, 265, 1978.
39. Weiss, H. J., The pharmacology of platelet inhibition, *Prog. Hemostasis Thromb.*, 1, 199, 1972.
40. Mills, D. C. B. and Smith, J. B., The influence on platelet aggregation of drugs that affect the accumulation of adenosine $3',5'$-cyclic monophosphate in platelets, *Biochem. J.*, 121, 185, 1971.
41. Bick, R. L., Treatment of bleeding and thrombosis in the patient with cancer, in *Management of the Patient with Cancer*, Nealon, T., Ed., W. B. Saunders, Philadelphia, 1976, 48.
42. Cohen, L. S., Clinical pharmacology of acetylsalicylic acid, *Semin. Thromb. Hemostas.*, 2, 146, 1976.
43. Bick, R. L., Adams, T., and Schmalhorst, W. R., Bleeding times, platelet adhesion and aspirin, *Am. J. Clin. Pathol.*, 65, 69, 1976.
44. O'Brien, J. R., Effects of salicylates on human platelets, *Lancet*, 1, 779, 1968.
45. Weiss, H. J., Aspirin ingestion compared with bleeding disorders — search for a useful platelet antiaggregant, *Blood*, 35, 333, 1970.
46. Bowie, E. J. W. and Owen, C. A., The value of measuring platelet "adhesiveness" in the diagnosis of bleeding diseases, *Am. J. Clin. Pathol.*, 60, 302, 1973.
47. Hirsh, J. and McBride, J. A., Increased platelet adhesiveness in recurrent venous thrombosis and pulmonary embolism, *Br. Med. J.*, 2, 797, 1965.
48. Hume, M., Platelet adhesiveness and other coagulation factors in thrombophlebitis, *Surgery*, 59, 110, 1966.
49. Bygdeman, S., Eliasson, R., and Johnson, S. R., Relationship between postoperative changes in adenosine-diphosphate induced platelet adhesiveness and venous thrombosis, *Lancet*, 1, 1301, 1966.
50. Fitzgerald, D. E. and Butterfield, W. J. H., A cause of increased platelet anti-heparin factor in a patient with Raynaud's phenomena and gangrene, treated by aspirin, *Angiology*, 20, 317, 1969.
51. Salzman, E., Harris, W. H., and deSanctis, R. W., Reduction in venous thromboembolism by agents affecting platelet function, *N. Engl. J. Med.*, 284, 1287, 1971.
52. Harris, W. H., Aspirin prophylaxis against thromboembolism disease, *Thromb. Haemostas.*, 38, 237, 1977.
53. Craven, L. L., Experiences with aspirin in the nonspecific prophylaxis of coronary thrombosis, *Miss. Val. Med. J.*, 75, 38, 1953.
54. Boston Collaborative Drug Surveillance Group, Regular aspirin intake and acute myocardial infarction, *Br. Med. J.*, 1, 436, 1974.
55. Dale, J., Prevention of arterial thromboembolism with acetylsalicylic acid in patients with prosthetic heart valves, *Thromb. Haemostas.*, 38, 66, 1977.

56. **Elwood, P. C., Cochrane, A. L., and Burr, M. L.**, A randomized controlled trial of acetylsalicylic acid in the secondary prevention of mortality from myocardial infarction, *Br. Med. J.*, 1, 436, 1974.
57. **Alledort, L.**, Platelets and thromboembolism, *Semin. Thromb. Hemostas.*, 2, 136, 1976.
58. **Kincaid-Smith, P.**, Modification of the vascular lesions of rejection in cadaveric renal allografts by dipyridamole and anticoagulants, *Lancet,* 1, 920, 1969.
59. **Sullivan, J. M., Harken, D. E., and Gorlin, R.**, Pharmacologic control of thromboembolic complications of cardiac-valve replacement, *N. Engl. J. Med.,* 284, 1391, 1971.
60. **O'Sullivan, E. F. and Renny, J. T. G.**, Antiplatelet Drugs in the Prevention of Postoperative Deep-Vein Thrombosis, in 3rd Congr. Int. Soc. Thromb. Hemostas., Washington, D. C., 1972, 438.
61. **Evans, G.**, Effects of drugs that suppress platelet surface interaction on incidence of amarrosis fugax and transient cerebral ischemia, *Surg. Forum,* 23, 239, 1972.
62. **Steele, P., Rainwater, J., and Genton, E.**, Controlled trial of sulfinpyrazone in rheumatic heart disease, *Thromb. Haemostas.,* 38, 194, 1977.
63. **Evans, G. and Gent, M.**, Effect of platelet suppressive drugs on arterial and venous thromboembolism, in *Platelet, Drugs, and Thrombosis, Proceedings,* S. Karger, Basel, 1975, 258.
64. **Steele, P. P., Weily, H. S., and Genton, E.**, Platelet survival and adhesiveness in recurrent venous thrombosis, *N. Engl. J. Med.,* 288, 1148, 1973.
65. **Kaegi, A., Pineo, F. G., and Shimizu, A.**, Arteriovenous-shunt thrombosis: prevention by sulfinpyrazone, *N. Engl. J. Med.,* 290, 304, 1974.

Chapter 15

THROMBOLYTIC THERAPY

Genesio Murano and Rodger L. Bick

TABLE OF CONTENTS

I.	Introduction	260
II.	Urokinase and Streptokinase	260
	A. Molecular Properties	260
	B. Pharmacologic Properties	260
III.	Indications	261
	A. Pulmonary Embolism	261
	B. Deep Vein Thrombosis	262
IV.	Complications of Therapy	264
	A. Bleeding	264
	B. Allergic Reactions	264
	C. Fever	264
	D. Phlebitis	264
V.	Laboratory Monitoring	265
VI.	Anticoagulation at Termination of Therapy	266
VII.	Conclusions	266
References		266

I. INTRODUCTION

In contrast to anticoagulant drugs (Chapter 14), which function by impeding further growth of an existing thrombus, thrombolytic agents have the unique virtue of inducing the dissolution of intravascular fibrin (thrombi) and the digestion of fibrinogen and other proteins, resulting in a more immediate recanalization of occluded vessels and improved microperfusion due to altered rheologic properties of blood.

The most dramatic effects of pharmacologically activated fibrinolysis are noted when therapy is instituted early in the disease (thrombi less than a few days old). Once thrombi are penetrated by fibroblasts and converted to scar tissue or have been covered by endothelium, the probability of full vessel rehabilitation is poor. It is, therefore, important to establish a definitive early diagnosis, usually best achieved by visualizing intravascular thrombi by ascending phlebography, arteriography, or by injecting ^{125}I-fibrinogen.

Thrombolytic therapy originated with the demonstration that certain enzymes will induce the dissolution of (1) preformed plasma clots, in vitro,[1] (2) experimentally induced intravascular thrombi in animals[2] and (3) superficial venous thrombi in human volunteers.[3] Of the various agents tested,[4] the two enzymes urokinase (UK) and streptokinase (SK) have received world-wide attention and have undergone limited, but rigorous, prospective clinical evaluation in the treatment of thrombosis.

This chapter briefly summarizes the results of some clinical trials and outlines the presently accepted therapeutic regimen in the treatment of deep vein thrombosis, and massive pulmonary embolism.[5-18] The use of thrombolytic agents in cerebrovascular disease, retinal venous thrombosis, myocardial infarction, arterial thrombosis, as well as the use of plasminogen in hyaline membrane disease, and the subject of chemical thrombolysis have received more limited attention (in many instances, with less encouraging results) and will not be discussed here.[18-21]

II. UROKINASE AND STREPTOKINASE

A. Molecular Properties

Urokinase is an enzyme produced by the kidney and found in the urine. It is a potent activator of the fibrinolytic system. Two molecular forms of urokinase are found in current therapeutic preparations: the high molecular weight (HMW) and the low molecular weight (LMW) form (55,000 and 34,000, respectively). The LMW species is derived from the HMW species by proteolysis.[4] Immunologically the two forms are similar. Depending on the method of preparation, either one or the other species (or in varying proportions) are isolated. Kidney tissue cultures and urine are sources of urokinase.

Streptokinase is a bacterial enzyme synthesized by group C beta hemolytic streptococci. Its molecular weight is 47,000.[4] Table 1 summarizes some of the properties of urokinase and streptokinase.

B. Pharmacologic Properties

Urokinase and streptokinase act on the endogenous fibrinolytic system by converting plasminogen to the potent proteolytic enzyme plasmin (Chapter 3, Section III). Plasmin, in turn, degrades fibrin clots as well as fibrinogen and other plasma proteins.[22] Plasmin is rapidly inactivated by a variety of naturally occurring plasma inhibitors.[23] Since plasminogen is present in the thrombus/embolus, lysis occurs within, as well as on the surface.[24]

Intravenous infusion of urokinase and streptokinase is promptly followed by increased fibrinolytic activity, and its effect may persist for up to 12 hr after discontin-

TABLE 1

Properties of Urokinase and Streptokinase

Property	Streptokinase	Urokinase	
Source	β-Hemolytic streptococci	Human urine	Human kidney tissue culture
Molecular weight	47,000	55,000	34,000
Stability	Stable	Stable	
Half-life	∼ 10 min (variable)	∼ 15 min	
Route of administration	Intravenous	Intravenous	
Pyrogenecity	Yes	No	
Antigenicity	Yes	No	
Dosage	Uniform-variable[a]	Uniform	
Retreatment	6 months	Ad-lib	
Market price	Reasonable	Expensive	

[a] Variable dose regimen is seldom applicable.

From Bell, W. R., *Semin. Thromb. Hemost.*, 2, 1, 1975. With permission.

uation. This activity is evidenced by a shortening of the euglobulin lysis time (EGLT), a decrease in plasma levels of plasminogen and fibrinogen, and an increase in the amount of circulating fibrin(ogen) degradation products (FDP)[14] (Table 2). Urinary and tissue culture urokinase have comparable fibrinolytic activities in humans.[17]

The activity of urokinase and streptokinase is expressed in international units and is a measure of their ability to induce the lysis of a fibrin clot via the plasmin system in vitro. The half-life of both enzymes is quite short (10 to 20 min).[14] The effective blood levels and disappearance rates of streptokinase vary with the availability of substrate (plasminogen).

The efficacy of urokinase and streptokinase in the lysis of pulmonary emboli[11-14,16] and the efficacy of in the lysis of deep vein thrombi[5,6,8,9,15,25] have been established by angiography, perfusion lung scans, pulmonary arterial and right heart pressure measurements, and ascending venography, before and after treatment.

III. INDICATIONS

A. Pulmonary Embolism

Based on results obtained in the National Heart and Lung Institute-sponsored urokinase pulmonary embolism trial (UPET) and urokinase-streptokinase pulmonary embolism trial (USPET),[11-14,16] the two thrombolytic agents urokinase and streptokinase are indicated in adults for the lysis of acute massive pulmonary emboli (Table 3).

For best results, treatment should be instituted as soon as possible after onset of pulmonary embolism and no later than 5 days after onset. Under these circumstances, angiographic and hemodynamic measurements demonstrate a more rapid improvement during the first 24 hr of therapy than with heparin.[11,12] However, it has not been established that treatment with urokinase or streptokinase decreases morbidity or mortality when compared to heparin therapy alone.

In these studies, urokinase was administered intravenously in a loading dose of 4400 Units/kg/hr over a period of 10-20 minutes, followed by a continuous infusion of 4400 Units/kg/hr for a period of 12 or 24 hr. Streptokinase was administered intrave-

TABLE 2

Effects of Intravenous Infusion of Urokinase or Streptokinase

Generalized intravascular proteolysis (GIP)

Decreased fibrinogen
Increased FDP/fdp   Prolonged TT[a]
Decreased plasminogen
Increased plasmin → shortened EGLT[b]
Decreased Factors V, VIII, etc.

[a] TT = Thrombin time.
[b] EGLT = Euglobulin lysis time.

TABLE 3

Indications for Fibrinolytic Therapy[a]

Acute massive pulmonary emboli[b] (UK/SK)
   Obstruction or significant filling defects involving two or more lobar pulmonary arteries or equivalent amount of emboli in other vessels
   Embolization accompanied by unstable hemodynamics, i.e., failure to maintain BP without supportive measures
Deep vein thrombosis[c] (SK)
   Extensive thrombi of deep veins (*not* superficial vein thrombophlebitis)

[a] Instituted within 5 days of onset of symptoms.
[b] Diagnosis confirmed by pulmonary arteriography.
[c] Diagnosis confirmed by ascending venography.

nously in a loading dose of 250,000 units* over a period of 20 min, followed by a continuous infusion of 100,000 units/hr for a period of 24 hr. At termination of thrombolytic therapy, patients received intravenous continuous heparin for 7 to 10 days, followed by oral anticoagulants for 2 to 6 months. Clinical parameters (pulmonary angiograms, lung perfusion scans, cardiorespiratory hemodynamics) were evaluated independently by a number of panelists, each rendering an independent judgment. To establish that the endogenous fibrinolytic system had been activated, the concentration of fibrinogen, plasminogen, FDP, and EGLT were measured in each patient (US-PET) preinfusion, during, and at termination of therapy.

As expected, the concentration of fibrinogen and plasminogen decreased, the EGLT shortened, and the concentration of FDP increased (Figure 1). Pulmonary angiograms, lung perfusion scans, and cardiorespiratory hemodynamics showed significant improvements (Table 4). It is noted that there was no dramatic difference in clinical or laboratory parameters between the 12-hr and 24-hr urokinase regimen. Clinically, urokinase and streptokinase were equally effective.

B. Deep Vein Thrombosis

Several published randomized clinical studies[5,6,9,15] have established that streptokinase is indicated for the lysis of acute, extensive thrombi of the deep veins (DVT) in adults (Table 3). Long-term benefits in DVT (as well as safety and effectiveness in septic thrombophlebitis) have not been established, although two reports[8,25] suggest somewhat better salvage of valvular function with streptokinase and heparin than with heparin alone.

In studies on DVT, streptokinase was administered intravenously in a loading dose of 250,000 Units, followed by a continuous infusion of 100,000 Units/hr for a period of 72 hr. At termination of thrombolytic therapy, patients were treated with heparin. Efficacy was judged by serial venography, evaluated by "blinded" readers.

Table 5 summarizes the results of these studies. As in the case of pulmonary embolism, best results were obtained when therapy was instituted within a few days of onset of the thrombotic event.

* Actual dose determined by the streptokinase resistance test (SKRT). Since human exposure to streptococci is common, antibodies to streptokinase (streptokinase resistance) are found normally. During the early phase of systemic streptokinase therapy, these antibodies neutralize an equivalent amount of streptokinase, rendering it unavailable for activating the lytic system. Thus a loading dose of streptokinase sufficient to neutralize the resistance is required.

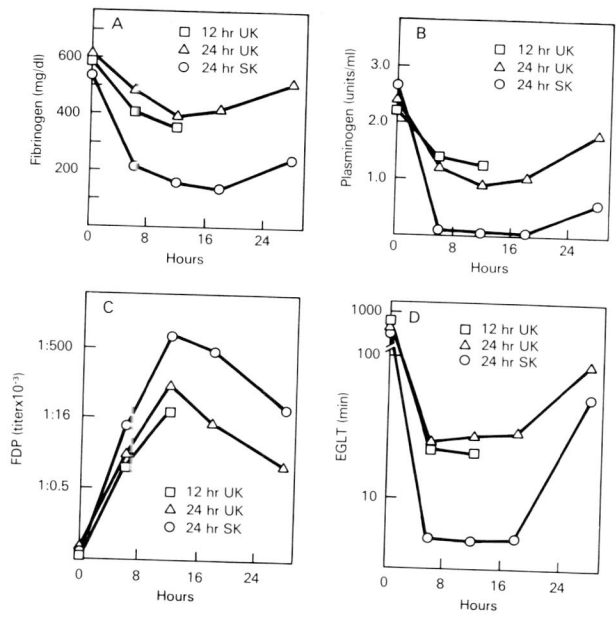

FIGURE 1. (A) Plasma fibrinogen concentration, (B) plasma plasminogen concentration, (C) serum fibrin(ogen) degradation products (FDP titer), (D) euglobulin lysis time (EGLT): pre-, during, and postthrombolytic therapy. Each point expresses a mean value, from USPET. (Adapted from Bell, W. R., *Semin. Thromb. Hemost.*, 2, 1, 1975. With permission.)

TABLE 4

Urokinase and Streptokinase in Pulmonary Embolism: Chances and Clinical Parameters

Parameter[c]	UPET[a]		USPET[b]		
	Heparin	12 hr urokinase	12 hr urokinase	24 hr urokinase	24 hr streptokinase
Improvement in angiographic score (0—4 point system)	0.54	1.78	1.66	1.76	1.70
Decrease in perfusion defect (relative %)	8.3	24.1	20.0	29.2	18.5
Decrease in pulmonary artery pressure (mm Hg)	1.1	6.2	7.28	7.53	5.3
Change in cardiac index (l/min/m^2)	−0.05	+0.02	+0.06	+0.30	+0.60

[a] Urokinase pulmonary embolism trial.
[b] Urokinase-streptokinase pulmonary embolism trial.
[c] Evaluations obtained between 18 and 30 hr after initiation of therapy. After several days there was no difference between the heparin and urokinase/streptokinase-treated patients.

From Fratantoni, J. C., Ness, P., and Simon, T. L., *N. Engl. J. Med.*, 293, 1073, 1975. With permission.

TABLE 5

Streptokinase in Deep Vein Thrombosis[a]

	No. of patients	
	Streptokinase	Heparin
Complete lysis	37	7
Incomplete lysis	36	56

[a] Evaluated by venography (summary of four clinical trials).[5,6,9,15]

IV. COMPLICATIONS OF THERAPY

A. Bleeding

Activation of the fibrinolytic system by urokinase or streptokinase results in seriously compromised hemostatic function. This is attributed to the generalized intravascular proteolysis (GIP) introduced by plasmin (Table 2). As a consequence, hemorrhage (in varying degrees) occasionally occurs. Severe spontaneous bleeding, including cerebral, retroperitoneal, and gastrointestinal has been documented in less than 5% of the patients treated. Several fatalities due to cerebral hemorrhage have occurred.

Less severe spontaneous bleeding, such as superficial hematoma, hematuria, and hemoptysis, has been observed during treatment, at approximately twice the frequency as that occurring during heparin therapy. In several instances, spontaneous bleeding has been traced to concomitant anticoagulant treatment, which is presently contraindicated. Oozing of blood from sites of percutaneous trauma is frequent; hence, all invasive procedures, especially arterial punctures and intramuscular injections must be avoided and intravenous punctures kept to a minimum before and during treatment with thrombolytic agents.

B. Allergic Reactions

Reactions representing possible anaphylaxis have been observed in about 3% of patients treated with streptokinase for venous thrombosis or pulmonary embolism. These ranged in severity from minor breathing difficulty to bronchospasm, periorbital swelling, or angioneurotic edema. Other milder allergic effects such as urticaria, itching, flushing, nausea, headache, or musculoskeletal pain have been observed in approximately 12% of patients, with no apparent relationship to dosage. Transient elevation or lowering of systolic blood pressure of greater than 25 mm Hg has been observed in less than 2% of patients. Relatively mild reactions, e.g., bronchospasms and skin rash, have been reported, although rarely, with urokinase.

C. Fever

Although streptokinase is nonpyrogenic in standard animal tests, approximately one third of patients treated with streptokinase have shown increases in body temperature of 1.5°F or more. The incidence of fever $\geq 104°F$ is about 3.5%. Febrile reactions with urokinase occur in about 3% of patients.

D. Phlebitis

Phlebitis near the site of intravenous infusion has been reported in less than 2% of patients treated with streptokinase. Tables 6 to 10 summarize contraindications, adverse reactions, and management.

TABLE 6

Contraindications for Fibrinolytic Therapy

1. Surgery within 10 days (liver/kidney biopsy, lumbar puncture, thora/paracentesis, multiple cutdowns)
2. Intra-arterial diagnostic procedure within 10 days
3. Ulcerative wound
4. Recent trauma (internal injuries)
5. Visceral or intracranial malignancy
6. Pregnancy and first 10 days postpartum
7. Ulcerative colitis, diverticulitis, bleeding (or potential) lesion of GI/GU tract
8. Severe hypertension
9. Acute/chronic hepatic or renal insufficiency
10. Uncontrolled hypocoagulable state
    Factor/platelet/vascular dysfunction
    Spontaneous fibrinolysis
11. Chronic lung disease with cavitation (tuberculosis)
12. Subacute bacterial endocarditis or rheumatic valvular disease
13. Recent (<2 months) cerebral embolism/thrombosis/hemorrhage
14. Any condition predisposing to unmanageable bleeding
15. Predisposition to allergic reactions (SK)
16. Predisposition to systemic infection (SK)
    Septic thrombophlebitis
    Infected AV cannula
17. Predisposition to cerebral embolism (atrial fibrillation)
18. Concurrent use of anticoagulants
19. In children

TABLE 7

Adverse Reactions to Streptokinase and Urokinase Therapy

Streptokinase	Urokinase
Bleeding	Bleeding
Allergic Rx	Mild allergic Rx
Fever	Fever (rare)
Phlebitis	

TABLE 8

Streptokinase/Urokinase: Bleeding RX and Management

	Type of bleeding	General management
	Cerebral	Discontinuation of SK-UK
2%[a]	Retroperitoneal	Packed red cells
	Gastrointestinal	Volume expanders
	Superficial hematoma	Whole blood
2 ×[a] Heparin	Hematuria	Aminocaproic acid
	Hemoptisis	
	Oozing (sites of percutaneous trauma)	

V. LABORATORY MONITORING

During thrombolytic therapy, the thrombin time (TT) is prolonged due to decreased fibrinogen and increased FDP (Table 2). This test, then, is recommended as a *practical* means of assessing the pharmacologic effect of fibrinolytic agents.* Table 11 outlines, in a general way, the procedure.

---

* Other laboratory modalities, such as the measurement of plasminogen, plasmin, FDP, and fibrinogen, may be used adjunctively; however, they furnish no additional information with regard to pharmacologic response and degree of clot resolution.

TABLE 9

Streptokinase/Urokinase: Allergic RX[a] and Management

	Type of reaction	General management
	Minor breathing difficulty (SK)	Mild reactions: concomitant antihistamine and/or corticosteroids
2.5%[b]	Bronchospasm (SK-UK) Periorbital swelling (SK) Angioneurotic edema (SK) Urticaria (SK-UK)	Severe reactions: immediate discontinuation of therapy with i.v. administration of corticosteroids (PRN)
12%[b]	Itching (SK-UK) Flushing (SK) Nausea (SK) Headache (SK) Musculoskeletal pain (SK)	

[a] Occur primarily with SK.
[b] Frequency.

TABLE 10

Streptokinase: Fever/Phlebitis and Management

Symptom	Management
Fever	
Temp. rise of 1.5°F (35%)	Symptomatic treatment "Acetaminophen" *not* Aspirin
Temp. rise >104°F (3.5%)	
Phlebitis	
Near infusion site (<2%)	Dilution of SK solution

TABLE 11

Thrombolitic Therapy Laboratory Monitoring

Thrombin time (TT) at 0 time
If patient was on heparin, wait for TT to return <2 × normal prior to commencing therapy
Prolonged TT during therapy indicates fibrinolytic state due to:

Fibrinogen↓
Plasmin ↑
FDP/fdp ↑

VI. ANTICOAGULATION AT TERMINATION OF THERAPY

At the end of thrombolytic therapy, treatment with heparin by continuous intravenous infusion is recommended. Heparin treatment should not be instituted until the thrombin time has decreased to *less than twice* the normal control value. Oral anticoagulants have been used (after heparin); however, their prophylactic efficacy is questionable.

VII. CONCLUSIONS

Data reported in the studies described indicate that both urokinase and streptokinase are (1) capable of inducing a fibrinolytic state in man and (2) definitely superior to heparin alone in accelerating the rate of clot dissolution. These agents can be *safely* employed in humans, provided therapy is supervised by a physician competent in the management of thrombohemorrhagic phenomena.

It is important to note that although no difference in mortality was detected between pulmonary embolism patients on thrombolytic agents and patients on heparin, it is apparent that particularly patients with massive pulmonary emboli received considerable benefit from the *rate* of return of their cardiopulmonary hemodynamics toward normal. Patients not responding to conventional anticoagulants are (in most instances) excellent candidates for thrombolytic therapy — an alternative to embolectomy.

REFERENCES

1. **Christensen, L. R.**, Streptococcal fibrinolysis: a proteolytic reaction due to a serum enzyme activated by streptococcal fibrinolysin, *J. Gen. Physiol.*, 28, 363, 1945.
2. **Johnson, A. J. and Tillett, W.**, The lysis in rabbits of intravascular blood clots by the streptococcal fibrinolytic system (streptokinase), *J. Exp. Med.*, 95, 449, 1952.
3. **Johnson, A. J. and McCarty, W.**, Some aspects of the mechanism of thrombolysis, *Thromb. Diath. Haemorrh.*, 5, 391, 1961.
4. **Bang, N. U.**, Physiology and biochemistry of fibrinolysis, in *Thrombosis and Bleeding Disorders*, Bang, N. U., Beller, F. K., Deutsch, E., and Mammen, E. F., Eds., Academic Press, New York, 1971, 292.
5. **Robertson, B. R., Nilsson, I. M., and Nylander, G.**, Thrombolytic effect of streptokinase as evaluated by phlebography of deep venous thrombi of the leg, *Acta Chir. Scand.*, 134, 203, 1968.
6. **Kakkar, V. V., Flanc, C., Howe, C. T., O'Shea, M., and Flute, P. T.**, Treatment of deep vein thrombosis. A trial of heparin, streptokinase and Arvin, *Br. Med. J.*, 1, 806, 1969.
7. **Hirsch, J.**, Dosage regimens for streptokinase treatment: evaluation of a standard dosage schedule, *Australas. Ann. Med.*, 19 (Suppl. 1), 12, 1970.
8. **Kakkar, V. V.**, Results of streptokinase therapy in deep venous thrombosis, *Postgrad. Med. J. Suppl.*, 49, 60, 1973.
9. **Tsapogas, M. J., Peabody, R. A., Wu, K. T., Karmody, A. M., Devaraj, K. T., and Eckert, C.**, Controlled study of thrombolytic therapy in deep vein thrombosis, *Surgery*, 74, 973, 1973.
10. **Brogden, R. N., Splight, T. M., and Avery, G. S.**, Streptokinase: a review of its clinical pharmacology, mechanism of action and therapeutic uses, *Drugs*, 5, 357, 1973.
11. **Sasahara, A. A., Hyers, T. M., and Cole, C. M.**, The urokinase pulmonary embolism trial, *Circulation, (Suppl. II)*, 47, 1, 1973.
12. **Fratantoni, J. C., Ness, P., and Simon, T. L.**, Thrombolytic therapy: current status, *N. Engl. J. Med.*, 293, 1073, 1975.
13. **Sasahara, A. A., Bell, W. R., Simon, T. L., Stengle, J. M., and Sherry, S.**, The phase II urokinase-streptokinase pulmonary embolism trial, *Thromb. Diath. Haemorrh.*, 33, 464, 1975.

14. **Bell, W. R.,** Thrombolytic therapy: a comparison between urokinase and streptokinase, *Semin. Thromb. Hemost.,* 2, 1, 1975.
15. **Seaman, A. J., Common, H. H., Rosch, J., Dotter, C. T., Proter, J. M., Lindell, T. D., Lawler, W. L., and Schlueter, W. J.,** Deep vein thrombosis treated with streptokinase or heparin: a randomized study, *Angiology,* 27, 549, 1976.
16. **Sherry, S.,** Streptokinase, urokinase: do they really work?, *Modern Med.,* (November 1), 72, 1976.
17. **Marder, V. J., Donahoe, J. F., Bell, W. R., Cranley, J. J., Kwaan, H. C., Sasahara, A. A., and Barlow, G. H.,** Comparison of in vivo biochemical effects of human urokinase prepared from urinary and tissue cultures sources, Abstr. 6th Int. Congr. Thrombosis Haemostasis, *Thromb. Hemostas.,* 38, 195, 1977.
18. **Paoletti, R. and Sherry, S., Eds.,** *Thrombosis and Urokinase,* Academic Press, New York, 1977.
19. **Mammen, E. F., Ed.,** *Thrombolytic Therapy,* Vol. 2, Sem. Thromb. Hemost., Stratton Int. Medical, New York, 1975, 1.
20. **Davidson, J. F., Samana, M. M., and Desnoyers, P. C., Eds.,** *Progress in Chemical Fibrinolysis and Thrombolysis,* Vol. 1, Raven Press, New York, 1975.
21. **Mammen, E. F., Ed.,** *Venous Thromboembolism,* Vol. 2, Sem. Thromb. Hemost., Stratton Int. Medical, New York, 1976, 203.
22. **McNicol, G. P.,** The fibrinolytic system, *Postgrad. Med. J. Suppl.,* 49, 10, 1973.
23. **Aoki, N., Moroi, M., Matsuda, M., and Tachiya, K.,** The behavior of α_2-plasmin inhibitor in fibrinolytic states, *J. Clin. Invest.,* 60, 361, 1977.
24. **Chesterman, C. N., Allington, M. J., and Sharp, A.,** Relationship of plasminogen activator to fibrin, *Nature (London) New Biol.,* 238, 15, 1972.
25. **Common, H. H., Seaman, A. J., Rosch, J., Porter, J. M., and Dotter, C. T.,** Deep vein thrombosis treated with streptokinase or heparin, *Angiology,* 27, 645, 1976.

GLOSSARY

ACA	Aminocaproic acid
ACT-INHIB	Activator-inhibitor
ADP	Adenosine diphosphate
AG-AB	Antigen-antibody
AHF	Antihemophilic factor
AHG	Antihemophilic globulin
AMP	Adenosine monophosphate
ANS	Autonomic nervous system
APTT	Activated partial thromboplastin time
ASA	Acetylsalicylic acid
ATP	Adenosine triphosphate
ATPase	Adenosine triphosphatase
ATT	Aspirin tolerance test
AV	Arterio-venous
BM	Basement membrane
BP	Blood pressure
cAMP	Cyclic adenosine monophosphate
COAX	Coagulant-anticoagulant axis
CPB	Cardiopulmonary bypass
CRM	Cross-reacting material
CVD	Collagen vascular disease
C1-INH	Inhibitor to first complement component
C1→9	Complement components
DIC	Disseminated intravascular coagulation
DVT	Deep vein thrombosis
EC	Endothelial cell
EDS	Ehler-Danlos syndrome
EDTA	Ethylenediaminetetraacetate
EEL	External elastic lamina
E(G)LT	Euglobulin lysis time
FDP	Fibrin(ogen) degradation products
FM	Fibrin monomer
GIP	Generalized intravascular proteolysis
HHT	Hereditary hemorrhagic telangiectasia
HUS	Hemolytic-uremic syndrome
Ig	Immunoglobulin
IEL	Internal elastic lamina
iP	Inorganic phosphate
ITP	Idiopathic thrombocytopenia purpura
IV	Intravenous
IVP	Intravenous push
OWR	Osler-Weber-Rendu (syndrome)
PE	Pulmonary embolism
PES	Pseudoxanthoma elasticum
PF	Platelet factor
PGI_2	Prostacyclin
PIVKA	Protein induced by vitamin K absence/antagonism
PSO_4	Protamine sulfate
PT	Prothrombin time
PTA	Plasma thromboplastin anticedent

PTT .... Partial thromboplastin time
RDS .... Respiratory distress syndrome
RT .... Reptilase time
SE .... Subendothelium
SFM .... Soluble fibrin monomer
SK .... Streptokinase
SKRT .... Streptokinase resistance test
SPD .... Storage pool disease
TBT .... Template bleeding time
TT .... Thrombin time
TTP .... Thrombotic thrombocytopenic purpura
TXA_2 .... Thromboxane
UK .... Urokinase
VKA .... Vitamin K antagonist
VWF .... von Willebrand factor

Index

INDEX

A

Acetylsalicylic acid
    effect on platelet function, 120
    use in thrombosis therapy, 216, 218
Acidosis/alkalosis, DIC associated with, 165
Acquired circulating anticoagulants, see Inhibitors
ACTH, degradation by plasmin in DIC, 167
Actinomycin D, association with hemorrhage, 221, 222
Acute febrile illness as thrombocytolytic state, 125
Adenosine, role in platelet aggregation, 23
Adenosine diphosphate, see ADP
Adenylate cyclase
    of platelet membranes, 21
ADP
    in platelets, 28
    platelet aggregation studies with, 110
    receptors for, 23
    role in platelet aggregation, 23, 24, 29
    role in storage pool disease, 111, 112
Adrenaline, increased Factor VIII activity caused by, 106
Adrenergic blocking agents, classification of platelet disorder induced by, 101
Adrenosen, control of bleeding by, 92
Adriamycin, primary fibrino(geno)-lysis caused by, 221, 222
Afibrinogenemia
    bleeding disorders in, 156
    decreased platelet retention in, 105
    platelet abnormalities in, 117
    platelet disorder classification, 100
    tests for, 86
Albinism, conditions associated with, 113, 114
Alcoholism, liver disease caused by, 185
Alkaline phosphatase, role in platelet aggregation, 22
Allergic reactions to streptokinase, 264, 266
Alpha granules of platelets, 18
Alport's syndrome, 116
Amebocytes, analogy to platelets, 97
Aminasin, antitumor effect in animals, 229
Aminocaproic acid, use in cardiopulmonary bypass, 193
Amniotic fluid embolism, DIC associated with, 164
AMP, see also Cyclic AMP
    inhibition of platelet aggregation, 23
Amyloidosis, association with acquired vascular defects, 93
Anabolic steroids, use with vitamin K antagonists, 249
Analgesics
    causing thrombocytopenia, 132
    inhibition of platelet function, 121
Anemia
    autoimmune hemolytic, association with immunologic thrombocytopenia, 131
    iron deficiency
        association with thrombocytosis, 135
        in Osler-Weber-Rendu disease, 91
        platelet disorder classification, 101
        thrombocytosis in, 125
    megaloblastic, as thrombocytolytic state, 125
    microangiopathic hemolytic, 175
    pernicious, platelet disorder classification, 101
    sideroblastic, platelet disorder classification, 100
Anesthetics, inhibition of platelet function, 121
Angioid streaks, in Ehler-Danlos syndrome, 90
Angiomata, large, association with thrombocytopenia, 84
Angioneurotic edema, hereditary, complement deficiency in, 68
Antibiotics
    causing thrombocytopenia, 132
    inhibition of platelet function, 121
    use with vitamin K antagonists, 249
Antibodies
    as complement stimulus, 67
    to clotting factors, 86
    to fibrinogen, 206
Anticoagulants
    effect on metastatic disease in cardiac patients, 231
    inhibition of platelet function, 121
    oral
        change to from heparin therapy, 248
        clinical aspects, 246
        clinical trials, 248
        contraindications, 247, 249
        drugs interacting with, 248, 249
        indications, 248
        mechanism of action, 246
        monitoring, 248
        types, 246
        use following thrombolytic therapy, 262
    use in malignancy, 216
Antidepressant drugs, classification of platelet disorder induced by, 101
Antigen-antibody complex
    DIC associated with, 164
    presence as activator of complement system, 67
Antihemophilic factor, 44
    role in Factor Xα formation, 55
Anti-inflammatory drugs, inhibition of platelet function, 121
Antineoplastics affecting hemostasis, 221, 222
α2-Antiplasmin, inhibitor of plasmin, 64
Antiplatelet antibodies in storage pool syndrome, 120

Antiplatelet drugs
  clinical aspects, 254
  clinical trials, 255
  dosage, 254
  indications, 255
  mechanism of action, 253
  side effects, 254
  tolerance test, 254
  use in cancer therapy, 216, 218
Antithrombin III
  decrease in, in certain disorders, 239
  function with heparin, 249, 250
  inhibition of coagulation, 61, 62
  levels in malignancies, 216, 217
Aortic aneurysm as thrombocytolytic state, 125
Aortic insufficiency, in Ehler-Danlos syndrome, 40
Aplastic anemia, association with thrombocytopenia, 84
Arachidonic acid, synthesis of prostaglandin endoperoxides from, 11
Arachnodactyly in Marfan's syndrome, 91
Arteries, structure, 6, 7
Arteriosclerosis at bifurcations, 7
Arthritis, rheumatoid
  as acquired vascular disorder, 92
  association with immunologic thrombocytopenia, 131
  Factor VIII inhibitors in, 207
Arthrombia, essential, platelet disorder classification, 100
L-Asparaginase, hypofibrinogenemia associated with, 222
Aspirin
  as cause of bleeding, 86
  as cause of vascular defect, 93
  clinical aspects of treatment, 254
  dosage, 254
  effect in von Willebrand's syndrome, 105
  effect on platelet aggregation, 29
  effect on platelet function, 120, 121
  indications, 255
  mechanism of action, 253
  platelet disorder induced by, classification, 101
  side effects, 254
  tolerance test, 105, 254
  use by thrombocythemia patients, 138
  use with heparin on warfarin, 255
Aspirin-like defect
  clinical features, 115
  diagnosis, 115
  pathophysiology, 115
  platelet disorder classification, 100
  release reaction abnormality in, 117
  role in storage pool disease, 112
  therapy, 116
Atherogenesis, factors predisposing to, 11
Atherosclerosis
  as thrombocytolytic state, 125
  platelet adhesion in, 239
  role of platelets in pathogenesis, 97

Athrombia, laboratory findings in, 111
ATP
  conversion to cAMP in platelet membrane, 21
  effect of epinephrine on in platelet aggregation, 24
  inhibition of platelet aggregation, 23
  production in platelets, 28
Autoerythrocytic sensitization syndrome, mechanism of, 93
  disorders in, 120
Autoprothrombin II-A, role in platelet aggregation, 24
A-V fistula, in Osler-Weber-Rendu disease, 92

B

Bacterial endocarditis, contraindication of thrombolytic therapy, 265
Bacterial infections, thrombocytopenia complicating, 129
Bacterial lipopolysaccharides, interaction with first component of complement, 67
Bacteremia, association with DIC, 164
Barbiturates, use with vitamin K antagonists, 249
Basement membrane
  exposure in trauma, 9
  of capillary endothelium, 6
  platelet adhesion, 10
Battered child syndrome, similarity of disease manifestations, 84
Bernard-Soulier syndrome
  clinical features, 109
  laboratory diagnosis, 109
  pathophysiology, 108
  platelet disorder classification, 100
  ristocetin-induced aggregation in, 106
  therapy, 109
Bile salts, role in thrombin formation, 51
Bleeding disorders, see also Hemorrhage; Vascular disorders
  Alport's syndrome, 116
  causes, 84
  drug-induced, 82, 84, 86
  Glanzmann's thrombasthenia, 111
  hemophilia, see Hemophilia
  hereditary on acquired defects, classification, 82, 83
  in DIC, 168
  intracerebral bleeding, cause of, 82
  manifestations of, 82—84
  Osler-Weber-Rendu disease, 91
  pseudoxanthoma elasticum, 91
  screening tests, 84—86
  von Willebrandis syndrome, 99—107
Bleeding time test
  diagnostic test, 98
  in Bernard-Soulier syndrome, 109
  in thrombasthenia, 111
  in von Willebrand's syndrome, 99, 105
Blood

circulating, changes in, role in thrombosis, 238
coagulation, see Coagulation
flow, changes in, role in thrombus formation, 238
group O, genetic linkage to HHT, 91
platelets, see Platelets
Blue sclerae in vascular disorders, 90, 91
Bone defects
  in Marfan's syndrome, 91
  in osteogenesis imperfecta, 91
Bone marrow
  disorders causing thrombocytopenias, 84
  examination in low platelet count, 85
  hypoplasia
    causes of, 128
    in Fanconi's syndrome, 126
  infiltration, thrombocytopenia in, 128
  platelet production by megakaryocytes, 30
  replacement, thrombocytopenia associated with, 208
  study, in platelet disorder, 98
  suppression, thrombocytopenia associated with, 219
Bradykinin, contraction of endothelial cells caused by, 7
Breast carcinoma
  inhibitors associated with, 219
  splenic metastases in, 220
Bruising
  aspirin ingestion associated with, 93
  as sign of collagen disease, 92
  defective lipid peroxidation associated with, 138
  in afibrinogenemia, 156
  in aspirin-like defect, 115
  in Bernard-Soulier syndrome, 109
  in storage pool disease, 114
  in vascular disorders, 90, 91
  in von Willebrand's syndrome, 104, 207
  platelet function defect associated with, 221
Burns, DIC associated with, 164, 165

C

Calcinosis, subcutaneous, in pseudoxanthoma elasticum, 91
Calcium
  chelators, inhibition of platelet aggregation, 21
  deficiency in storage pool disease, 113
Calcium ions
  chelation affecting platelet shape, 29
  role in Factor IX formation, 56
  role in Factor Xa formation, 54, 55
  role in platelet aggregation, 21
  role in thrombin formation, 45, 51
cAMP, see Cyclic AMP
Cancer, see Malignancy; particular cancers
Cannula, infected, thrombolytic therapy contraindicated, 265
Capillaries, structure, 6, 7

γ-Carboxyglutamic acid
  occurrence in Factor IX, 56
  occurrence in prothrombin and Factor X, 53
  role in fibrin formation, 46
  role in thrombin formation, 51, 52
  structure, 47
Carcinoma, thrombocytosis associated with, 135
Carcinomatosis as thrombocytolytic state, 125
Cardiopulmonary bypass
  antifibrinolytic agents used in, 193
  antiplatelet drugs prior to surgery, blood loss related to, 196
  bleeding during, causes of, 197, 198
  case history requirements, 194
  coagulation factor deficiencies during, 191
  differential diagnosis, 199
  disseminated intravascular coagulation associated with, 192, 194
  fibrino(geno)lysis during, 191
  hemorrhage in
    incidence, 188
    management, 198
    potential causes, 193
    prevention, 194—197
  heparin doses in, 250
  heparin rebound in, 193, 194
  hypofibrinogenemia in, 191, 192
  hypothermic perfusion in, 193
  physical findings in patients, preoperative, 195
  platelet function in, 189, 190
  preoperative findings, 194—198
  techniques, 188
  thrombocytopenia in, 188
  vascular defects, 190, 191
Cardiovascular drugs, inhibition of platelet function, 121
Central nervous system bleeding in Alport's syndrome, 116
Cerebral embolism, contraindication of thrombolytic therapy, 265
Cerebral ischemic attacks
  drugs used in treatment, 122
  use of sulfinpyrazone in, 255
  use of vitamin K antagonists in, 248
Chediak-Higashi syndrome, platelet disorder classification, 100
Chediak-Steinbrinck-Higashi anomaly, clinical features, 114
Chemotherapy
  anticoagulant treatment in conjunction with, 231
  as treatment of dysproteinemias, 120
  cytotoxic, DIC associated with, 165
  DIC affected by, 217
  hemostasis affected by, 221
  normalization of coagulation following, 214
  thrombocytopenia associated with, 208, 219
Chloral hydrate, use with vitamin K antagonists, 249
Chloramphenicol, use with vitamin K antagonists, 249
Chlorothiazides, suppression of megakaryocytes, 128

Chlorpropamide, use with vitamin K antagonists, 249
Christmas disease, see Hemophilia
Chronic liver disease, see Liver disease
Cinchona alkaloids causing thrombocytopenia, 132
Circulating blood, changes in, role in thrombosis, 238, 239
Circumcision, hemophilia observed in, 150, 152
Cirrhosis
    as thrombocytolytic state, 125
    fibrinolytic activity in, 62, 230
    platelet aggregation changes in, 120
    platelet disorder classification, 100
Clofibrate, use with vitamin K antagonists, 249
Clot formation, see Coagulation
Coagulation
    early steps in, 56—58
    effect of on development of metastases, 228
    factors, see also Factor I, Factor II, etc.
        changes in, in thrombosis, 239
        deficiencies, 44
        deficiencies during cardiopulmonary bypass, 191
        diagnosis of abnormalities, 85
        listed, 45
        synonyms, 45
    fibrin formation, 46—49
    hypercoagulability, see Hypercoagulability
    inhibitors, decrease in certain disorders, 239
    inhibitory mechanisms, 59—62
    proteins, as hemostatic compartment, 82
    stimulation in trauma, 6
    thrombin formation, 49—52
Collagen
    acquired diseases, association with vascular defect, 92
    configuration, relationship to induction properties, 11
    decrease in, in Ehler-Danlos syndrome, 90
    defect, in osteogenesis imperfecta, 91
    enzyme transfering amino-sugar to, 21
    impaired adhesion of platelets, 100, 109
    in internal elastic lamina, 6
    layer surrounding blood vessels, 7
    platelet adhesion to, 29
    platelet interaction, 10
    role in activation of Factor XII, 57
    role in changes in vessel wall, 240
    role in platelet adhesion, 9
    role in platelet aggregation, 23, 27, 29
Colon carcinoma
    splenic metastases in, 220
    streptokinase treatment, study of, 231
    thrombosis associated with, 216
Complement system
    activated first component inhibitor, role in plasmin formation, 64
    activation by plasmin, 63, 68
    components, functions of, 69
    deficiencies in, effects of, 68, 70
    degradation of complement by plasmin in DIC, 167
    interrelationships with coagulation and fibrinolysis, 68—70
    mechanisms, 67
    role in platelet aggregation, 20, 21
    role of Hageman factor in activation, 159
Compliance vessels, veins as, 6
Connective tissue disorder, manifestations of, 84
Consanguinity in thrombasthenia patients, 111
Consumption coagulopathy, see Disseminated intravascular coagulation
Coronary artery disease, increased Factor VIII activity in, 106
Corticosteroids, use with vitamin K antagonists, 249
Coumarins as oral anticoagulants, 246
Crush injuries, DIC associated with, 164, 165
Cryofibrinogens, increased levels in malignancy, 214
Cryoprecipitate, use in afibrinogenemia treatment, 157
Cushing's syndrome
    association with vascular defect, 92
    blood tests for, 85
    increased Factor VIII activity in, 106
Cyanotic congenital heart disease
    as thrombocytolytic state, 125
    hemostasis derangements during CPB, 193
    platelet disorder classification, 101
    platelet factor 3 deficiency, 120
Cyclic AMP
    biochemical reactions involving, 22
    effect of dipyridamole on, 253
    inhibition by epinephrine in platelet aggregation, 24
    role in platelet aggregation, 21
Cyclo-oxygenase deficiency, platelet disorder classification, 100
Cytosine arabinoside, association with thrombocytosis, 137
Cytosol of platelets, 18

D

Daunomycin, primary fibrino(geno)lysis caused by, 222
Deep vein thrombophlebitis, see Thrombophlebitis
Defibrination syndrome, see Disseminated intravascular coagulation
Dense bodies of platelets, see Platelets
Dermatitis herpiformis, Factor VIII inhibitors in, 207
Dermatomyositis as acquired vascular disorder, 92
Diabetes
    as thrombocytolytic state, 125
    decreased fibrinolytic activity in, 240
    increased Factor VIII activity in, 106

increased fibrinolytic inhibitors in, 240
platelet adhesion in, 239
DIC, see Disseminated intravascular coagulation
Diethylstilbestrol, effect on platelet production, 128
DiGuglielmo's syndrome
in effective thrombopoiesis in, 129
platelet disorder classification, 100
Diphenylhydantoin, use with vitamin K antagonists, 249
Dipyridamole
dosage, 254
inhibition of platelet aggregation, 121
mechanism of action, 253
side effects, 254
tolerance test, 254
use in thrombosis therapy, 216, 218
use with other drugs, 255
Disseminated intravascular coagulation
acute, hemorrhage in, 217
associated conditions, 164—166
association with malignancy, 214, 228
association with myeloma, 208, 209
association with Osler-Weber-Rendu disease, 92
association with thrombocytopenia, 84
as thrombocytolytic state, 125
bleeding in, 168
blood tests for, 85
causes, 164, 165
chemotherapy affecting, 217
clinical manifestations, 164, 165, 168
comparison with primary fibrino(geno)lysis, 184
decreased platelet retention in, 105
diagnosis, 166, 168—171
during cardiopulmonary bypass, 192, 194
Factor IX concentrates causing, 155
heparin therapy, 252
in adenocarcinoma of prostate, 215
microangiopathic hemolytic anemia as cause, 217
pathophysiology, 165—168
platelet disorder classification, 100
radioimmunoassay in diagnosis, 170
radiotherapy as cause, 217
related syndromes, 174—177
role of Hageman factor in, 159
sepsis as cause, 217
shock in, 168
shock lung, similarity, 175
storage pool syndrome associated with, 120
therapy, 172—174
therapy in cancer patients, 218
thrombocytopenia in, 129
transfusion as cause, 218
Disulfiran, use with vitamin K antagonists, 249
Diverticulitis, contraindication of thrombolytic therapy, 265
DNA synthesis, impaired, platelet production abnormality associated with, 129
Dohle bodies, in May-Hegglin anomaly, 117

Doppler ultrasonography, use in thrombosis diagnosis, 247
Drugs
affecting platelet function, 120, 121
bleeding disorders induced by, 82, 84, 86
Factor VIII inhibitors following exposure to, 207
immunosuppressive, in treatment of ITP, 134
interaction with vitamin K antagonists, 248, 249
marrow hypoplasia caused by, 128
Dwarfism in Fanconi's syndrome, 126
Dysfibrinogenemia
clinical manifestations, 156
diagnosis, 157
in liver disease, 184
in liver metastases, 219
mechanism of clotting abnormality in, 48
pathophysiology, 156, 158
treatment, 157
Dysproteinemia
abnormal platelet function in, 119
bleeding due to, 84

E

Ecchymoses
in acute DIC, 217
in Factor V deficiency, 157
in Factor XIII deficiency, 159
in liver disease, 185
in prothrombin deficiency, 157
in uremia, 119
in vascular disorders, 90
in von Willebrand's syndrome, 207
Ecto-ATPase, role in platelet aggregation, 21
Ectopia lentis in Marfan's syndrome, 91
Ehler-Danlos syndrome, 90
coagulation abnormalities in, 117
platelet disorder classification, 100
Ehrlich's sarcoma in mice, metastasis study of, 229
Elastic tissue
abnormal, in pseudoxanthoma elasticum, 91
increase in, in Ehler-Danlos syndrome, 90
Elastin in internal elastic lamina, 7
Electrocauterization for control of epistaxis, 92
Endocarditis
bacterial, contraindication of thrombolytic therapy, 264, 165
nonbacterial thrombotic, association with carcinomas, 230
Endothelial cells
relationship to Factor VIII components, 103
role in Factor VIII biology, 102
Endothelium
damage to, effects of, 174, 175
role in hemostasis, 7
structure, 6
Endotoxins, role in platelet aggregation, 27

Enzymes of platelet plasma membranes, function, 21, 27
Epinephrine
　effect on platelet count, 125
　role in platelet aggregation, 23, 24, 27, 29
Epistaxis
　detection by fibrinogen chromatography, 241
　formation, 46
　in aspirin-like defect, 115
　in Bernard-Soulier syndrome, 109
　in essential thrombocythemia, 137
　in Factor VII or Factor X deficiency, 157
　in liver disease, 185, 186
　in Osler-Weber-Rendu disease, 91
　in storage pool disease, 114
　in liver metastases, 219
　levels in malignancy, 214
　polymerization, 19
Fibrinogen
　affinity of plasmin for, 63
　antibodies to, 206
　chromatography, use in thrombosis diagnosis, 241
　clotting agents, 24
　conversion to fibrin, 44, 45, 46
　degradation products, see Fibrinogen/fibrin degradation products
　increased turnover in malignancy, 214
　increase in, in certain disorders, 239
　increase in, in malignancy, 230
　inhibitors to, 206
　in platelet interior, 19
　levels in liver disease, 184
　release from α-granules, 28
　role in platelet aggregation, 20, 23
　structure, 46, 48, 66
　subspecies, detection by chromatography, 241
Fibrinogen Detroit
　mechanism of clotting abnormality, 48
　pathophysiology, 156
Fibrinoligase, see Factor XIIIα
Fibrinogen/fibrin degradation products
　as coagulation inhibitors, 61
　chemistry and function, 65, 66
　creation in DIC pathophysiology, 166, 167
　in vascular disorders, 90, 91
　in von Willebrand's syndrome, 104, 207
Erythrocytes, production, relationship to platelet production, 124
Estrogens
　control of bleeding by, 92
　increased levels in liver disease, 185
　thrombocytopenia produced by, 125, 128
Etchlorvynol, use with vitamin K antagonists, 249
Ethacrynic acid, use with vitamin K antagonists, 249
Ethanol, effect on platelet production, 128
External elastic lamina in vascular structure, 7
Eye defects in Marfan's syndrome, 91

F

Factor I
　deficiency, 156, 157
　role in hypercoagulability, 214
Factor II
　association with platelet membranes, 19
　decreased synthesis in liver disease, 184
　defect, diagnosis of, 85
　deficiency, congenital, 157
　inhibitors to, 206
　role in CPB hemorrhage, 192
　vitamin K antagonists affecting synthesis, 246
Factor V
　decreased levels in liver disease, 185
　defect, diagnosis of, 85
　deficiency characterization, 44
　deficiency, congenital, 157
　degradation by plasmin in DIC, 167
　increase in, in certain ailments, 239
　increase in, in malignancy, 230
　inhibitors to, 206
　in platelets, 19
　role in CPB hemorrhage, 192
　role in hypercoagulability, 214
　role in thrombin formation, 51
Factor VII
　association with platelet membranes, 19
　decreased synthesis in liver disease, 184
　deficiency characterization, 44
　deficiency, congenital, 157
　defect, diagnosis of, 85
　increase in, in certain ailments, 239
　nonproteolytic activation, 59
　role in Factor Xα formation, 54
　role in fibrin formation, 45
　structure, 54, 55
　synthesis, 46
　vitamin K antagonists affecting synthesis, 246
Factor VIII
　antibodies, development in hemophilia patients, 153
　antibody preparation, 101
　antigen synthesis, 102
　antigen synthesis and release, 7
　as antihemophiliac factor, 150
　as clotting factor, 44
　association with platelet membranes, 19
　components, terms for, 101, 102
　concentrate, use in management of hemophilia, 153
　decreased levels
　　in liver disease, 185
　　in platelet release abnormalities, 116
　deficiency, diagnosis of, 85
　deficiency, platelet disorder classification, 100
　deficiency rate in hemophiliacs, 152
　degradation by plasmin in DIC, 167
　increased activity, causes of, 105, 106
　increase in, in certain ailments, 239
　increase in, in malignancy, 230
　inhibitors to, 206
　macromolecular complex, 151
　pathophysiology, 150, 151

properties, 55, 102
reduced activity in von Willebrand's syndrome, 99, 100, 101
relationship of components to endothelial cell, 103
role in CPB hemorrhage, 192
role in fibrin formation, 45
role in formation of Factor Xα, 55
role in hypercoagulability, 214
role in platelet aggregation, 27
Factor IX
  abnormalities, diagnosis of, 85
  association with platelet membranes, 19
  decreased levels in liver disease, 185
  decreased synthesis in liver disease, 184
  deficiency characterization, 44
  deficiency, in hemophilia B, 150, 154
  deficiency, platelet disorder classification, 100
  degradation by plasmin in DIC, 167
  inhibitors to, 207
  role in fibrin formation, 45
  role in hypercoagulability, 214
  vitamin K antagonists affecting synthesis, 246
Factor IXα
  formation, 56
  role in formation of Factor Xα, 55
  structure, 56
  synthesis, 46
Factor X
  activation by Factor VII, 54, 55
  association with platelet membranes, 19
  decreased synthesis in liver disease, 184
  deficiency characterization, 44
  deficiency, congenital, 157
  defect, diagnosis of, 85
  derivation of Factor Xα from, 52, 53
  generation of thrombin, rate of, 249
  inhibition by antithrombin III, 249
  role in coagulation in mucinous adenocarcinoma, 215
  role in fibrin formation, 45
  role in platelet aggregation, 24
  structure, 53
  vitamin K antagonists affecting synthesis, 246
Factor X$\alpha\alpha$, formation, 53
Factor Xα
  activation of Factor XIII, 49
  as inhibitor, 60
  formation, 52—56
  role in thrombin formation, 51
  synthesis, 46
Factor X $\alpha\beta$, formation, 53
Factor XI
  activation, role of collagen in, 11
  decreased levels in liver disease, 185
  deficiency characterization, 44
  deficiency, diagnosis of, 85
  deficiency, in hemophilia C, 150, 155
  degradation by plasmin in DIC, 167
  inhibitors to, 207
  role in fibrin formation, 45
  role in hypercoagulability, 214

Factor XIα
  formation, 56
  structure, 57
  surface function, 58
Factor XII
  activation by collagen, 9
  conversion to Factor XIIα, 57
  deficiency, 159
  deficiency characterization, 44
  deficiency, diagnosis of, 85
  enzymes activating, 57
  levels in liver metastases, 219
  nonproteolytic activation, 59
  role in complement activation, 68
  role in fibrin formation, 45
  role in kinin generation, 66, 67
  structure, 57
Factor XIIα
  action of plasmin on, 63
  conversion of Factor XII to, 57
Factor XIII
  activation to enzymatic form, 49
  as intraplatelet procoagulant, 20
  conversion to Factor XIIIα
  deficiency characterization, 44
  deficiency, congenital, 159
  deficiency in malignancy, 219
  inhibitors to, 207
Factor XIIIα, role in cross-linking process of fibrin formation, 47—50
Fanconi's syndrome, anomalies in, 126
Fatty acids, role in platelet aggregation, 27
FDP, see Fibrinogen/fibrin degradation products
Felty's syndrome, altered platelet distribution in, 129
Fibrin
  affinity of plasmin for, 63
  antithrombin effect, 61
  cascade formation, 44
  conversion of fibrinogen to, 44, 45
  degradation products, see Fibrinogen/fibrin degradation products
  dissolution, 65
  formation
    cross-linking process, 48
    polymerization, 47
    proteolysis, 46
    stabilization, 48
    tumors associated with, 214
  lysis, see Fibrinolysis
  plate technique in diagnostic testing, 86
  viscosity, variations in, 47
Fibrin monomer
  increased levels in malignancy, 214
Fibrinolysis, see also Fibrinogen/fibrin degradation products
  activator activity, decreased, in thrombophlebitis, 241
  decreased activity in certain disorders, 240
  during cardiopulmonary bypass, 191
  hypofibrinolysis mechanisms, 240
  increase in enzymes in malignancy, 214

inhibitors, 240
in malignant tissues, 228, 230
interrelationship with complement system, 68—70
mechanism of dissolution, 65
plasmin formation, 63
therapy based on, see Thrombolytic therapy
Fibrinopeptides
release in fibrin formation, 45
structure, 46, 48
Fibrinoplastic substance, role in clotting, 19
Fibrin stabilizing factor, see Factor XIII
Fitzgerald factor deficiency, 85, 160
Fletcher factor deficiency, 85, 160
Fletcher trait, association with thromboembolism predisposition, 64
Floppy mitral valve in Ehler-Danlos syndrome, 90

G

Galactosyl-hydroxylysine groups, role in collagen-platelet interaction, 11
Gall bladder, cancer of, thrombosis associated with, 216
Gastrointestinal bleeding
control by Adrenosen, 92
in acute DIC, 217
in essential thrombocythemia, 137
in Factor VII or Factor X deficiency, 157
in hereditary disorder
in Osler-Weber-Rendu disease, 91, 92
in pseudoxanthoma elasticum, 91
in uremia, 119
in vascular disorders, 90
in von Willebrand's syndrome, 104
thrombosis occurring with, 137
Gastrointestinal tract, carcinoma of
fibrinolysis in tissue, 228
postoperative thrombosis associated with, 216
Gaucher's disease, altered platelet distribution in, 129
Genitourinary bleeding
control by Adrenosem, 92
in acute DIC, 217
in essential thrombocythemia, 137
in Factor VII or Factor X deficiency, 157
in Osler-Weber-Rendu disease, 92
in vascular disorders, 90
Genitourinary drugs, inhibition of platelet function, 121
Giant cavernous hemangiomata, similarity to HHT, 92
Gingival bleeding
association of platelet function defects with, 221
in Ehler-Danlos syndrome, 90
in liver disease, 186
in malignancies, 168
in vascular disorders, 90
Glanzmann's thrombasthenia

bleeding due to, 84
clinical features, 111
decreased platelet retention in, 105
diagnosis, 111
pathophysiology, 110
platelet disorder classification, 100
therapy, 111
Glass-bead retention assays
disorders in which decreased retention found, 105
in Bernard-Soulier syndrome, 109
in storage pool disease, 114
in thrombasthenia, 111
in von Willebrand's syndrome, 106
platelet function testing by, 99, 105, 106
Glomerular disease, drugs used in treatment, 122
Glucagon, use with vitamin K antagonists, 249
Glucose in platelet metabolism, 28
Glucose-6-phosphate dehydrogenase deficiency, platelet disorder classification, 100, 118
Glutethiomide, use with vitamin K antagonists, 249
Glycocalyx of platelets, 18—20
Glycogen storage disease
bleeding disorder in, 117
platelet disorder classification, 100
Glycolysis process in platelets, 28
Glycoprotein, enzyme transfering amino-sugar residue to, 21
Glycosyl transferase
in platelet plasma membrane, 21
role in platelet-collagen interaction, 10
Golgi complex
of megakaryocytes, 122
of platelets, 18
Gout as thrombocytolytic state, 125
Gram-negative organisms, association with DIC, 164
Gram-positive organisms, association with DIC, 164
Griseofulvin, use with vitamin K antagonists, 249
Growth hormone, degradation by plasmin in DIC, 167
Guanidosuccinic acid
role in defective platelet function, 119
role in hemorrhage in malignant paraprotein disorders, 208

H

Hageman factor, see also Factor XII
deficiency, 159
role in complement activation, 159
Hageman trait, association with thromboembolism predisposition, 64
Haloperidol, use with vitamin K antagonists, 249
Hamartomata, association with Osler-Weber-Rendu disease, 92
Heart valves, prosthetic
antiplatelet agents used in connection with, 255

as thrombocytolytic state, 125
drugs preventing thrombosis on, 122
platelet destruction associated with, 129
Hemagglutination inhibition assay system, 106
Hemarthroses
   Factor VIII inhibitors associated with, 207
   in afibrinogenemia, 156
   in Factor VII or Factor X deficiency, 157
   in thrombasthenia, 111
   in vascular disorders, 90
Hematomata
   in Factor V deficiency, 157
   in Factor XIII deficiency, 159
   in prothrombin deficiency, 157
Hematuria
   in liver disease, 186
   in storage pool disease, 114
   in von Willebrand's syndrome, 104
Hemodialysis as therapy in uremia, 119
Hemoglobimuria, paroxysmal nocturnal,
      ineffective thrombopoiesis in, 129
Hemolytic-uremic syndrome
   clinical features, 175
   similarity to TTP, 130
Hemophilia
   A
      carriers, detection of, 151
      clinical aspects, 152
      diagnosis, 152
      distinction from von Willebrand's disease,
         150, 151
      Factor VIII inhibitors, incidence of, 206
      laboratory and clinical features, 107
      management, 152—154
   B
      clinical aspects, 154
      Factor IX inhibitors in, 207
      genetic variants, 154
      identification, 150
      management, 155
      pathophysiology, 154
   C
      clinical aspects, 155
      identification, 150
      management, 155
      pathophysiology, 154
      sex incidence, 155
   Christmas disease, see B, supra
   classical, see A, supra
   Factor VIII deficiency in
      pathophysiology of Factor VIII, 150, 151
      recognition, 150
      test for, 86
   genetic factors, 150, 152
   hemostatic compartments involved in, 82
   history, 150
   joint bleeding in, 84
   sex incidence, 150
Hemoptysis
   in Osler-Weber-Rendu disease, 92
   in osteogenesis imperfecta, 91
Hemorrhage

drugs associated with, 221
in cardiopulmonary bypass, 188, 193—197
in DIC, 164, 165, 217
   mechanism of, 167
   multiple, 168
in liver disease, 183, 185, 187
in malignancy, 217—219
in malignant paraprotein disorders, 208
in primary hyperfibrino(geno)lysis, 182
in uremia, 208
in Waldenstron's microglobulinemia, 208
therapy, in malignant paraprotein disorders,
   209
Hemorrhagic diathesis
   as sign of vascular disorder, 92
   in vascular disorders, 90
Hemorrhagic thrombocythemia, platelet disorder
      classification, 100
Hemostatic compartments, classification for
      diagnosis, 82
Henoch-Schonlein syndrome
   blood tests for, 85
   purpura associated with, 93
Heparin
   administration methods, 250
   clinical aspects of use, 250
   clinical trials, 252
   dose calculation, 249, 250
   effect on cell growth, 229
   half-life, 251
   inhibition by PF-4, 19
   mechanism of action, 249, 250
   mini-heparin therapy
      in DIC, 173, 174, 218
      indications, 252, 253
      in thrombosis, 216
      subcutaneous injection, 250
   monitoring, 251
   role in inhibition of coagulation, 61, 62
   therapy change to vitamin K antagonists, 248
   therapy, in DIC, 172, 173
   treatment affecting hepatic metastases, 229
   treatment before chemotheraphy in lung
         cancer, 231
   use as anticoagulant, 22
   use before cytotoxic chemotherapy, 165
   use following thrombolytic therapy, 262, 267
   use in cardiopulmonary bypass, 193, 194
   use in malignancy, 216
Hepatic metastases, see Liver
Hepatocytes, site of biosynthesis of fibrin *a*
      chains, 49
Hereditary hemorrhagic telangiectasia, 91, 92
Hermansky-Pudlek syndrome
   clinical features, 113
   platelet disorder classification, 100
Heyokinase of platelet membranes, 21
HHT, see Oslor-Weber-Rendu disease
Hip surgery
   aspirin use in, 255
   heparin prophylaxis in, 254
Histamine, contraction of endothelial cells caused

by, 7
Histoplasmosis, thrombocytopenia in, 128
Hodgkin's disease
  altered platelet distribution in, 129
  as thrombocytolytic state, 125
  thrombocytosis associated with, 135
Homocystinuria
  as thrombocytolytic state, 125
  platelet hyperfunction in, 118
Hughes-Storen syndrome, activation phase factor in, 160
Hunter's syndrome
  coagulation abnormalities in, 117
  platelet disorder classification, 100
Hurler's syndrome
  coagulation abnormalities in, 117
  platelet disorder classification, 100
Hydroxyphenolacetic acid, inhibition of platelet function, 119
Hypercoagulability
  association with malignancy, 214
  laboratory diagnosis, 241
  pathophysiology, 214, 215
Hyperfibrino(geno)lysis, see Primary hyperfibrino(geno)lysis
Hyperglobulinemia, clotting defects in, 86
Hypersplenism in malignancy, 220
Hypertension
  contraindication of thrombolytic therapy, 265
  malignant, contraindication of oral coagulants, 247
Hyperthyroidism
  association with immunologic thrombocytopenia, 131
  increased Factor VIII activity caused by, 106
Hypnotics causing thrombocytopenia, 132
Hypoalbuminemia, Factor VIII deficiency associated with, 219
Hypofibrinogenemia
  bleeding in, 156
  in cardiopulmonary bypass, 191, 192
  in liver disease, 184
  L-asparaginase therapy associated with, 221
  tests for, 86
Hypofibrinolysis mechanisms, 240
Hypogenitalism in Fanconi's syndrome, 126
Hypoglycemia, increased Factor VIII activity following, 106
Hypoplasia
  acquired, 127, 128
  congenital, 126, 127
Hypothermic anesthesia, thrombocytopenia in, 129

I

Idiopathic thrombocytopenic purpura
  as thrombocytolytic state, 125
  clinical features, 132, 133
  forms of, 131
  manifestations of, 84
  platelet disorder classification, 100
  ristocetin-induced aggregation in, 102
  treatment, 133, 134
^{125}I-fibrinogen scans, use in thrombosis diagnosis, 247
Imipramine, inhibition of serotonin uptake, 25
Immunoglobulins
  as complement activation stimulus, 67
  as inhibitors, 206
  drug-induced, 130
  role in platelet aggregation, 20
Impedence plethysmography, use in thrombosis diagnosis, 247
Indanedione derivatives as oral anticoagulants, 246
Infectious mononucleosis
  ristocetin-induced aggregation in, 106
  thrombocytopenia complicating, 130
Infiltrative diseases, classification of thrombocytopenia associated with, 127
Inflammation
  in course of complement function, 67
  role of Factor XII in, 66
Inhibitors
  in lupas erythematosus, 208
  in malignant paraprotein disorders, 219
  in tumors, 219
  to Factor V, 206
  to Factor VIII, 206, 207
  to Factor IX, 207
  to Factor XI, 207
  to Factor XIII, 207
  to fibrinogen, 206
  to prothrombin, 206
  to von Willebrand factor, 207
  types, 206
Injury
  bleeding following
    in hemophilia, 152, 154
    in hypofibrinogenemia, 156
    in prothrombin deficiency, 157
  clotting at site, 61
  coagulation factors in, 239
  contraindication of thrombolytic therapy, 265
  DIC associated with, 164, 165
  effect on Factor Xα formation, 56
  fibrinolytic activity in, 62
  minor, bleeding in, 82
  poor healing following, in Factor XIII deficiency, 159
  tissue factor release upon, 54
Insulin, degradation by plasmin in DIC, 167
Internal elastic lamina of blood vessels, 6
Intra-articular bleeding
  in afibrimogenemia, 156
  in Factor VII and Factor X deficiencies, 157
  in Factor XIII deficiency, 159
  of hemophiliacs, 152, 154
Intracerebral bleeding by hemophiliacs, 152

Intracranial bleeding
　　in acute DIC, 217
　　in osteogenesis imperfecto, 91
Intramuscular bleeding of hemophiliacs, 152, 154
Intraperitoneal bleeding in acute DIC, 217
Intrauterine infection as cause of
　　thrombocytopenia, 126
Intravascular hemolysis
　　DIC associated with, 164, 165
　　increase in coagulation factors in, 239
Insulin, role in complement activation, 68
Ionizing radiation, thrombocytopenia resulting
　　from, 128
Iron deficiency anemia, see Anemia
Isotopes used in labeling in platelet life span
　　study, 124

J

Jaundice associated with pancreatic carcinoma,
　　230
Joint bleeding in hemophilia, 84
Joints
　　hyperexetensible, in Marfan's syndrome, 91
　　hypermobile, in Ehler-Danlos syndrome, 90

K

Kallikrein
　　activation of plasminogen, 64
　　role in Factor XII conversion, 57
　　role in kinin generation, 66
Kasabach-Merritt syndrome, relationship to
　　HHT, 92
Kinins
　　action on by plasmin, 63
　　function, 67
　　generation, 66
　　　interrelationship with complement system, 70
　　　role of Hageman factor in, 159
Kininogen
　　classes of, 66
　　role in Factor XI activation, 56, 57

L

Laennec's type cirrhosis, in Oster-Weber-Rendu
　　disease, 92
Laki Lorand Factor, see Factor XIII
Latex, role in platelet aggregation, 27
Leukemia
　　acute
　　　platelet surface reactivity in, 230
　　　ristocetin-induced aggregation in, 106
　　acute myelocytic, drug-induced DIC in, 221
　　association with thrombocytopenia, 84
　　blood tests for, 85
　　chronic lymphocytic, association with
　　　immunologic thrombocytopenia, 131
　　chronic myelogenous, thrombocythemia in, 137
　　DIC associated with, 165, 166
　　hairy cell, platelet disorder classification, 101
　　ineffective thrombopoiesis in, 129
　　microangiopathic hemolytic, DIC caused by,
　　　217
　　myelocytic, platelet disorder classification, 100
　　thrombocytopenia in, 128
Leukemic reticuloendotheliosis, platelet disorder
　　classification, 101
Leukocytes, role in plasmin synthesis, 63
Leukocytosis, blood tests for, 85
Lipids, role in thrombus formation, 239, 240
Lipoprotein as tissue factor, 7
Liver
　　cirrhosis, see Cirrhosis
　　metastases
　　　antithrombin III levels in, 216, 217
　　　dysfibrinogenemia in, 219
　　　Factor XII deficiency in, 219
　　　Factor XIII deficiency in, 219
　　　heparin treatment in rats, 229
　　　prekallikrein levels in, 219
　　　prothrombin complex deficiencies associated
　　　　with, 219
　　parenchymal cells, prothrombin synthesis in, 49
Liver disease
　　alcoholism causing, 185
　　coagulation protein changes, 184
　　diagnosis, 185, 186
　　estrogen levels in, 185
　　hemorrhage in, 183, 185, 187
　　platelet changes in, 185
　　primary hyperfibrino(geno)lysis in, 182, 185
　　therapy, 86, 187
　　vascular defects in, 185
Lung carcinoma
　　association with recurrent phlebitis, 230
　　heparin treatment before chemotherapy, 231
　　splenic metastases associated with, 220
　　thrombosis associated with, 216
Lungs, metastases to, in animals, 228
Lupus erythematosus
　　antibodies to clotting in, 86
　　anticoagulants associated with, 208
　　as acquired vascular disorder, 92
　　association with immunologic
　　　thrombocytopenia, 131
　　association with von Willebrand's syndrome,
　　　108
　　as thrombocytolytic state, 125
　　Factor VIII inhibitors in, 207
　　Factor XI inhibitors in, 207
　　platelet disorder classification, 100
Lymphoma
　　altered platelet distribution in, 129
　　fibrinolytic activity in, 62
　　lymphocytic, association with immunologic
　　　thrombocytopenic, 131

Lymphoproliferative malignancies in Wiskott-Aldrich syndrome, 113
Lymphosarcoma, anticoagulants used in, 231
Lysosomal enzymes, release from α-granules, 28

M

$α_2$ Macroglobulin, role in plasmin formation, 64
Malaria, thrombocytopenia complicating, 130
Malignancy
  acute DIC in, 217
  anticoagulants affecting, 231
  antithrombin III levels in, 216, 217
  antitumor therapy affecting hemostasis, 216
  coagulation factors, increase in, 239
  contraindication of thrombolytic therapy, 265
  development of metastases, see Metastases
  DIC associated with, 165, 166, 168, 228
  Factor XIII deficiency in, 219
  fibrin formation in tissue, 228
  fibrinolytic activity in, 219, 228
  hemorrhage in, 217—219
  hemostasis disturbances in, 230
  hypercoagulability and thrombosis associated with, 214, 216
  hyperfibrino(geno)lysis in, 201
  increase of fibrinolysis inhibitors in, 240
  metastasis, see Metastases
  paraprotein disorders, defective hemostasis in, 208, 209
  platelet function defects, 220
  postoperative thrombophlebitis associated with, 216
  primary hyperfibrino(geno)lysis in, 219
  procoagulant activity in cells, 228
  splenic metastases in, 220
  surgery for, heparin prophylaxis in, 252, 253
  therapy of DIC, 218
  thrombocytopenia in, 219
  thrombocytosis associated with, 215, 230
  thrombotic thrombocytopenia purpura in, 220
Malignant melanoma, hemorrhage in acute DIC associated with, 217
Malignant paraprotein disorders, see Paraprotein disorders
Marfan's syndrome
  clinical features, 90
  coagulation abnormalities in, 117
  platelet disorder classification, 100
Maturation defects, association with thrombocytopenia, 84
May-Hegglin anomaly, 100, 117
Mefenemic acid, use with vitamin K antagonsists, 249
Megakaryoblasts, structure, 122
Megakaryocytes
  abnormalities in Bernard-Soulier syndrome, 109
  drugs suppressing, 128
  effect of estrogen on, 125
  Factor VIII-related antigen content, 102
  formation, 122, 123
  in ITP, 133
  platelet production, 30, 122
  process forming giant platelets, 117
  site of biosynthesis of fibrin a chains, 49
Megakaryopoiesis in liver disease, 185
Megaloblastic anemia, association with thrombocytopenia, 84
Melphalan, effects on hemostasis, 221, 222
Menimgococcus, association with DIC, 164
Menopause, increased Factor VIII activity associated with, 106
Menorrhagia
  in aspirin-like defect, 115
  in Bernard-Soulier syndrome, 109
  in Osler-Weber-Rendu disease, 92
  in von Willebrand's syndrome, 104
Meprobamate, use with vitamin K antagonists, 249
Metastases
  animal experiments, 228, 229
  development, 228
  extrapulmonary, development, 229
  heparinization of rats affecting, 229
  in rhabdomyosarcoma in mice, 229
  liver, see Liver
  pancreatic carcinoma, 230
  plasmin injection affecting, 229
  pulmonary, in animals, 228
Methylphenidate, use with vitamin K antagonists, 249
Methylxanthines, role in platelet aggregation, 21
Microangiopathic disorders, drugs used in treatment, 122
Microangiopathic hemolytic anemia, red cell changes in, 175
Microcephaly in Fanconi's syndrome, 126
Microophthalmia in Fanconi's syndrome, 126
Microtubules of platelets, 18
Mithramycin, effects on hemostasis, 222
Mitochondria of platelets, 18, 28
Molluscoid pseudotumors in Ehler-Danlos syndrome, 90
Monoclonal immunoglobulin spike, association with von Willebrand's syndrome, 108
Mononucleosis
  ristocetin-induced aggregation in, 106
  thrombocytopenia complicating, 130
Mucinous adenocarcinomas, association with thrombus formation, 215
Muco-cutaneous hemorrhage in storage pool disease, 114
Mucopolysaccharidosis, coagulation abnormalities in, 117
Mucosal bleeding
  conditions associated with, 84
  in aspirin-like defect, 115
  in Factor V deficiency, 157
  in Factor VII or Factor X deficiency, 157
  in malignancies, 168
  in thrombasthenia, 111

in vascular disorders, 90
in von Willebrand's syndrome 104
Multiple myeloma, see Myeloma
Mumps, thrombocytopenia complicating, 130
Myelocytic leukemia, platelet disorder
  classification, 100
Myelofibrosis
  thrombocythemia in, 137
  thrombocytopenia in, 84
Myeloid metaplasia, platelet disorder
  classification, 100
Myeloma
  abnormal platelet function in, 208, 209
  clotting defects in, 86
  disseminated intravascular coagulation
    associated with, 208, 209
  Factor VIII inhibitors in, 207
  hemorrhage in, 208, 209
  thrombocytopenia in, 208
  treatment of hemorrhage in, 209
Myeloproliferative disorders
  bleeding in, 119
  decrease in fibrinolytic enzymes in, 214
  decreased platelet retention in, 105
  platelet aggregation disorders in, 221
  platelet lipid peroxidation in, 138
  thrombocythemia in, 135, 137
  thrombocytosis in, 215
Myelosuppression, association with
  thrombocytopenia, 84
Myocardial disease, anticoagulant therapy
  affecting metastases, 231
Myocardial infarction
  decreased fibrinolytic activity in, 240
  decrease in Antithrombin III following, 239
  drugs used in treatment, 122
  fibrinolysis inhibitors in, 240
  increased fibrinogen dimer and polymer in, 242
  soluble fibrin monomer in, 170
  vitamin K antagonists used in, 248

N

Neo-synephrine, epistaxis controlled by, 92
Neuraminidase, effect on serotonin uptake, 25
Norepinephrine, role in platelet aggregation, 27
Nucleotidase of platelet membranes, 21

O

Obstetrical accidents
  DIC resulting from, 164, 165
    treatment, 172
Oculocutaneous albinism, conditions associated
  with, 113
Opsonization as result of complement function,
  67
Oral anticoagulants, see Anticoagulants
Oral contraceptives

decrease in antithrombin III associated with,
  239
effect in von Willebrand's syndrome, 105
increased Factor VIII activity caused by, 106
increased fibrinogen dimer and polymer
  associated with, 242
increased fibrinolytic inhibitors associated with,
  240
soluble fibrin monomer in users, 170
use with vitamin K antagonists, 249
Osler-Weber-Rendu disease
  described, 91, 92
  telangiectasia in, 84, 91
Osteogenesis imperfecta
  clinical features, 91
  coagulation abnormalities in, 117
  platelet disorder classification, 100
Osteogenic sarcoma, thrombocytosis associated
  with, 135
Osteoporosis in heparin therapy, 250
Ovary, carcinoma of
  anticoagulant therapy, 231
  thrombosis associated with, 216
Ox brain thromboplastin time in hemophilia B,
  154

P

Pain, role of Factor XII in, 66
Pancreatic carcinoma
  association with endocarditis, 230
  intravascular clotting in, 215
  metastasis, 230
  thrombocytosis in, 215
  thrombophlebitis associated with, 230
Pancytopenia in Fanconi's syndrome, 126
Papain, role in platelet aggregation, 27
Papaverine, inhibition of platelet aggregation, 23
Parahemophilia, congenital, 157
Paraprotein disorders
  association with acquired vascular defects, 93
  bleeding in, 119
  malignant
    defective hemostasis in, 208, 209
    inhibitors in, 219
    platelet function abnormalities in, 220
    thrombosis associated with, 216
Paroxysmal nocturnal hemoglobinuria, platelet
  disorder classification, 100
Pemphigus vulgaris, Factor VIII inhibitors in, 207
Peptic ulcer, use of oral anticoagulants in
  contraindicated, 247
Periateritis nodosa, association with vascular
  disorder, 84
Peripheral loss, association with
  thrombocytopenia, 84
Peritoneal dialysis as therapy in uremia, 119
Petechiae
  as sign of collagen disease, 92
  cause of, 82

in acute DIC, 217
in liver disease, 185
in vascular disorders, 90
PGI$_2$, see Prostacyclin
Phenol, inhibition of platelet function, 119
Phentolamine, role in platelet aggregation, 25
Phlebitis, see also Thrombophlebitis
    reaction in streptokinase treatment, 264
Phosphatase of platelet membranes, 21
Phosphodiesterase of platelet membranes, 21
Phospholipids
    role in Factor Xα formation, 55
    role in Factor XII activation, 57
    role in thrombin formation, 51
PIVKA
    derivatives, synthesis in liver disease, 184
    effect on fibrin formation, 46
Placental abruption, DIC associated with, 164
Plasma cell myeloma
    increased Factor VIII caused by, 106
    platelet disorder classification, 100
Plasma membrane of platelets, 18
Plasmapheresis as treatment of dysproteinemias, 120
Plasma transglutaminase, see Factor XIIIα
Plasmin
    action on plasma proteins in DIC, 167
    complement activation by, 68
    designation as fibrinolytic enzyme, 62
    formation, 63, 65
    function as enzyme, 63
    generation in DIC pathophysiology, 165
    injection decreasing metastases, 229
    proteolysis of fibrin and fibrinogen, 65
Plasminogen
    activation, role in primary hyperfibrino(geno)lysis, 182
    activator activity, decreased, effect of, 240
    activators, 7, 63, 64
    conversion to plasmin, 63
    measurement in diagnosis of thrombosis, 241
    structure, 63
Platelets
    abnormal function in cardiopulmonary bypass, 189, 190
    abnormalities in Bernard-Soulier syndrome, 109
    abnormalities in Wiskett-Aldrich syndrome, 113, 114
    adhesion-aggregation reaction, 10
    adhesion and cohesion, 28, 29
    adhesion disorders, 99—110
    adhesion, increased, in acute thrombosis, 238
    adhesion to endothelial cells in trauma, 9
    age, effects of, 32
    aggregation
        abnormal, in multiple myeloma, 209
        abnormalities in myeloproliferative disorders, 221
        aspirin affecting, 29
        calcium chelators as inhibitors, 21
        diagnostic tests, 85
        enzymes involved in, 21
        epinephrine function, 24
        inhibition by nucleotides, 23
        molecules involved in, 20
        primary, disorders of, 110, 111
        ristocetin affecting, 19, 101
        role of ADP in, 23, 29
        role of complement in, 20, 21
        secondary, disorders of, 111
        stimulation in trauma, 6
        thrombin-induced, 24
    altered distribution, 127, 129
    antibodies
        drug-induced, 130
        tests for, 133
    antigens, immunization to, thrombocytopenia associated with, 130
    as hemostatic compartment, 82
    association of dysfunction with uremia, 118
    cofactor, as clotting factor, 44
    count
        for diagnostic purposes, 98
        in pregnancy, 125
        in thrombocytopenia, 125
    dense bodies
        number of, in storage pool disease, 113, 114
        PF-4 in, 19
        serotonin storage in, 25
        substances contained in, 27
    dense tubular system, 19, 25
    destruction, 126, 129
    disorders
        diagnosis, 98, 99
        hereditary and acquired, classification, 100
        in malignancy, 20
        von Willebrand's syndrome, 99-107
    drugs affecting function, 120, 121
    dysfunction
        bleeding due to, 84
        drug-induced, 82, 84
        in liver disease, 185
    early studies, 97
    enzyme abnormalities in Glanzmann's thrombasthenia, 110
    factor 3
        deficiency, 116
        phospholipids derived from, 51, 55
        release in liver disease
    Factor V, binding to particles, 19
    Factor XI activation, role of collagen in, 11
    factors associated with, 19, 20
    fibrinogen deficiency in Glanzmann's thrombasthenia, 110
    function
        abnormalities, in malignant paraprotein disorders, 208
        in hemostasis, 30
        role of Factor VIII in, 151
    functional disorders, see disorders, supra
    giant

association with renal dysfunction, 116
in May-Hegglin anomaly, 117
origin, 117
syndrome, 100, 108, 109
α-granules, 28
increase in, in malignancy, 230
inhibition of aggregation by PGI_2, 11
interaction with subendothelium, 10
isotopes used to label for life span determination, 124
kinetics, 124, 126
life span determination, isotopes used to label, 124
lipid content, abnormal, in storage pool disease, 113
lipid peroxidation in myeloproliferative disorders, 138
membrane abnormality in Glanzmann's thrombasthenia, 110, 111
membrane glycoprotein content, in Bernard-Soulier syndrome, 109
metabolism, 28
microtubules, 25
mitochondria, 18, 28
nonmetabolic ADP content deficiency, clinical syndromes involving, 113
open canalicular system, 18, 25, 27
organelle zone, 27, 28
peripheral zone, 18-25
PF substances of, 19
plasma membranes
 biochemical properties, 21
 enzymes of, 21
 morphology, 21
 receptors on, 23
 surface charge, 23
production, 30
 drugs affecting, 128
 impaired DNA synthesis affecting, 129
 in thrombocytopenia, 123
 process, 122-124
prostaglandin synthesis, 115
pseudopod formation, 25, 27
responses, inflammatory and immunologic, evaluation procedure, 97
responsiveness, 31
retention, glass-bead column assays for, see Glass-bead retention assays
role in atherosclerosis pathogenesis, 97
role in vascular action, 9-11
senile, destruction of, 124
shape change
 on cohesion, 29
 on exposure to ADP, 110
size variation, 32
sol-gel zone, 25, 26
splenic pool, effect on of spleen enlargement, 129
storage granules, 25
structural changes during organelle retraction, 26
structure, 18, 19

survival, 124
 period, 31
 shortened, role in Wiskott-Aldrich syndrome, 113
thrombosthenin content, 25, 26
thrombosthenin function in pseudopod formation, 27
turnover, increased, in malignancy, 214
zones, 18
Pneumoencephalography, increased Factor VIII activity following, 106
Polyarteritis nodosa as acquired vascular disorder, 92
Polycythemia rubra vera
 platelet disorder classification, 100
 thrombocythemia in, 137
 thrombocytosis following phlebotomy, 135, 137
Polylysine, role in platelet release system, 25
Postpartum women
 antibodies to clotting factors, development, 86
 contraindication of thrombolytic therapy, 265
 Factor VIII inhibitors in, 207
 hemorrhage in von Willebrand's syndrome, 104
 thrombosis risk in, 238, 239
Prednisone, increased Factor VIII activity caused by, 106
Pregnancy
 contraindication of thrombolytic therapy, 265
 effect in von Willebrand's syndrome, 104, 105
 increased coagulation factors in, 239
 increased Factor VIII activity caused by, 106
 increased fibrinolytic inhibitors in, 240
 platelet count during, 125
 use of heparin in, 251
 use of vitamin K antagonists in contraindicated, 246
Prekallikrein
 decreased synthesis in liver disease, 184
 levels in liver metastases, 219
 plasma, identification with Fletcher factor, 160
Preleukemic syndromes, platelet disorders in, 100, 221
Primary fibrino(geno)lysis, drugs causing, 221, 222
Primary hyperfibrino(geno)lysis
 association with chronic liver disease, 182, 185
 comparison with DIC, 182, 184
 coagulation factor abnormalities resulting from, 86
 during cardiopulmonary bypass, 191, 192
 in malignancy, 201, 219
 pathophysiology, 182, 183
Promyelocyticleukemia, association with DIC, 165, 166
Propranolol, inhibition of epinephrine uptake in platelet aggregation, 24
Prostacyclin, role in platelet aggregation, 11
Prostaglandin
 inhibition of synthesis by aspirin, 253
 role in platelet aggregation, 11
 synthesis and metabolism, 115
Prostatic carcinoma

DIC in, 215
    hemorrhage in acute DIC, 217
    splenic metastases in, 220
    surgery, heparin prophylaxis in, 252, 253
    therapy affecting abnormal hemostasis, 216
Prosthetic heart valves, see Heart valves
Prosthetic surfaces, drugs preventing thrombosis on, 122
Protamine, use in cardiopulmonary bypass, 193, 194
Protein-C
    inhibition of coagulation, 60
    synthesis, 46
Prothrombin
    complex concentrate as hemotherapeutic agent, 86
    complex, deficiencies associated with liver metastases, 219
    complex factors, decreased synthesis in liver disease, 184
    consumption time in Bernard-Soulier syndrome, 108
    conversion to thrombin, 44, 52
    deficiency, congenital, 157
    inhibitors to, 206
    structural similarity to Factor X, 53
    structure, 49
Prothrombins, role in thrombin formation, 49
Pseudodysfibrinogenemia in liver disease, 185
Pseudoxanthoma elasticum
    clinical features, 91
    coagulation abnormalities in, 117
    platelet disorder classification, 100
Psoriasis, Factor VIII inhibitors in, 207
Psychiatric associations of autoerythrocytic sensitization syndrome, 93
Psychiatric drugs, inhibition of platelet function, 121
Pulmonary embolism
    decreased fibrinolytic activity in, 240
    heparin therapy, 252
    increased fibrinogen dimer and polymer in, 242
    in hip fracture patients, aspirin therapy, 255
    soluble fibrin monomer in, 170
    thrombolytic therapy, 261, 263
    use of vitamin K antagonists in, 248
Pulmonary fibrosis, increase of fibrinolysis inhibitors in, 240
Pulmonary infarction in essential thrombocythemia, 137
Pulmonary metastases in animals, 228
Purpura
    allergic, association with vascular defects, 93
    as sign of collagen disease, 92
    association with thrombocytopenia, 84
    cause of, 82
    fulminans, in coronary artery bypass surgery, 191
    in acute DIC, 217
    in liver disease, 185
    in vascular disorders, 90

Q

Quinidine, use with vitamin K antagonists, 249
Quinine
    thrombocytopenia induced by, 130
    use with vitamin K antagonists, 249

R

Radiation therapy
    DIC caused by, 217
    normalization of coagulation following, 214
    thrombocytopenia associated with, 208, 219
Radioimmunoassay in diagnosis of DIC, 170
Regional enteritis, Factor VIII inhibitors in, 207
Renal dialysis as thrombocytolytic state, 125
Renal failure in DIC, 168
Renal insufficiency, contraindication of thrombolytic therapy, 265
Reptilase, role in fibrin formation, 47
Reserpine, inhibition of serotonin uptake, 25
Respiratory distress syndrome, 176
Retained fetus syndrome, DIC associated with, 164
Reticulin defect, in osteogenesis imperfecta, 91
Reticulocytosis, blood tests for, 85
Rhabdomyosarcoma in mice, metastases in, 229
Rheumatic heart disease, thromboembolism in, sulfinpyrazone treatment, 255
Rheumatoid arthritis
    as acquired vascular disorder, 92
    association with immunologic thrombocytopenia, 131
    Factor VIII inhibitors in, 207
Rickettsial infections, thrombocytopenia complicating, 129
Rifampin, use with vitamin K antagonists, 249
Ristocetin
    effect on platelet aggregation, 101, 105, 106
    in platelet function evaluation, 99
    prevention by antibody in Bernard-Soulier syndrome, 109
    role in platelet aggregation, 19, 27, 29
Rocky Mountain spotted fever, thrombocytopenia complicating, 130
Rubella in newborn, thrombocytopenia in, 128

S

Sarcoidosis, altered platelet distribution in, 129
Sarcoma, fibrinolytic activity in, 219, 228
Scleroderma as acquired vascular disease, 92
Scurvy
    abnormal platelet function in, 120
    association with vascular defect, 85
    blood tests for, 85
    platelet disorder classification, 101
Sepsis, association with DIC, 164, 172, 217

Septicemia, association with DIC, 164, 165
Serotonin
    contraction of endothelial cells caused by, 7
    deficiency in storage pool disease, 113
    role in platelet aggregation, 24, 25, 27
Shistocytosis, blood tests for, 85
Shock lung, similarity to DIC, 175
Shunt thrombosis, sulfinpyrazone prophylaxis, 255
Sialic acid, role in coagulation, 215
Sickle cell anemia, amino acid substitution in, 157
Sideroblastic anemias, platelet disorder classification, 100
Skin
    abnormalities in pseudoxanthoma elasticum, 91
    bleeding from
        in thrombasthenia, 111
        in von Willebrand's syndrome, 104
    fragility, in Ehler-Danlos syndrome, 90
    necrosis caused by oral anticoagulants, 248
Smoking
    effect on platelets, 125
    thrombocytolytic state associated with, 125
Smooth muscle
    effect on of kinins, 67
    layer in blood vessels, 6, 7
Snake venom
    clotting of fibrinogen, 24, 27
    role in fibrin formation, 47
Spleen
    enlargement, in thrombocytopenia, 84
    metastases in malignancies, 220
    platelet pool affected by enlargement, 129
    site of biosynthesis of fibrin a chains, 49
Splenectomy
    as treatment for ITP, 134
    platelet count following, 135
    response to in thrombocytopenia, 114, 135
Staphylococcal coagulase, clotting of fibrinogen, 24
Staphylokinase as activator of plasminogen, 63
Stomach cancer
    association with endocarditis, 230
    splenic metastases in, 220
    thrombosis associated with, 216
Storage pool disease
    antiplatelet antibodies in, 120
    classification, 111
    clinical features, 113
    decreased platelet retention in, 105
    diagnosis, 114
    disseminated intravascular coagulation in, 120
    pathophysiology, 112
    therapy, 114
Strabismus in Fanconi's syndrome, 126
Streptokinase
    as activator of plasminogen, 63
    complications of therapy, 264, 265, 266
    deep vein thrombosis treatment, 262, 264
    dosage, 262
    efficacy, 261
    in colon carcinoma treatment, study of, 231
    indications, 261, 262
    intravenous infusion, effects of, 262
    molecular properties, 260
    pharmacologic properties, 260, 261
    source of, 260
    use in pulmonary embolism, 261, 263
    use in thrombolytic therapy, 260
Streptomycin, inhibitors to Factor V associated with, 206
Stypren time test, 157
Subendothelium
    exposure at at bifurcations, 7
    interaction with platelets, 10
    interaction with platelets in Bernard-Soulier syndrome, 109
    role in hemostasis, 6, 9
Sulfinpyrazone
    dosage, 254
    indications, 255
    inhibition of platelet aggregation, 121
    mechanism of action, 253
    side effects, 254
    tolerance test, 254
Surgery
    bleeding following, 82
        in hemophilia, 152, 154
        in hypofibrinogenemia, 156
        in prothrombin deficiency, 157
    cardiopulmonary bypass, see Cardiopulmonary bypass
    contraindication of thrombolytic therapy, 265
    decreased fibrinolytic activity following, 240
    fibrinolytic activity in, 62
    for malignancy, normalization of coagulation following, 214
    heparin prophylaxis in, 252, 253, 254
    platelet destruction caused by, 129
    poor healing following, in Factor XIII deficiency, 159
    postoperative increase in coagulation factors, 239
Sympathetic blocking agents, inhibition of platelet function, 121
Systemic lupus erythematosus, see Lupus erythematosus

T

TAR baby syndrome, clinical features, 114
Telangiectasia
    hereditary hemorrhagic
        association with von Willebrand's syndrome, 104
        platelet defects in, 118
    in liver disease, 185
    in Osler-Weber-Rendu disease, 84
    in vascular disorders, 90
Thiazides as cause of thrombocytopenia, 128
Thrombasthenia, see Glanzmann's

thrombasthenia
Thrombin
    activation of Factor XIII, 49
    as inhibitor, 60
    conversion of fibrinogen to fibrin, 44, 45, 47, 49
    formation, 44, 45, 49—52
    generation by Factor X, 249
    generation in DIC pathophysiology, 165, 167
    receptors, 24
    role in platelet aggregation, 24, 27
    substrate specificity, 52, 53
    synthesis, 46
Thrombocythemia
    association with myeloproliferative disorders, 135, 137
    bleeding problems, 137
    causes of, 136
    definition, 134
    diagnosis, 137
    in myelofibrosis, 137
    platelet disorder classification, 100
    treatment, 138
    use of antiplatelet drugs by patients, problem of, 138
Thrombocytolytic states, 125
Thrombocytopathies, classification, 111
Thrombocytopenia
    altered distribution of platelets, effect of, 129
    amegakaryocytic, 126—128
    as complication of infections, 129
    association with Alport's syndrome, 116
    association with rubella in newborn, 128
    causes of, 84, 122
    causes of marrow hypoplasia resulting in, 128
    classification, 127
    drug-induced, 82, 84, 130—132
        as cause of thrombocytosis, 136
    drugs causing, 128
    estrogens producing, 125
    fetal, thiazide diuretics as cause, 128
    following splenectomy, 114, 135
    idiopathic thrombocytopenic purpura, see Idiopathic thrombocytopenic purpura
    immunologic, 127, 130—134
    in Bernard-Soulier syndrome, 108, 109
    in bone marrow infiltration disorders, 128
    in cardiopulmonary bypass, 188, 189
    in DIC, 129
    ineffective thrombopoiesis as cause, 129
    in liver disease, 185
    in malignancy, 219, 220
    in May-Hegglin anomaly, 117
    in multiple myeloma, 208
    in Wiskott-Aldrich syndrome, 113
    isoimmune, 130
    marrow response to, 123
    megakaryocytic, 127—134
    mithramycin as cause, 221
    nonimmunologic destructive, 127, 129
    occurrence prior to thrombocytopenic, 135
    pathophysiology, 126
    platelet abnormalities in, 31
    platelet count, 125
    platelet disorder classification, 100
    platelet production, 122, 123
    posttransfusion, 131
    ristocetin as cause, 101
    screening tests, 85
    splenic enlargement associated with, 84
    TAR baby syndrome, 114
Thrombocytosis
    acute blood loss associated with, 135
    association with malignancy, 135, 215, 230
    association with renal polycythemia, 124
    causes, 135, 136
    iron deficiency anemia associated with, 135
    occurrence of thrombocytopenia prior to, 135
Thromboembolism
    antiplatelet therapy, 255
    as thrombocytolytic state, 125
    heparin inhalation therapy, 250
    heparin therapy, 252
    in rheumatic heart disease, sulfin pyrazone treatment, 255
    predisposition to, factors influencing, 64
    use of vitamin K antagonists in prevention, 248
Thrombokinase, conversion of prothrombin to thrombin, 44
Thrombolytic therapy
    contraindications, 265
    enzymes used in, 260
    heparin treatment following, 267
    indications, 261, 262
    laboratory monitoring, 265, 266
    principle of, 260
Thrombometer test in von Willebrand's syndrome, 99
Thrombopathies, classification, 111
Thrombophlebitis
    association with pancreatic carcinoma, 230
    deep vein
        antithrombin III levels in, 240
        aspirin prophylaxis, 255
        coagulation factors, increase in, 239
        decreased fibrinolytic activity in, 240
        heparin therapy, 252
        increased fibrinogen dimer and polymer in, 242
        platelet adhesion in, 238
        role of vascular damage in, 241
        soluble fibrin monomer in, 170
        sulfinpyrazone treatment, 255
        use of vitamin K antagonists in, 248, 249
    postoperative, in malignancy, 216
    recurrent, development of lung cancer associated with, 230
    septic, streptokinase therapy, 262, 265
Thromboplastin
    clinical use, 82
    role in Factor Xα formation, 54
    role in thrombin formation, 44

Thrombopoiesis
    abnormal, in storage pool disease, 113
    ineffective, thrombocytopenia associated with, 127, 129
    role in platelet production, 123, 124
Thrombopoietin, control of megakaryocytopoiesis, 30
Thromboscintograms, use in thrombosis diagnosis, 247
Thrombosis
    acute, platelet adhesion in, 238
    antiplatelet drugs used in therapy, 216
    arising at bifurcations, 7
    association with malignancy, 214, 216
    cerebrovascular, increased fibrinogen dimer and polymer in, 242
    coagulation factor changes in, 239
    deep vein
        streptokinase therapy, 262, 264
    diagnostic methods, 247
    diffuse, in DIC, 164, 165, 168
    factors in, 238—240
    incidence in lower extremities, 241
    laboratory diagnosis, 241
    management of, 216
    pathophysiology, 214, 215
    role of platelet adhesion in, 239
    vessel wall changes in, 240
Thrombosthenin
    ATP bound to, 28
    structure and function, 25, 26, 27
Thrombotic thrombocytopenic purpura
    clinical feature of, 130, 176
    in malignancy, 220
Thromboxane
    synthesis, 11
    synthetase deficiency, platelet disorder classification, 100
Tissue factor
    lipoprotein as, 7
    role in Factor Xa formation, 54
Tolbutamide, use with vitamin K antagonists, 249
Tonsillectomy, hemophilia observed in, 152
Transfusion
    as therapy in thrombasthenia, 111
    as therapy in von Willebrand's syndrome, 99
    DIC caused by, 218
    hemolysis associated with as cause of DIC, 164
    thrombocytopenia following, 131
Transglutaminase, see Factor XIII
Transplants, effect of dipyridamole in, 255
Trauma, see Injury
Trypsin
    role in clotting in pancreatic carcinoma, 215
    role in platelet aggregation, 27
    structural similarity of coagulation factors, 56
Tuberculosis
    contraindication of thrombolytic therapy, 265
    thrombocytopenia in, 128
Tumors
    acquired circulating anticoagulants in, 219

Aminasin, effect of, 229
association with fibrin formation, 214
DIC associated with, 165
fibrinolytic activity in, 228
hemorrhage in acute DIC, 217
procoagulant activity in cells 228
TXA_2, see Thromboxane
Typhus, thrombocytopenia complicating, 130

U

Ulcerative colitis
    coagulation factors in, 239
    contraindication of thrombolytic therapy, 265
    Factor VIII inhibitors in, 207
Umbilical cord bleeding
    in afibrinogenemia, 156
    in Factor VIII deficiency, 159
Uremia
    bleeding due to, 84
    clinical features, 119
    decreased platelet retention in, 105
    diagnosis, 119
    hemorrhage in, 208
    pathophysiology, 118
    platelet disorder classification, 100
    platelet dysfunction associated with, 118
    therapy, 119
Urokinase
    as activator of plasminogen, 63
    complications of therapy, 264, 265, 266
    dosage, 261
    efficacy, 261
    indications, 261, 262
    intravenous infusion, effects of, 262
    molecular properties, 260
    pharmacologic properties, 260, 261
    source of, 260
    use in pulmonary embolism, 261, 263
    use in thrombolytic therapy, 260
Uterus, site of biosynthesis of fibrin a chains, 49

V

Vacuoles of platelets, 18
Valvular heart disease, decreased platelet retention in, 105
Vascular basement membranes, role in Factor XII activation, 57
Vascular defects, drug-induced, 82, 84
Vascular disorders
    acquired, 92, 93
    coagulation factor inhbitors in, 207, 208
    diagnosis, 90
    DIC associated with, 165
    hereditary, 90—93
    in cardiopulmonary bypass, 190
    in liver disease, 185

manifestations of, 90
Vascular permeability
   increased, resulting from complement function, 68
   kinins affecting, 67
Vascular tree
   as hemostatic compartment, 82
   structure, 6
Vascular wall structure, 6
Vasculidities, association with vascular disorders, 84
Vasculitis as reaction to oral anticoagulants, 248
Vasoconstriction
   in response to stimuli, 7
   in trauma, 9
Veins
   as compliance vessels, 6
   smooth muscle layer, 6, 7
   structure, 6, 7
Venography, use in thrombosis diagnosis, 247
Venous thrombosis, drugs used in treatment, 122
Vesicles of platelets, 18
Vessel wall, changes in, role in thrombus formation, 240
Viruses
   infections
      association with DIC, 164, 165
      thrombocytopenia complicating, 129
   role in platelet aggregation, 27
Vitamin E, use with vitamin K antagonists, 249
Vitamin K
   antagonism by actinomycin D, 221
   antagonists, use as anticoagulants, 246—249
   effect on cell membrane function, 229
   Factor IX dependence, 56
   function in fibrin formation, 46
   prothrombin as dependent, 49
   therapy in liver disease or drug-induced bleeding, 86
VKA, see Vitamin K
Von Willebrand factor
   assays for, 105
   function, 102
   inhibitor to, 207
   role in platelet aggregation, 20
   synthesis and release, 103
Von Willebrand's syndrome
   acquired, 107
   clinical features, 104, 207
   distinction from hemophilia, 150, 151
   laboratory and clinical features, 107
   laboratory diagnosis, 105, 106
   pathophysiology, 99—104
   platelet disorder classification, 100
   response of patient to cryoprecipitate, 108
   therapy, 106, 107
   variants, 103

W

Waldenstrom's macroglobulinemia
   bleeding in, 119
   Factor VIII inhibitors in, 207
   hemorrhage in, 208
   platelet disorder classification, 100
Warfarin
   effect on cell membranes, 229
   use in connection with chemotherapy, 231
   use in coronary artery bypass, 193
   use in malignancy, 216
Waring blender syndrome, 129
Wilson's disease, platelet defects in, 118
Wiskott-Aldrich syndrome
   clinical features, 113
   platelet abnormalities in, 126
   platelet disorder classification, 100

Z

Zymosan, role in complement activation, 68